Immunohistochemistry

IBRO HANDBOOK SERIES:
METHODS IN THE NEUROSCIENCES

General Editor: **A. D. Smith**
 Department of Pharmacology
 University of Oxford

Volume 1: **Tracing Neural Connections with Horseradish Peroxidase**
 Edited by M-Marsel Mesulam

 0 471 10028 5   280 pages (cloth)   1982
 0 471 10029 3   280 pages   (paper)   1982

Volume 2: **Brain Microdissection Techniques**
 Edited by A. C. Cuello

0 471 10523 6   approx   pages   (cloth)   due early 1983
0 471   approx   pages   (paper)   due early 1983

Volume 3: **Immunohistochemistry**
 Edited by A. C. Cuello

Volumes in Preparation

Receptor Binding Methods
N. Birdsall and E. C. Hulme

**Histochemical and Ultrastructural Identification
of Monoamine Neurons**
Edited by J. B. Furness and M. Costa

Chemical Lesions
Edited by G. Jaim-Etcheverry

Intracellular Perfusion of Excitable Cells
Edited by P. G. Kostyuk and O. A. Krishtal

Chronic Animal Preparation for Unit Recording
R. Lemon

Immunohistochemistry

Edited by
A. C. Cuello
Departments of Pharmacology and Human Anatomy
University of Oxford, UK
and
Tutor and Fellow, Lincoln College, Oxford

A Wiley–Interscience Publication

JOHN WILEY & SONS
Chichester · New York · Brisbane · Toronto · Singapore

Library of Congress Cataloging in Publication Data:
Main entry under title:
Immunohistochemistry.
  (IBRO handbook series; v. 3)
  'A Wiley–Interscience publication.'
  Includes index.
  1. Immunochemistry—Technique. 2. Histochemistry—
Technique. 3. Cytochemistry—Technique.
I. Cuello, A. C. II. Series. DNLM: 1. Histocytoche-
mistry.
2. Immunologic techniques. 3. Immunochemistry.
QY 250 132
QR183.6.146 1983   574.8'212   82–161156

ISBN 0 471 10245 8 Cloth
ISBN 0 471 90052 4 Paper

British Library Cataloguing in Publication Data:
Immunohistochemistry.—(IBRO handbook series:
  methods in the neurosciences; v. 3)
  1. Immunohistochemistry—Techniques
  2. Neurochemistry
  I. Cuello, A. C.
  612'.814   QR183.6

ISBN 0 471 10245 8 Cloth
ISBN 0 471 90052 4 Paper

Text set in 10/12 pt Linotron 202 Times, printed and
bound in Great Britain at The Pitman Press, Bath

Contents

Contributors

G. J. Boer	*Netherlands Institute for Brain Research, Ijdijk 28, 1095 KJ Amsterdam, The Netherlands*
D. M. Boorsma	*Department of Dermatology, Academic Hospital Free University, De Boelelaan 1117, 1081 HV Amsterdam, The Netherlands*
R. M. Buijs	*Netherlands Institute for Brain Research, Ijdijk 28, 1095 KJ Amsterdam, The Netherlands*
V. Chan-Palay	*Department of Neurobiology, Harvard Medical School, Boston, Massachusetts 02115, USA*
M. Costa	*Centre for Neuroscience, Department of Human Physiology and Morphology, School of Medicine, The Flinders University of South Australia, Australia*
A. C. Cuello	*Neuroanatomy/Neuropharmacology Group, Departments of Pharmacology and Human Anatomy, University of Oxford, South Parks Road, Oxford OX1 3QT, UK*
J. R. De Mey	*Laboratory of Oncology, Janssen Pharmaceutica, Research Laboratories, B-2340 Beerse, Belgium*
M. del Fiacco-Lampis	*Department of Anatomy, University of Cagliari, Via G.T. Porcell 2, Cagliari, Sardinia, Italy*
J. B. Furness	*Centre for Neuroscience, Department of Human Physiology and Morphology, School of Medicine, The Flinders University of South Australia, Australia*
*G. Galfré	*MRC Laboratory of Molecular Biology, Cambridge, UK*
H. J. Geuze	*Centre for Electron Microscopy, Medical School, State University of Utrecht, Utrecht, The Netherlands*
J. J. Haaijman	*Institute for Experimental Gerontology TNO, P.O. Box 5815, 2280 HV Rijswijk, The Netherlands*
T. Hökfelt	*Department of Histology, Karolinska Institute, S-10401 Stockholm, Sweden*
T. H. Joh	*Laboratory of Neurobiology, Cornell University Medical College, 1300 York Avenue, New York, NY 10021, USA*

* Please see end of contributor list for present (temporary) address.

H. W. J. Joosten — *Department of Anatomy and Embryology, University of Nijmegan, P.O. Box 9101, 6500 HB Nijmegan, The Netherlands*

C. Milstein — *MRC Laboratory of Molecular Biology, Cambridge, UK*

G. Paxinos — *Department of Psychology, The University of New South Wales, Kensington, New South Wales, Australia 2033*

Chr. W. Pool — *Netherlands Institute for Brain Research, Ijdijk 28, 1095 KJ Amsterdam, The Netherlands*

J. V. Priestley — *Neuroanatomy–Neuropharmacology Group, University Department of Human Anatomy, South Parks Road, Oxford OX1 3QX, UK*

M. E. Ross — *Laboratory of Neurobiology, Cornell University Medical College, 1300 York Avenue, New York, NY 10021, USA*

R. A. Rush — *Department of Physiology, School of Medicine, The Flinders University of South Australia, Australia*

M. Schachner — *Department of Neurobiology, University of Heidelberg, Im Neuenheimer Feld 504, 6900 Heidelberg 1, Federal Republic of Germany*

L. Skirboll — *Department of Histology, Karolinska Institute, S-10401 Stockholm, Sweden*

J. W. Slot — *Centre for Electron Microscopy, Medical School, State University of Utrecht, Utrecht, The Netherlands*

M. V. Sofroniew — *Neuroanatomy/Neuropharmacology Group, Department of Human Anatomy, University of Oxford, South Parks Road, Oxford OX1 3QX, UK*

H. W. M. Steinbusch — *Department of Anatomy and Embryology, University of Nijmegan, P.O. Box 9101, 6500 HB Nijmegan, The Netherlands*

D. F. Swaab — *Netherlands Institute for Brain Research, Ijdijk 28, 1095 KJ Amsterdam, The Netherlands*

F. Vandesande — *Zoological Institute, Naam Sestraat 59, B-3000 Leuven, Belgium*

F. W. van Leeuwen — *Netherlands Institute for Brain Research, Ijdijk 28, 1095 KJ Amsterdam, The Netherlands*

A. A. J. Verhofstad — *Department of Anatomy and Embryology, University of Nijmegan, P.O. Box 9101, 6500 HB Nijmegan, The Netherlands*

J-Y. Wu — *Department of Cell Biology, Baylor College of Medicine, Texas Medical Center, Houston, Texas 77030, USA*

* Present address:

G. Galfré   *Institute of Animal Physiology, MRC Molecular Biology, Hills Road, Cambridge CB2 2QH*

Foreword

LAURIE GEFFEN

Centre for Neuroscience, The Flinders University of South Australia,
Bedford Park, S.A. 5042, Australia

It is difficult to think of any technique that has had a more profound influence on the development of neurobiology in the last decade than immunohistochemistry. Unlike microelectrode recording, the other great technical advance that has profoundly influenced the course of modern neuroscience, immunohistochemistry, was not originally developed to solve neurobiological problems but found its first applications in histopathology to detect microbial antigens and auto-antibodies and later in endocrinology to localize the site of synthesis of various hormones.

The principle that antibodies can be used as histochemical reagents if suitable markers were linked to antibody molecules without impairing the capacity of the antibody to react with specific antigens was recognized nearly 50 years ago (Marrack, 1934). Of the various dyes that were tried as markers, only the fluorescent dyes provided the requisite sensitivity, the first being fluorescein isocyanate-labelled antibodies that were used to localize pneumococcal antigens in infected tissues (Coons *et al.*, 1942).

In the post-war years, the application of immunohistochemistry in histopathology increased greatly with improvements in conjugation, tissue fixation, and lamp and filter systems for fluorescent microscopes. Perhaps the most significant development for later application of the technique to neurobiology was the demonstration by Marshall (1951) of the localization *in vitro* of a native molecule (adrenocorticotrophic hormone) in normal tissue (hog pituitary) using fluorescent-labelled antibodies raised against a partially purified antigen. Localization of endogenous antigens *in vivo* was accomplished four years later by an 'indirect' technique whereby rabbit antiserum against a rat renal antigen was injected into rats and the presence of rabbit γ globulin in frozen sections of rat kidney was detected using fluorescence-labelled chicken antibodies against rabbit globulin (Mellors, Siegen, and Pressman, 1955).

In the 1960s a number of heavy metal markers such as ferritin were introduced to permit the visualization of antibodies in the electron microscope. Heavy metals did not prove ideal for immunohistochemistry for various technical reasons although elegant new colloidal gold methods look promising. By far the most popular methods for combined immunohisto-chemistry and cytochemistry are those involving enzyme-linked antibodies, in particular horseradish peroxidase. Methods using enzyme-conjugated anti-bodies were developed independently by Nakane and Pierce (1966) and Avrameas and Uriel (1966) although they have largely been superseded by the ingenious peroxidase–antiperoxidase (PAP) technique of Sternberger *et al.* (1977).

Thus, by the late 1960s, all the technology necessary for the application of immunohistochemistry and immunocytochemistry to neurobiology was avail-able. The first neuronal antigen to be localized was the enzyme dopamine β-hydroxylase that was shown by immunofluorescence to be present through-out peripheral sympathetic neurones (Geffen, Livett, and Rush, 1969). Within a few years, immunohistochemistry became a major tool for mapping neurotransmitter pathways in the central nervous system, pioneered by three groups, those of Hartman and Udenfriend (1972), Hökfelt, Fuxe, and Goldstein (1973), and Pickel, Joh, and Reis (1976). While initial efforts were focused on monoamine synthesizing enzymes, the range of antisera quickly broadened to include other transmitter synthesizing enzymes, neuropeptides and even monoamines themselves.

Apart from neurotransmitters and their associated enzymes, the field has rapidly expanded to include antisera against other constituents of synapses and markers specific for particular classes of neurons and glia. While such studies began in the mid 1960s with the immunofluorescence studies of Rauch and Raffel (1964) on myelin basic protein, and Hyden and McEwen (1966) on S-100 glial protein, the introduction to neurobiology of the monoclonal antibody technique of Kohler and Milstein (1975) gave enormous impetus to the localization of specific antigens that were not amenable to purification in sufficient amounts to raise conventional antisera.

It is a particular pleasure to be associated with this volume in view of the collaboration I had with Claudio Cuello when he first entered the field in 1975. He has gathered authoritative contributions from most of the leading laboratories in the world, not least his own, and it is especially pleasing to note the truly international representation of the authors of the individual chapters. After more than a decade of extra-ordinary progress, the field is sorely in need of a Handbook that consolidates the wide range of immuno-histochemical techniques. I confidently predict this volume and its future editions will become the standard reference source for neurobiologists.

REFERENCES

Avrameas, S. and Uriel, J. (1966). 'Methodé de marquage de antigènes et d'anticorps avec des enzymes et son application en immunodiffusion.' *C.R. hebd. Seanc. Acad. Sci. (D) Paris*, **262**, 2543–2545.

Coons, A. A., Creech, H. J., Jones, R. N., and Berliner, E. (1942). 'The demonstration of pneumococcal antigen in tissues by the use of fluorescent antibody.' *J. Immunol.*, **45**, 159–170.

Geffen, L. B., Livett, B. G., and Rush, R. A. (1969). 'Immunohistochemical localization of protein components of catecholamine storage vesicles.' *J. Physiol., Lond.*, **204**, 593–605.

Hartman, B. K. and Udenfriend, S. (1972). 'The application of immunological techniques to the study of enzymes regulating catecholamine synthesis and degradation.' *Pharmacol. Rev.*, **24**, 311–330.

Hökfelt, T., Fuxe, K., and Goldstein, M. (1973). 'Immunohistochemical studies on monoamine-containing cell systems.' *Brain Res.*, **62**, 461–469.

Hyden, H. and McEwen, B. (1966). 'A glial protein specific for the nervous system.' *Proc. Natl. Acad. Sci. (USA)*, **55**, 354–358.

Marrack, J. (1934). 'Nature of antibodies.' *Nature, Lond.*, **133**, 292–293.

Marshall, J. M. (1951). 'Localization of adrenocorticotrophic hormone by histochemical and immunohistochemical methods.' *J. exp. Med.*, **94**, 21–30.

Mellors, R. C., Siegel, M., and Pressman, D. (1955). 'Analytical pathology. I. Histochemical demonstration of antibody localization in tissue, with special reference to the antigen components of kidney and lung.' *Lab. Invest.*, **4**, 69–89.

Nakane, P. K. and Pierce, G. B. (1966). 'Enzyme-labeled antibodies: preparation and application for the localization of antigens.' *J. Histochem. Cytochem.*, **14**, 928–931.

Pickel, V. M., Joh, T. H., and Reis, D. J. (1976). 'Monoamine synthesizing enzymes in central dopaminergic, noradrenergic and serotonergic neurons. Immunocytochemical localization by light and electron microscopy.' *J. Histochem. Cytochem.*, **24**, 792–806.

Rauch, H. C., and Raffel, S. (1964). 'Immunofluorescent localization of encephalitogenic protein in myelin.' *J. Immunol.*, **92**, 452–455.

Sternberger, L. A., Hardy, P. H., Cuculis, J. J., and Meyer, H. G. (1970). 'The unlabeled antibody–enzyme method of immunohistochemistry. Preparation and properties of soluble antigen–antibody complex (horseradish peroxidase–antihorseradish peroxidase) and its use in identification of spirochetes.' *J. Histochem. Cytochem.*, **18**, 315–333.

Preface for IBRO Handbook Series

During the last fifty years there have been two changes in the way in which scientists have studied the nervous system. First of all, the traditional and largely independent major scientific disciplines of physics, chemistry, physiology, pharmacology, and pathology gave rise to the more specialized sub-disciplines of neurophysiology, neurochemistry, neuropharmacology, etc., and the science of experimental psychology was born. Then, after about another generation, it became clear that a deeper understanding of the brain could not be achieved by separate and unrelated studies in each of these sub-disciplines. Rather, a unified approach was needed in which the specialized methods were applied in a co-ordinated way to solve a particular problem. Indeed, combinations of methods could often yield results not obtainable by the application of any individual technique. Thus, scientists studying the nervous system began to call themselves neurobiologists or neuroscientists because they did not wish to be identified with any particular experimental discipline. Very soon meetings took place (e.g. in 1955 the First International Meeting of Neurobiologists) and organizations (Neuroscience Research Program, MIT) were founded to give formal recognition of this new approach to the study of the brain. In 1958 the decision was taken in Moscow to establish the International Brain Research Organization (IBRO), which became incorporated as an independent organization through a bill in the Parliament of Canada at Ottawa in 1961.

IBRO now has 2000 members, most of whom hold senior positions in research or teaching, in 52 countries of all political complexions. Through its National Corporate members, many of which are Academies of Sciences or national societies for neuroscience, the body of neuroscientists reflected in IBRO must be of the order of 15,000. One of the programmes of IBRO, all of which aim to serve the international community of neuroscientists, is the publication programme. IBRO publications include *IBRO News*, *Neuroscience*, and the *IBRO Symposia Series*. With the present *Handbook Series*, IBRO aims to fill a major gap in the world literature. The neuroscientist needs to be able to turn to whichever specialized method is most suited to the problem he is currently studying. The series on *Methods in the Neurosciences* will help to provide expert advice on exactly how to carry out the experiments, on what difficulties can occur, and on the limitations of the method.

It is planned as a continuing series, so that new volumes can be published as and when new methods are developed, tested, and found useful. It is my hope that books in this series will have a significant impact on neuroscience throughout the world, by helping to provide the tools with which the scientist can tackle his problems.

A. David Smith
Director of Publications, IBRO
University Department of Pharmacology
South Parks Road
Oxford OX1 3QT

Preface

When Dr A. D. Smith (Director of the IBRO Series for Methods in the Neurosciences) invited me to edit a book on *Immunohistochemistry* it appeared a gigantic enterprise. This area of research has clearly exploded during the last few years, not only methodologically but also in the enormous amount of new and revolutionary ideas brought about by the application of immunohistochemical techniques (see Foreword). I considered the main tendencies and potential applications of immunohistochemical techniques in neuroscience and contacted a number of colleagues, many of whom were able to contribute to this enterprise, and I am most grateful to them for their enthusiastic support. At about the same time, I had the good fortune to participate in the First European Molecular Biology Organisation's Course on immunohistochemistry, organized by Dick Swaab and colleagues (Fred van Leeuwen, Chris Pool, Gerard Boer and others) which was held at the Brain Research Institute in Amsterdam. That particular course was very significant in the completion of this book, because there we had the chance to have lengthy discussions and to practice procedures in a most stimulating atmosphere. Many of the present contributions result from papers discussed during that course.

This book would not have been accomplished without the enthusiastic help of my colleagues of the Neuroanatomy/Neuropharmacology Group at the Departments of Pharmacology and Human Anatomy, Oxford and in particular without the skilful secretarial help of Mrs Ella Iles. The advice received from Dr Stephen Thornton of John Wiley and Sons was also very welcome.

The support of friends, in particular Ruben Gutman, and my wife, Martha, has been invaluable throughout this enterprise.

As a result of the efforts of all the authors of this volume to spell out the practical and theoretical aspects of immunohistochemical techniques for application in the neurosciences, it is my hope that our colleagues in the field will be helped in unravelling the biochemical anatomy of the nervous system.

A. Claudio Cuello
1982

Immunohistochemistry
Edited by A. C. Cuello
© 1983 IBRO

CHAPTER 1

On the way to a Specific Immunocytochemical Localization

CHR. W. POOL, R. M. BUIJS, D. F. SWAAB, G. J. BOER, AND F. W. VAN LEEUWEN

Netherlands Institute for Brain Research, IJdijk 28, 1095 KJ Amsterdam, The Netherlands

I INTRODUCTION

The anatomical connections between brain structures have already been studied for a long time by powerful techniques, such as silver impregnation, staining of degenerating fibres, and ortho- or retrograde transport of labelled substances or enzymes. The finding that the transformation of information between neurons in the brain is a process of chemical rather than electrical transmission (Dale, 1935; Eccles *et al.*, 1954) focussed the attention of the neuroanatomists also on the substances that might be involved in this process. Staining techniques were soon developed to demonstrate some of these putative transmitters, e.g. the Falck–Hillarp reaction for amines (Falck *et al.*, 1962), the enzyme–cytochemical methods for the cholinergic systems, and the Gomori staining for neurosecretory systems. However, these techniques exhibit the drawback that they are rather non-specific or not applicable to other systems. The introduction of immunocytochemistry (ICC) in brain research as a tool to study the localization of known or putative transmitter substances seemed to solve most of these problems and has therefore led to the discovery of a number of neuronal pathways previously completely unknown (cf. review by Livett, 1978). Now that the first excitement about the enormous potentialities of ICC techniques is over, it seems necessary to focus our attention also on some of the technical limitations of ICC techniques. This chapter deals mainly with two questions concerning the use of ICC technology in (brain) research: (1) The selection of the tissue-processing and ICC staining-procedures best suited for solving a given problem. Since, however, general rules can hardly be given in this respect, the results presented in this chapter (Section II) are mainly derived from our experiences with the ICC localization of peptides in the brain. (2) Aspects of specificity in ICC, Sections III–XI, being focussed on the question: What compound(s) is/are actually stained by a given immunocytochemical staining procedure?

II SELECTION OF THE TISSUE PROCESSING AND IMMUNOCYTOCHEMICAL STAINING PROCEDURES

Apart from the availability of a potent and specific first antiserum, a great number of factors influence the final outcome of an ICC staining procedure, as is illustrated in Figure 1. It will be clear that the chance of a successful ICC study will be increased considerably when an insight is obtained into the role of each of these factors. However, since 'staining' in each ICC procedure is

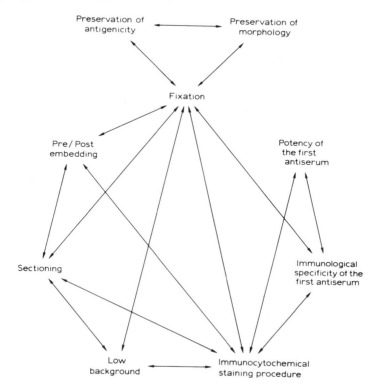

Figure 1 Diagram representing the mutual relationships between the factors influencing the final outcome of an immunocytochemical staining procedure

the result of a complicated set of interrelationships between these factors (represented by the arrows in Figure 1) the exact contribution of each individual factor cannot be determined. For instance, a test on the applicability of different tissue fixations for the maintenance of tissue morphology cannot be determined independently from their involvement in the conservation of detectable immunoreactivity of the tissue antigens. At the same time the detection level of immunoreactivity will be determined by the specificity and potency of the first antiserum, both again dependent on the sensitivity of the ICC procedure used.

In this section some of the difficulties in selecting the proper tissue processing and ICC staining procedures will be discussed. Despite their apparent close relationship an attempt has been made to discuss them in two separate sections.

II.1 Selection of the Tissue Processing Procedure

With respect to the selection of the proper tissue processing procedure, attention has to be focussed on the preservation of immunoreactivity, as well as tissue structure. However, almost any form of tissue processing (fixation and embedding) will change the immunoreactivity of the antigens, while in non- or mildly fixed tissue the embedding—as well as the long ICC incubation procedures—will harm the morphology. Therefore, a compromise will be necessary, from which the final outcome will largely depend on the aim of the ICC study (e.g. a localization at the light microscopical or at the ultrastructural level).

Freezing of the tissue,.followed by sectioning on a cryostat, usually offers the best preservation of immunoreactivity and is therefore very suitable for antigens that lose their immunoreactivity very easily (or for antigens that are difficult to fixate, such as cAMP or melatonin (Ong and Steiner, 1977; Vivien-Roels *et al.*, 1981). In such sections, however, cell membranes are usually still intact, and consequently hamper the penetration of the antibodies. The use of a detergent, such as Triton X-100, during the antiserum incubations in order to improve penetration, will result, in these unfixed sections, in an appreciable loss of the tissue structure. Thinner sections might solve the penetration problem, but are not practical for the study of the course of fibres within the CNS.

For the LM localization of peptides good results have been obtained with respect to the maintenance of immunoreactivity and morphology, by using buffered fixatives based on formalin with or without picric acid, or glutaraldehyde (Vandesande and Dierickx, 1979; Sofroniew and Weindl, 1978; Buijs *et al.*, 1978; Sternberger, 1979). The duration of the fixation, however, also seems to be an important variable (Swaab *et al.*, 1975; Buijs *et al.*, 1978). Although it was possible to demonstrate vasopressin in the human supraoptic and paraventricular nucleus vaguely, after they had been stored in 4% formalin in our museum for more than 50(!) years at room temperature (Swaab, 1982), the stainability of this peptide in the human brain kept in formalin fixative, was diminished clearly after only 1 month of fixation. However, these findings will certainly not hold for all peptide antigens in the brain. For instance, enkephalin immunoreactivity could very well be demonstrated in rat lateral septi that had been fixed for 2 h in 2.5% glutaraldehyde, 1% paraformaldehyde (Buijs, 1982), while using the same fixative no staining was observed in the neural lobe (van Leeuwen, 1983).

It is conceivable that the qualitative demonstration of an antigen in low concentrations will cause more problems than where it is present in high amounts. For example, with the tissue processing and ICC staining procedures already used for a long time to study the hypothalamo-neurohypophyseal system, the extrahypothalamic oxytocin and vasopressin fibres could not be demonstrated (Sofroniew and Weindl, 1978; Buijs *et al.*, 1978).

Vasopressin fibre pathways in the rat hypothalamus neurohypophyseal system were equally well maintained in formalin or glutaraldehyde-fixed tissue, while the vasopressin-containing fibres in the rat lateral septum could only be demonstrated after glutaraldehyde fixation (Figure 2).

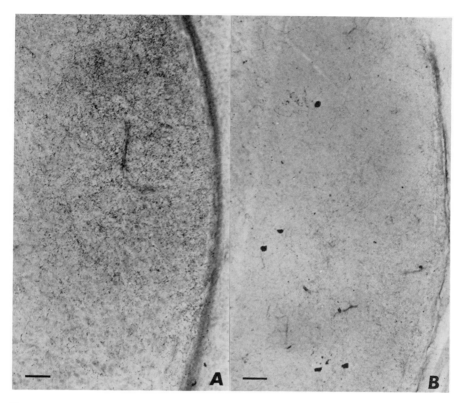

Figure 2 Two vibratome sections of the rat lateral septum incubated with anti-vasopressin 1:1000 and subsequently following the incubation scheme as given in Appendix I. (A) Lateral septum from a rat brain which has been fixed by immersion with 2.5% glutaraldehyde:1% paraformaldehyde. (B) Lateral septum fixed in 4% paraformaldehyde. Notice the difference in the number and staining intensity of the vasopressin-containing fibres. (Bar = 50 μm)

In EM studies, some loss of antigenicity is gladly taken in exchange for preservation of ultrastructure. In spite of the fact that in immuno-EM studies on the adenohypophysis OsO_4 has been used successfully (Beauvillain *et al.*, 1975; Li *et al.*, 1977; Dacheux, 1981) the use of this fixative is generally accompanied by a loss of all immunoreactivity. Formalin fixation generally yields tissue with poor ultrastructural preservation; however, the use of formalin in combination with glutaraldehyde gives much better results. If glutaraldehyde in the usual concentration of 2.5% seriously diminishes the immunoreactivity of the peptide, one may try concentrations of 0.05–0.2%, which usually does not harm the immunoreactivity of a peptide very much (McLaughlin *et al.*, 1975; Pickel *et al.*, 1976; Chan-Palay and Palay, 1977; see also Chapter 11).

For both LM and EM studies, one can choose to embed the fixed tissue, prior to the sectioning and ICC staining (post-embedding staining), or to section the unembedded material using a vibratome or cryostat and use these sections in an ICC staining procedure (pre-embedding staining). As has been stated before, embedding of the tissue in paraffin or epon usually results in a decrease of the immunoreactivity. For instance EM post-embedding staining results in an extraction of membranes (and consequently in a considerable loss of structural details) as OsO_4 generally cannot be used as a fixative. In addition, the long incubation times with the first antiserum, often required in this procedure, might result in a high level of non-specific staining (Buijs and Swaab, 1979). Consequently, a post-embedding ICC staining method is generally not the first choice when a very good preservation of ultrastructural details is needed. An alternative is the use of the pre-embedding staining technique, by which the material can be fixed by OsO_4 after the ICC staining, but prior to embedding. The use of this pre-embedding staining method, however, includes the possibility that due to the vigorous H_2O_2–diamino-benzidine reaction, the diaminobenzidine (DAB) deposits might be spread over other membranous structures, resulting in a false localization of the antigen. An approach that might solve the drawbacks of both the pre- and post-embedding staining procedures in EM, is the use of ultrathin frozen sections in combination with an immunocytochemical protein A–gold stain-ing, which permits even the localization of different antigens in one ultrathin section (see Chapter 12). A drawback in this procedure is that the very small pieces of tissue necessary in this procedure do not allow the survey that is often so necessary in a heterogeneous organ like the brain.

In conclusion, both for the LM and EM localization of cell bodies and the tracing of their fibres in the brain, vibratome or thick frozen sections (Hunt *et al.*, 1980; see Chapter 11) are a good choice. Triton X-100 is generally added to the first antiserum in a concentration of 0.1–2.0% (Sofroniew and Glasmann, 1981) to allow a better penetration of the antibodies (see Appendix I). An additional advantage of using this detergent is the dimi-nished background staining, due to a less non-specific adherence of the antibodies to the tissue. The preparation of a vibratome section, however, requires relatively strongly fixed tissue and although this procedure can be used for determining whether the antigen (a peptide) is present in synaptic structures (McLaughlin *et al.*, 1975; Pickel *et al.*, 1976; Buijs and Swaab, 1979; Figure 3) for a careful cytological study requiring alternating sections of

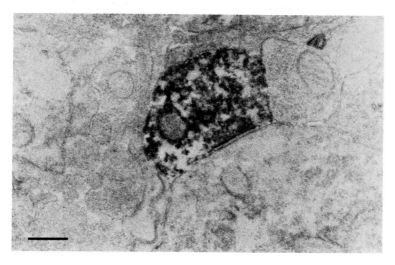

Figure 3 Vasopressin-containing terminal forming a synapse with an unlabelled dendrite in the lateral septum. (Bar = 0.25 μm)

the same structure (e.g. cell body), ultrathin cryosectioning or post-embedding staining (see Appendix II) of the material becomes a necessity.

II.2 Selection of the Immunocytochemical Staining Procedure

In immunocytochemistry several procedures, both immunological and non-immunological, are available to visualize antibodies that have bound to a tissue section. The indirect staining procedures are regarded as more sensitive than the direct procedures. Most workers accept that among the indirect procedures peroxidase–antiperoxidase is the most sensitive technique, followed by the peroxidase conjugate and the fluorescent conjugate in that order (Sternberger, 1979; Vandesande, 1979, see also Chapter 4). However, the validity of this assumption has been questioned (Boorsma *et al.*, 1976; see also Chapter 3). Indirect methods have the advantage that the same procedure can be used in combination with different (first) antisera, provided they are all raised in the same species. Although fluorescence techniques exhibit the advantage of a higher resolution at the LM level, peroxidase markers in peptide ICC are more widely used due to the stability of the DAB reaction product. An additional advantage of the immunoperoxidase technique is that the same material can relatively easily be used for both LM and EM (see Chapters 4 and 11). As will be discussed later in this chapter, this is important since different procedures used to visualize the same first antibodies may result in completely different immunocytochemical reactivity (see Sections VI and VII). The importance of using the same ICC staining procedures both at the EM and LM level may also be illustrated by the various attempts to visualize 'LM-markers' at the EM level and vice-versa. Nakane and Hartman (1980) for instance successfully applied fluorescent markers in scanning EM, while Gu *et al.* (1981) developed a technique to visualize electron-dense gold particles at the LM level.

III   THE APPROACH TO SPECIFICITY IN ICC

Specificity in ICC starts with obtaining some insight into the factors that influence the final outcome of an ICC staining procedure (Figure 1). However, as has already been discussed in the previous section, one of the main difficulties in each ICC study is that in most cases the specific contribution of each individual factor cannot be determined. Therefore, in order to gain at least some insight in, for example, the possible loss of antigenic determinants during the tissue fixation or in the immunological specificity of the first antiserum, the choice of the control experiments—as well as the sequence in which these experiments are carried out—is very important. The flowchart given in Figure 4 summarizes the steps usually followed to gain an insight into the specificity of an ICC staining procedure. This 'conventional' approach can be divided into three parts. During the first part the tissue processing and antiserum incubation conditions are selected in such a way that after incubation of a section (known to contain the component to be localized) with an antiserum raised against that component, a positive reaction is found. If by the start of an ICC study neither the quality of the antiserum nor the presence of the antigen in the tissue is known, it will be necessary to use a tissue that is known to contain this component. Only with some insight, both into the immunological characteristics of the anti-serum and into the procedures necessary to study immunocytochemically the localization of this compound, can the 'switch' to unknown tissues be made.

During the second step the first antiserum is pre-adsorbed with the component to be localized. Lack of reaction of this adsorbed antiserum in the tissue section forces the conclusion that the reaction between the tissue and the antiserum was caused only by antibodies that are able to react with the component used for the adsorption. This type of specificity has been called *method specificity* (see legend to Figure 4; van Leeuwen, 1981) and is commonly taken as the ultimate proof for specificity in ICC (Petrusz *et al.*, 1976, 1977). However, in order to prove 'monospecificity in ICC' (see Section XI) an additional step is necessary to ascertain whether no tissue components other than the antigen used in the adsorption test, (cross)-react with the antibodies responsible for the positive ICC reaction (i.e. *serum specificity*; see legend to Figure 4; van Leeuwen, 1981; Vandesande, 1979). The main reason

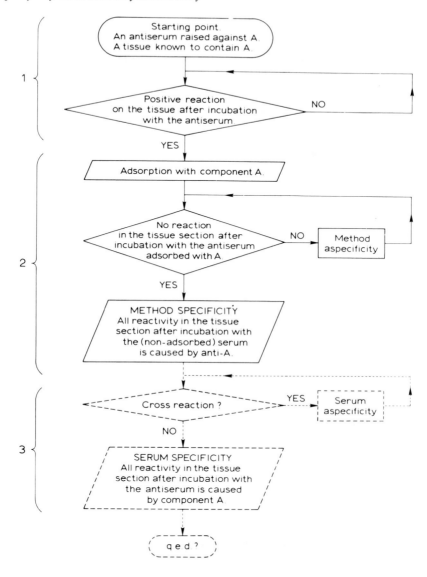

Figure 4 Flowchart of control experiments commonly used to investigate the specificity in an immunocytochemical staining procedure. In this approach *method specificity* is defined as the absence of staining caused by mechanisms other than the interaction between antibodies and the antigen to be localized, and *serum specificity* as the situation that the primary antibodies only react with the antigen to be localized and not with other (tissue) components (van Leeuwen, 1981)

that this step is often neglected is that usually no information is available about the presence of possible cross-reacting compound(s) in the tissue under study (Vandesande, 1979).

The immunocytochemical specificity as defined following this sequence of control experiments is mainly dependent on the specificity of the adsorption step. During this adsorption only the antibodies that react with the component to be localized have to be removed from the antiserum. Therefore, antigen preparations of high purity are required. This is often impossible to fulfil for antigens isolated from biological material (see Chapters 5, 6, and 7). However, even if an antigen preparation was available which only contained the component to be localized, the pre-adsorption test still only shows that the immunoreactive compound(s) in the tissue and this component share antigenic determinants. Method specificity obtained this way certainly does not allow definite conclusions with respect to the identity of the antigen(s) present in the tissue. An additional problem may arise during the adsorption step in the flowchart of Figure 4, when the animal already produced antibodies capable of reacting with tissue component(s) prior to immunization. Examples have been described, e.g., by Kurki *et al.* (1977) and Gordon *et al.* (1978), who were able to characterize immunocytochemically intermediate (10 nm) filaments using 'normal' human or rabbit serum, and Trenchev and Holborow (1976) who described auto-actin antibodies in 80% of their rabbits.

In conclusion, there are at least three drawbacks with respect to the use of the sequence of ICC controls as given in the flowchart in Figure 4.

(a) it often makes excessive demands on the purity of the antigen to be used for the adsorption in step 3;
(b) it does not supply sufficient information on the identity (or number) of immunoreactive compounds present in the tissue; and
(c) it leads to an unsolvable method aspecificity in the case of contaminating pre-immune antibodies.

During the last few years an approach towards specificity has been described differing at least in two important aspects from the procedure described above; firstly, the adsorption test with the antigen to be localized no longer plays such a crucial role; and secondly a positive identification of the immunoreactive compounds actually present in the tissue under investigation forms an intrinsic part of the whole procedure. The sequence of steps necessary for such an ICC specificity study is given in Figure 5. Despite the fact that all problems with respect to the general application of this approach are certainly not yet solved, it was still decided to use this approach as a basis for this chapter on specificity in ICC. Within this framework, Section IV will deal with the theoretical implications of the flowchart in Figure 5, while in Sections V–X the more practical aspects will be described. Section XI, finally, provides a small glossary in which some of the expressions used throughout this chapter are explained.

IV   A FLOWCHART OF IMMUNOCYTOCHEMICAL CONTROLS

In this section the flowchart given in Figure 5 serving as a guideline to Sections V–IX will be discussed. The various stages are illustrated with

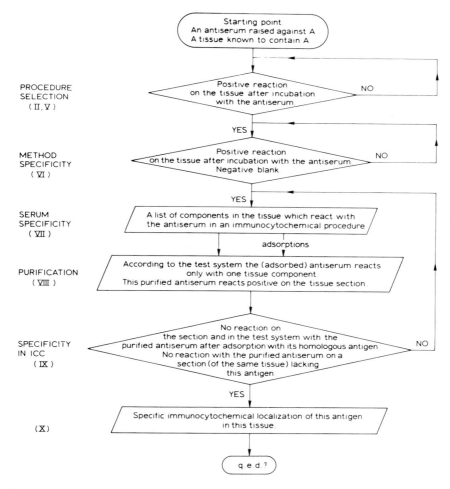

Figure 5   Flowchart summarizing the proposed sequence of control experiments to provide specificity in immunocytochemistry (specific only for one defined antigen, the antigen under investigation). This scheme (which is discussed in detail in Section IV) serves as a guideline to Sections IV–IX. For definitions of method specificity and serum specificity see Section XI

control experiments necessary to obtain a specific ICC localization of a component A in a certain tissue.

The initial demands made on the tissue and on the antiserum serving as starting points in the search for specificity in ICC are given in the first frame (see also Section III).

An antiserum raised against A
A tissue known to contain A

After incubation of the antiserum with a section of this tissue there are two possible outcomes:

positive reaction   no reaction

Since the tissue is known to contain the antigen, 'no reaction' can be designated as *false-negative*. Possible causes of this false-negativity may be found at the level of:

(a) the tissue section
(b) the procedure used to identify the first antibody
(c) the first antibody.

Points which are discussed in Section V.

Positive reaction on the tissue section

Having arrived at a stage where we obtained a positive reaction with a potent antiserum raised against component A, on a section known to contain this antigen, the next step is to examine the reactivity on a section from the same tissue after incubation with a 'non-immune serum' (i.e. serum with no immunoreactivity towards any of the tissue components) while all other steps are kept the same. This 'blank-value' is meant to ascertain whether the immunocytochemical reagents alone cause staining of the tissue, a situation which is called *method specificity* (see Section XI; Sternberger, 1979). (Notice that this definition is different from that given in the legend of Figure 4.)

After incubation with such a non-immune serum there are again two possible outcomes:

no reaction   positive reaction

Since no reactive antibodies are supposed to be present in the non-immune serum, a positive reaction found with this serum can be designated as *false-positive*. Causes for false-positive results at this stage may again be found at the level of (see Section VI):
(a) the tissue section
(b) the procedure used to identify the first antibody, or
(c) the first antiserum itself
Having eliminated the factors that may cause false positivity, the following conditions have to be met;

> Positive reaction on the section with the antiserum
> Negative blank (= Method specificity)

At this moment all attempts in an ICC specificity study have to be focussed on the question:
What component(s) in the tissue are actually responsible for the positive (immunological) reaction of the (first) antiserum?
    Which is a first step towards a 'serum-specific' ICC localization procedure (see Section XI).
    The criteria for a test which may reveal the *serum specificity* of an immunocytochemical staining procedure will be discussed in Section VII. In addition, some of the techniques currently used or being developed for this purpose will be described there.
    However, irrespective of what method is used, this step in an ICC serum specificity study should always result in:

> A list of components present in the tissue under study, which react with the antiserum in the immunocytochemical procedure.

When these compounds have been identified, the unwanted antibodies have to be removed from the antiserum. Some of the techniques currently used for this purpose and the interpretation of the final outcome of such *adsorption experiments* will be dealt with in Section VIII.

When all necessary antiserum purifications have been carried out we have arrived at a stage where:

(a) according to the test system we have a purified antiserum which reacts only with one tissue component
(b) this purified antiserum reacts positively on the tissue section

---

The *final test for serum specificity in ICC* must be performed both on the tissue section and in the model test system, and must give an insight into the validity of the serum specificity as was found in the model test system for the ICC reaction on the tissue section. These final tests and the implications of their outcome for the specificity of the ICC reaction on the tissue section will be described in Section IX.

Ideally, this next step in the flowchart should be:

(a) no reaction on the section and in the test system with the purified antiserum after adsorption with its homologous antigen (A), and
(b) no reaction with the purified antiserum on a section of the same tissue lacking this antigen

---

If at this stage these requirements cannot be fulfilled simultaneously, the staining results on the (normal) section with the purified antiserum (step 3) can be considered 'immunocytological' rather than 'immunocytochemical'. In order to obtain a more immunocytochemical result a jump backwards in the flowchart (see Figure 5) will be necessary (see also Section IX).

The question whether

A specific immunocytochemical localization of the component (A) in the tissue

---

can ultimately be obtained using this sequence of control experiments will be discussed in Section X.

---

q.e.d.?

V FALSE-NEGATIVITY

The starting point for the control of specificity in ICC is a positive reaction in a tissue (see step 1 of the Flowchart in Figure 5). However, the situation may occur that in a section from tissue which is known to contain a certain component no staining is found after incubation with an antiserum that is supposed to contain antibodies against that component, a phenomenon which is called false-negativity. As already mentioned in Section IV, causes for such false-negative results may be found in (a) the tissue section, (b) the immunocytochemical procedure used to detect the first antibody, or (c) the first antiserum itself.

V.1 Tissue Section

There are three possible mechanisms which might result in a false-negative ICC reaction caused by *the tissue section*, the first being a *loss of soluble antigens* during the tissue processing or ICC incubation procedures, which may be prevented by fixation of the tissue prior to the staining procedure (see Section II). However, in addition to an immobilization of the tissue components fixation may also lead to *modifications of antigenic determinants*. Many examples can be given in this respect (Swaab *et al.*, 1975; Steinbusch et al., 1978; Sternberger, 1979). In addition diminution of immunoreactivity has also been reported to occur during embedding procedures (Sternberger, 1979). A third possible cause for false-negativity at the tissue section level is the *inaccessibility of the antigen* during the antiserum incubation steps. This is especially important when thick sections are used, as for instance in pre-embedding immunocytochemical staining procedures (see Section II).

V.2 Procedure Used to Identify the First Antibody

The procedure used to visualize the first antibody may also be a cause for false-negativity. A negative ICC reaction, in spite of an immunoreactive compound in the section and a first antibody which reacts with this antigen, might occur when the PAP procedure is used to visualize the immune complexes. A high concentration of first antibodies in the tissue section, caused by a high concentration of the antigen, might result in binding both antigenic sites of the (second) bridge antibody and consequently in a *failure to bind the PAP complex* (Figure 6). Dilution of the first antiserum usually solves this problem (Bigbee *et al.*, 1977). However, also in the case of a two-step procedure the antiserum used to visualize the bound first antibodies .may be a cause for false-negativity. In sections incubated with serum samples from an oxytocin-immunized rabbit and subsequently stained with a commercially available horse anti-rabbit IgG fluorescein conjugate (PKF 17-2F3)

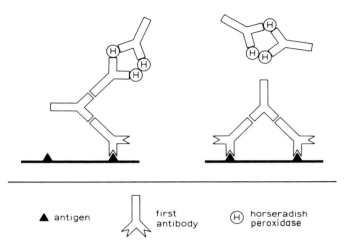

Figure 6   Diagram representing the 'Bigbee effect'. Due to a high local concentration of first antibodies in the tissue section both antigenic sites of the second (bridge) antibody are 'used', resulting in a failure to bind the PAP complex

hardly any reaction was observed with antiserum samples collected at the end of the 1.5-year immunization period. However, when these samples were applied in a PAP procedure using a different anti-rabbit IgG preparation, they turned out to have excellent staining abilities (Figure 7). This shows that in indirect staining procedures the final ICC reactivity may differ depending upon the *specificity (IgG subclass?) of the second antibody* (see Sections VIII and X).

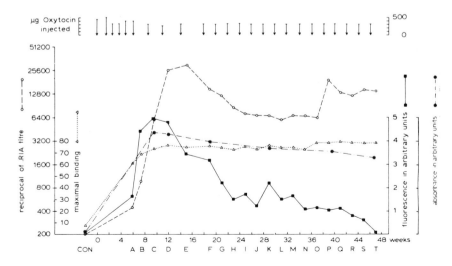

V.3 First Antiserum

False-negativity may also be due to a first antiserum that is less potent than expected, this may be due to:

(1) *The immunization procedure*

The most commonly used animal for immunization purposes is the rabbit. The selection of the species is important. Rabbits, for instance, may produce low (or no) titre antisera when immunized with a 'rabbit-related' antigen. The use of other animals (sheep, goat, rat, chicken) then has to be considered as well as the use of denatured antigens (Lazarides, 1976; Jockusch *et al.*, 1978). Peptides (or other compounds with a molecular weight below 4000 d) generally have poor immunogenic properties. In order to obtain 'high titre' antisera these compounds should be coupled covalently to large proteins like serum albumin or thyroglobulin (Skowsky and Fisher, 1972). Thyroglobulin seems to be superior in terms of percentage of rabbits that respond and in the radioimmunoassay (RIA) titre which is obtained (Skowsky and Fisher, 1972). In order to avoid interference due to the antibodies raised against the carrier protein (Vandesande, 1979; Steinbusch *et al.*, 1978), it seems appropriate to use proteins that are as little as possible related to the proteins of the tissue studied. Thyroglobulin or, even better, sunflower globulin (Grouselle *et al.*, 1978) seems to be a better choice than albumin.

False-negativity caused by the first antiserum may also be due to:

(2) *The selection of an improper antiserum sample*

Precipitation techniques (Ouchterlony, immunoelectrophoresis) or radio-immunoassays (RIA) are frequently mentioned as methods to select antisera for ICC studies. However, the general validity of these techniques for the determination of potency and/or specificity (see Section VII) of an antiserum

---

Figure 7 The course of antibody development in a rabbit (0–2) immunized with oxytocin (Sigma Grade V; lot 103c–2910) coupled to bovine thyroglobulin according to Skowsky and Fisher (1972). Each arrow indicates one immunization whereby the length represents the amount of oxytocin that was injected. Plasma samples were collected 1 week after each antigen injection. In each sample radioimmunoassay (a,b) and immunocytochemical (c,d) properties were measured: (**a**) maximal binding (percentage of oxytocin tracer to an excess of antibody ($\triangle$..........$\triangle$); (**b**) titre (the antibody dilution to which 50% of the oxytocin tracer was bound (see also Dogterom *et al.*, 1976) ($\bigcirc$----$\bigcirc$); (**c**) the potency in an indirect immunofluorescence procedure and ($\blacksquare$——$\blacksquare$); (**d**) the potency in a PAP-procedure ($\star$——$\star$). (**c**) and (**d**) were measured on neurohypophyseal sections of male Wistar rats using the different antiserum samples in the same dilution (1:80 for the IMF and 1:200 in the PAP procedure)

in an ICC procedure is non-existent and may therefore lead to the selection of an antibody that is potent in one of these techniques but causes a false-negative result in an ICC staining procedure. The considerable discrepancy between the reactivity of an antiserum in an indirect immunofluorescence procedure, in a PAP procedure, and in a RIA, is shown in Figure 7. Seven weeks after the start of the (oxytocin) immunization an excellent antiserum is obtained to use in both ICC staining procedures, while the same antiserum samples are worthless for radioimmunoassay. However, after 10–12 weeks the (high) potency in the RIA remains, the reactivity of the antiserum in the PAP procedure diminishes only slightly, while on the other hand the immunofluorescence values rapidly drop to useless values. Two conclusions have to be drawn from these findings:

(a) The characteristics of an antiserum vary during the immunization period. This means that the reactivity in an ICC staining procedure can be enhanced by using serum amounts collected at a proper time. Pooling of antisera collected at different time intervals during an immunization thus decreases mostly their capacity in ICC. In order to obtain large samples of antiserum, it is our experience that three times 50–60 ml blood can easily be collected from the same rabbit within 5 days, if intraperitoneal plasmapheresis is performed (Pool *et al.* (1982)).

(b) Whether an antiserum will be qualified as 'good' depends largely on the technique used. The 'best' antisera for immunocytochemical studies therefore have to be selected with the same ICC procedure as will be used on the tissue sections.

VI   METHOD SPECIFICITY

The moment a positive reaction in a tissue section is obtained after incubation of an antiserum followed by an ICC staining procedure, the question arises whether this reaction is only due to an immunological binding of antibodies from this serum (= method specificity; see Section XI), or (also) based on a false-positive reaction of the immunocytochemical reagents. The causes for false-positivity may again be found at the level of (1) the tissue section, (2) the procedure used to visualize the first antibody and (3) the first antiserum itself. In order to evaluate each of these possibilities different control incubations should be carried out.

VI.1   Tissue Section

The role of false-positivity caused by *the tissue section* will become obvious after inspecting an unstained section. Possible causes described for this type of false-positivity are:

(a) the presence of a *pigment in the cell* which resembles the DAB precipitate (when an immunoperoxidase method is used) like neuromelanin in the substantia nigra (Figure 8a);

(b) *autofluorescence* (in the case of an immunofluorescence procedure) as caused by lipofuscin which is conspicuous in tissue from older human beings (Figure 8b). One might try to solve this problem either by using a different fluorochrome and/or filter combination (although other conjugates (rhodamin) usually exhibit a lower emission than the FITC conjugates and the emission spectrum of lipofuscin is extremely large), or by switching to an immunoenzyme procedure.

VI.2 Procedure Used to Identify the First Antibody

False-positivity due to the procedure used to demonstrate the first antibody will become obvious when the first antiserum incubation is omitted. Some known examples are:

(a) *Pseudoperoxidase activity* (in the case of an immunoperoxidase procedure) caused by the haem groups in erythrocytes (Figure 8c). This can be prevented effectively by perfusing the animal or, if this is not possible (e.g. for human tissue), by pre-incubation with a methanol–hydrogen peroxide mixture (Streefkerk, 1972), or 100% methanol alone, which has the same effect in our hands (see Appendix I). Although Geyer (1973) mentioned lipofuscin as a source of pseudoperoxidase activity we did not find it to cause false-positivity in formalin-fixed human brains.

(b) *Endogenous peroxidase activity* as present, e.g., in neurons of the subfornical organ (Buijs, 1978, Figure 8d). This activity may be inhibited by methanol nitroferricyanide containing 1% sodium and 1% acetic acid (Strauss, 1971).

(c) In immunoelectron microscopy, in case of an immunoperoxidase staining, the *osmiophilia of cell organelles* (e.g. lipid droplets) (van Leeuwen, 1982, van Leeuwen *et al.*, 1983).

(d) Conjugates or other secondary antibodies may bind electrostatically to basic proteins in the tissue section (*protein/protein interaction*) (see e.g. Vandesande, 1980). Such non-specific binding appeared difficult to eliminate and may even be enhanced during the preparation of labelled antibodies. Hebert *et al.* (1967), for instance, showed that non-specific staining of FITC conjugates increased linearly with the FITC/protein ratio. At least some of this non-specific reactivity may be prevented by pre-incubation of the tissue with pre-immune serum from the animal which served as a source for the second antibody (Sternberger, 1979).

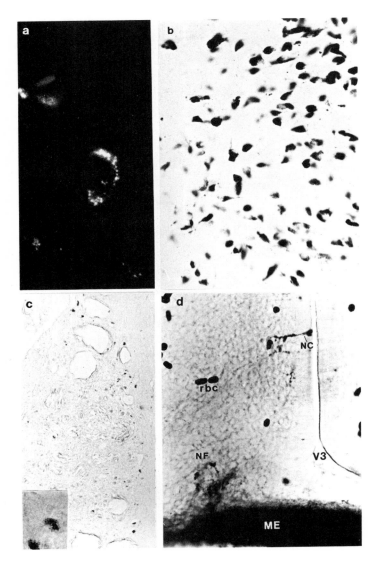

Figure 8 False-positive reactions. (**a**) Lipofuscin autofluorescence of paraventricular nucleus neurons in an unstained 6 μm paraffin section of a formalin-fixed human hypothalamus (male, 70 years old, 80.118; preparation E. J. Fliers (NIBR)). (**b**) Neuromelanin in the substantia nigra of a 61-year-old male. Unstained 100 μm vibratome section (preparation J. ter Borg, NIBR). (**c**) Endogenous peroxidase in cells at the border of the subfornical organ in the adult Wistar rat. 6 μm paraffin section incubated with the hydrogen peroxide. DAB medium only. (**d**) Pseudoperoxidase in red blood corpuscles (RBC). Hypothalamus of a fetal day 20 Wistar rat brain

VI.3 The First Antiserum

The same protein–protein interactions may of course occur during the incubation with *the first antiserum* and can only be recognized by incubating the section with a non-immune serum (see Section III), while all further incubation steps are kept unchanged. Pre-immune serum, antiserum raised against an antigen not present in the tissue under study, or the (first) antiserum pre-adsorbed with the injected immunogen may be used for this purpose. These control serum incubations approximate probably best the non-immune serum conditions when applied in a dilution, such that the concentration of immunoglobulins is the same as in the first antiserum used for the tissue incubation.

False-positive staining observed after incubation with a 'non-immune' serum may be caused by:

(a) *Free aldehydes* still present in the tissue due to the fixation procedure. For this reason Sternberger (1979) proposed a pre-incubation step with a (non-related) non-immune serum (see above), while incubations with Na-borohydrid (Lillie and Pizzolato, 1972; de Brabander *et al.*, 1979) or with small molecules or proteins containing free amino groups have also been applied for this purpose (see Appendices I and II).
(b) *Ionic interactions of IgG's* with basic proteins (e.g. Fc binding sites; Aarli *et al.*, 1975; Kraehenbuhl and Jamieson, 1974) might be reduced by enhancing the ionic strength of the buffer which is used to dilute the antiserum and for the rinsing steps (Capel, 1974; Grube, 1980).
(c) *Hydrophobic interactions*, e.g. of immunoglobulins with embedding media, may be prevented by the addition of a detergent like Tween or Triton X-100 to the incubation and washing media (see Appendix I).

Staining which persists after a non-immune serum incubation (e.g. with an adsorbed (first) antiserum) may point either to:

(1) the presence of contaminating antibodies induced by impurities in the immunogen in quantities sufficient to induce antibody formation but insufficient to allow a complete removal of these antibodies, or
(2) to contaminating antibodies already present in the serum before the immunization procedure started.

However, since in both cases this staining is based on an immunological reaction between antibodies of the first antiserum and the tissue, it cannot,

---

stained for vasopressin. Neurosecretory fibres (NC) are stained on the third ventricle (V3), in the region of the arcuate nucleus and in the median eminence (ME) (preparation D. N. Velis (NIBR))

according to the definition of method specificity given above (and in Section XI) be called false-positive but falls within the framework of serum specificity (Section VII) and should be studied accordingly.

VII   SERUM SPECIFICITY

In this section attention will be paid to the question of which tissue components are immunocytochemically stained in the tissue under study, the first step towards a type of specificity which is called serum specificity (step 3 of the flowchart in Figure 5; Section XI; Sternberger, 1979).

As has already been mentioned in Section III, antibodies are directed against antigenic sites of the immunogen and not against the molecule as an entity. Therefore, apart from the difficulties caused by the possible presence of small (highly antigenic) contaminations (see Section V), ICC serum specificity can never be derived solely from the characteristics of the injected immunogen. Related (but different) molecules in the tissue may share antigenic sites with this immunogen and therefore be a cause for a serum aspecific reaction. For the same reason, a positive immunocytochemical reaction with a monoclonal or 'affinity purified' antibody (see Sections VIII and X) or no staining after adsorption of the antiserum with the immunogen, perhaps provide some information on the antibodies responsible for the ICC staining, but certainly not about the nature of the immunoreactive tissue compound(s). It is therefore that, in order to prove serum specificity in ICC, the use of other ICC serum specificity tests will be necessary, enabling a positive identification of the ICC reactive compounds present in the tissue itself.

Requirements for an ICC serum specificity test

Since apart from the characteristics of the first antiserum a great number of additional factors influence the intensity and specificity of an ICC reaction (Figure 1), serum specificity in ICC should be studied under conditions that are as much as possible comparable to those used during the immunocyto-chemical staining of the tissue. An ICC serum specificity test should, in addition, allow control for improved specificity after an antiserum purifica-tion. On the basis of these conditions the following criteria for an ICC serum specificity test can be formulated:

VII.1   The (Antiserum) Incubation Conditions have to be Identical to those used in the Tissue Section

This condition is very important, especially since it has been shown that, e.g., precipitation and radioimmunoassay (RIA) techniques (frequently used to define serum specificity) may not in all cases reveal the potency and specificity of a (first) antiserum in an ICC procedure (Section V; Figure 7; Swaab *et al.*, 1977; van Raamsdonk *et al.*, 1979; Vandesande, 1979; Cumming, 1980).

VII.2 The Condition of the Antigens in the Test should be Identical to that in the Tissue

Changes in immunoreactivity of the tissue compounds can be induced by differences in the pre-treatment of the tissue (Section II), which implies that in an ICC specificity test the tissue should be processed in a way similar to that used for the preparation of the tissue sections. As will be shown later, this condition is very difficult to fulfil in model systems and the final outcome given by each type of ICC serum specificity test should, therefore, be checked afterwards in the tissue section itself (see Section VIII).

VII.3 All Tissue Antigens should be Included

In order to gain an insight into the possible immunoreactivity of all compounds present in the tissue under study no prior selection (e.g. by an extraction procedure) should be made in the test.

VII.4 Non-immunological Characterization of the Antigens should be Possible

When an immunoreactive tissue compound has been found, the next step will be to establish at least some of its characteristics such as: is it a protein, what is its molecular weight or isoelectric point. In some cases it may also be possible to characterize the antigen on the basis of biological activity (hormones, enzymes) (Geuze *et al.*, 1979). The establishment of these characteristics is necessary to prove the identity of the immunoreactive tissue compound for comparison with the antigen of primary interest. Moreover, some insight into the characteristics of the immunoreactive compounds may be convenient when they have to be isolated, e.g. in order to be able to use them in an antiserum purification procedure (see Section VIII).

VII.5 Quantification should be Possible

Even if the primary question (the localization of a certain component in a tissue section) is a qualitative one, quantification of the antigen/first antibody reaction in the test is important, for instance, to allow an accurate determination of the changes in ICC reactivity after purification of an antiserum (Section VIII).

At the present moment no antiserum test procedure is available which meets all these requirements but some of the successful attempts to develop ICC antiserum test systems which fulfil at least most of the criteria mentioned above will be discussed. In general, these serum specificity tests are aimed at either:

(a) characterizing immunocytochemically the coupling abilities of the first antiserum to a number of antigens known, supposed or expected to be present in the tissue, or
(b) determining directly what compounds from the tissue of investigation are actually coupling with the first antiserum.

Two of the most commonly used model tests which follow the first approach are the defined antigen substrate sphere (DASS) system, as originally described by Capel (1974) and the enzyme-linked immunosorbent assay (ELISA) as developed by Engvall and Perlmann (1971). In both techniques the proteinaceous compound to be tested is immobilized on a matrix (CNBr-activated agarose and polyethylene tubes respectively) and immuno-staining is performed identical to that on a tissue section (Figure 9). Both techniques allow a quantification of the first antiserum binding (condition 5). For DASS this has been done by microfluorometric readings after an immunofluorescence procedure (Capel, 1974; Deelder and Ploem, 1975) and by (micro)spectrophotometric determination of the peroxidase enzyme activity after HRP-conjugate (Streefkerk *et al.*, 1975; Pool, 1980; Appendix III) and PAP-incubation (see Appendix III). ELISA has also been performed using enzyme-conjugated antibodies or the PAP-procedure.

In connection with the determination of serum specificity in ICC, the DASS system has, for instance, successfully been applied by Swaab and Pool (1975) to determine quantitatively the reactivity of an oxytocin antiserum with the structurally related vasopressin (see also Figure 14).

The DASS and ELISA techniques fulfil requirements 1 and 5 described above, and consequently allow the determination of the reactivity of the antiserum in an ICC procedure towards compounds known or supposed to be present in the tissue under study. However, the immunoreactivity towards unknown tissue antigens will never be recognized this way. A test for the positive identification of antigens actually present in the tissue under investigation requires the solubilization and subsequent separation of all tissue components followed by a test on their reactivity in an immunocytochemical staining procedure.

Tissue material can probably best be solubilized by the use of SDS (sodium dodecyl sulphate) and/or urea. Large proteins and hydrophobic components are then included as well. Moreover, such a procedure appears not to disturb the antigen–antibody reaction (Stumph *et al.*, 1974). However, a single solubilization procedure does not allow the control on possible fragmentation

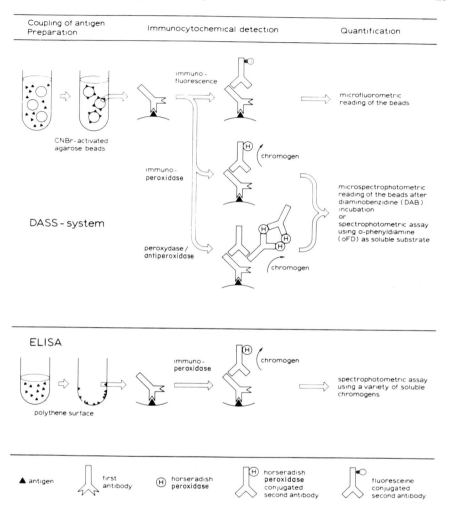

Figure 9 Serum specificity tests using isolated antigens. (**a**) In the defined antigen substrate sphere (DASS) system, proteinaceous compounds are covalently coupled to agarose beads which subsequently can be used in routine immunocytochemical staining procedures. In case of an immunofluorescence procedure the immunoreactivity can be determined by microfluorometric readings on individual beads, while after an immunoperoxidase staining procedure either microspectrophotometer readings on the beads or spectrophotometer determination of the absorbance of the supernatant may be used (see also Appendix III). (**b**) In the enzyme-linked immunosorbent assay (ELISA), the proteinaceous compound is adsorbed to a polyethylene surface, whereafter an immunoperoxidase staining is performed. The presence of immune reactivity can be detected by spectrophotometer readings with a variety of soluble chromogens (see for reviews O'Beirne and Cooper, 1979; and Smith and Gehle, 1980)

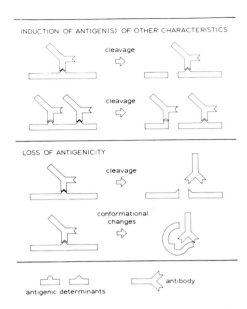

Figure 10 Schematic representation of possible changes in immunoreactivity upon tissue treatment. Cleavage of the original antigen can lead to the 'production' of two or more immunoreactive compounds (e.g. dependent upon the number of antigenic sites originally present on this antigen), or to total loss of immunoreactivity when the antigenic sites themselves are influenced by this cleavage. Conformational changes of the antigen can lead to sterical hindrance for the antibodies resulting in a false-negative immunoreaction

of immunoreactive compounds, either resulting in a loss of immunoreactivity or (in case of two or more antigenic determinants on the same molecule) in the production of immunoreactive compounds originally not present in the tissue (Figure 10). Preferably different tissue processing procedures should therefore be used: for instance, a combination of an ethanol/acetic acid or HCl extraction followed by an SDS/urea treatment of the remaining insolutes.

So far, the techniques used as ICC specificity test applying the steps of solubilization of the tissue, separation of the tissue compounds followed by an ICC reaction (Figure 11) all make use of an SDS electrophoresis in the second step. They differ, however, in the way the separated compounds are immobilized in order to perform the ICC staining procedures. An immobilization of a discontinuous spectrum of tissue components by slicing the gel after an SDS electrophoresis and coupling the tissue components from these slices onto polystyrene test tubes, followed by ELISA (SDS gel electrophoresis derived ELISA; GEDELISA) has been described by Lutz *et al.*

(1979) (Figure 11a). The immobilization of the continuous spectrum of SDS electrophoretically separated tissue compounds in the gel itself, followed by a routine ICC staining procedure (SDS gel electrophoresis immunoperoxidase method; SGIP) (Figure 11b), has been described by van Raamsdonk *et al.* (1977). Finally the transfer of the separated tissue compound, from the SDS gel onto filter paper (blot technique) followed by ICC staining or an autoradiographic procedure using I-labelled protein A (Figure 11c) has been described by Renart *et al.* (1979) and Towbin *et al.* (1979), respectively.

From these techniques GEDELISA seems to meet most of the criteria for an ICC specificity test as given above. Its use is mainly limited by the shortcomings of the ELISA technique. The physical adsorption of the antigen to the solid phase will not be the same for all proteinaceous compounds, and up to 30% of the antigen or antigen–antibody complexes may be lost during the washing and incubation steps (Engvall, 1980), while also the limited capacity of the adsorption of the (plastic) tubes may be a disturbing factor. An additional disadvantage of GEDELISA may be the loss of the high resolution of the SDS electrophoresis due to the slicing of the gel. This problem does not occur in the SGIP technique, in which the separated proteins are immobilized directly in the gel matrix by fixation with an ethanol–acetic acid mixture. However, also in this case it is not known whether this fixation procedure immobilizes all types of antigens. Unlike GEDELISA, the SGIP technique itself is not suitable for a quantification of the reactivity of the first antiserum (van Raamsdonk *et al.*, 1977). This quantification can, however, be introduced by combining SGIP with the DASS system. Antigens can be eluted from sliced gels and coupled covalently to CNBr-activated agarose beads. With these beads the reactivity of the antiserum can be determined quantitatively towards the same antigens initially identified in a SGIP procedure, thereby combining the advantages of a continuous spectrum of tissue components and avoiding the difficulties due to a physical adsorption of the antigens to the solid phase (Pool, 1980). A circumstantial advantage of SGIP is that it allows the use of the same protein spectrum (successive gel sections) for incubation with different antisera (van Raamsdonk *et al.*, 1977). The assessment of an antiserum affinity towards a continuous separation spectrum of tissue components is also inherent in the blot technique. Although, in principle, this approach can be made quantitative, so far it has not been worked out.

The SDS gel electrophoresis which is used in the three techniques described above, however, does not allow enough separation of proteinaceous material with molecular weights below 5 kD. Consequently, neither of these techniques can be used to gain an insight into, e.g., the distribution of immunoreactive peptides present in the tissue homogenates. Although this lack of resolving power may be overcome by the use of other separation techniques such as gel isoelectric focussing (Boer, 1979; van der Sluis *et al.*, 1983) or even

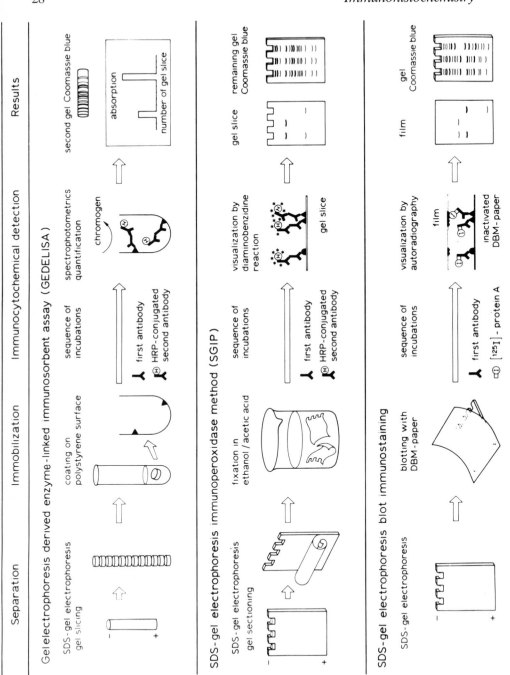

two-dimensional electrophoresis also the immobilization of these small compounds is a serious problem to be encountered (Boer, 1979; van der Sluis *et al.*, 1981). A new fixation technique using glutaraldehyde-impregnated filter paper is promising in this respect, and has already successfully been applied for the ICC staining of gel isoelectrofocussed standard peptides (van der Sluis *et al.*, 1983) (see Section VIII, Figure 13; Appendix IV).

VIII ANTISERUM PURIFICATION

See procedure for affinity purification of serum antibodies in Chapter 13, Section II.2.

When it has been assessed that an antiserum reacts with more than one component present in the tissue under study, the decision should be made whether this 'unwanted' reactivity has to be removed from the antiserum or not; for instance on the basis of the necessity for each particular study to use a 'one-tissue component specific' ICC localization procedure. Basically such an antiserum purification (step 4 in Figure 5) can be performed in two different ways:

(a) by *elution of antibodies* from immune complexes formed with the antigen to be localized ('affinity purified antibodies'); or

(b) by *the removal of the unwanted antibodies* by (pre-)incubation with the appropriate contaminating antigens.

The main difference between these two approaches is that the immuno-adsorbent in the first method has to be a preparation in which the antigen to be localized should be the only immunoreactive compound, while the second

---

Figure 11 Serum specificity tests based on the detection of ICC reactive compounds in an SDS gel electrophoretically separated tissue homogenate. (**a**) In GEDELISA, the separating gel is sectioned, fractions are subsequently eluted, and an ELISA is performed to detect immune reactivity (see also Figure 10). A second gel routinely stained with Coomassie blue is necessary to identify the antigens (Lutz *et al.*, 1979). (**b**) in the SGIP procedure longitudinal cryostat sections are made of the separating gel, and the proteins in the section are immobilized by a cold ethanol/acetic acid treatment. Gel sections flattened on glass slides can then be processed in an immunoperoxidase staining procedure in which the immune complexes can be visualized with oxidized diaminobenzidine. The remaining part of the unsectioned gel, stained with Coomassie blue, serves as the identification matrix. Several samples (lanes) can be treated simultaneously from the same gel, allowing the direct compari-son with 'standard' proteins or other tissue samples. (**c**) The blotting with diamino-benzyloxymethyl (DBM) paper allows the covalent binding of proteins diffusing out of the gell. The paper-bound components are then tested for immunoreactivity with a ^{125}I-protein A method using autoradiography. A second—routinely stained—gel is used for comparison (Renart *et al.*, 1979)

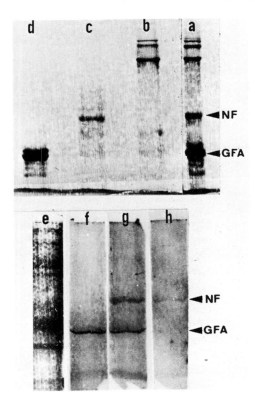

Figure 12 Preparation of the immunogens: (a) Rough neurofilament (NF), glial fibrillary acid (GFA) protein preparation as used in a preparative SDS electrophoresis. (b) SDS re-electrophoresis of the high molecular fraction. (c) SDS re-electrophoresis of the NF preparation (used for the immunization). (d) SDS re-electrophoresis of the GFA preparation (used for the immunization). The use of the SGIP procedure to identify immunoreactive compounds in a tissue homogenate. (e) Coomassie blue stained protein pattern of a SDS electrophoretically separated SDS/urea hippocampus extract. (f) Section of this gel incubated with the antiserum raised against glial fibrillary acid protein (GFA; see (d)). (g) Section of this gel incubated with an antiserum raised against neurofilament protein (see (c)). Notice next to the positive reaction of this antiserum with the NF band also a strong reaction with the GFA band. (h) Section of this gel incubated with the same anti-NF serum after adsorption with the GFA. This work was done in collaboration with Dr W. van Raamsdonk (Dept of Zoology, University of Amsterdam) and Dr C. Heyting (Netherlands Institute for Cancer Research)

method requires antigen preparations that do not contain the antigen to be localized. This implies that in all cases, prior to each adsorption, the immunocytochemical purity of the immunoadsorbent has to be known. This can be obtained by one of the antigen identification techniques described in

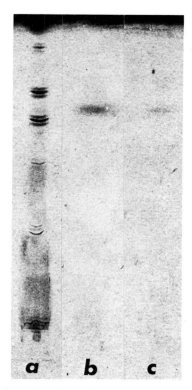

Figure 13 Isoelectric focussing in polyacrylamide gel slabs in pH range 2–11, followed by fixation with glutaraldehyde and PAP-staining, using an anti-oxytocin serum, (a) protein test mixture 9 (Serva); (b) oxytocin (Organon, Batch r.m. 435 AK, 100 ng); (c) oxytocin (Organon, Piton-S, 45 mU). (Preparation P. J. van der Sluis, NIBR)

Section VII. An example of such a test is shown in Figure 13. In case 100% pure antigen preparations are available in sufficient amounts both antiserum purification techniques might equally well be used. However, since this situation is an exception rather than a rule, the strategy followed for the antiserum purification will largely be dependent upon the (immunological) purity of the antigen preparations available. The conditions for the use of method (b) (the removal of unwanted antibody populations) are met most easily, while in addition cross-reacting antibodies (i.e. antibodies that react next to the antigen to be localized also with another antigen in the tissue) cannot be removed using the first method. For these reasons we will confine ourselves in this section only to this type of antiserum purification.

In order to remove a distinct population of antibodies from an antiserum a solid-phase immunoadsorbent should be used, since otherwise the tissue antigen may compete successfully with the antigen still present in soluble immunocomplexes in the adsorbed serum. This is especially important for small antigens (such as peptides), since they usually do not form precipitating immunocomplexes at all. The solid-phase media most commonly used for proteinaceous antigens are CNBr-activated agarose beads (see e.g. Vandesande, 1979). These antigen-coupled beads also exhibit an additional advantage: the amount of antibody bound to the beads can be determined quantitatively using the procedures described for the DASS system (see Section VII and Appendix III). This means that the amount of beads necessary minimally for an adsorption, as well as the final outcome of each adsorption, can be assessed quantitatively. The former may be of importance in the case of scarce antigens, while the latter enables a direct comparison of the reactivities of the non-adsorbed, adsorbed, and control serum towards this antigen (Figure 14). However, in order to evaluate the effect of the changed immunoreactivity for the tissue the reactivity of the adsorbed antiserum should be checked on a tissue section and in the model ICC serum specificity test (e.g. with the GEDELISA technique or the SGIP/DASS combination) where the reactivity towards each of the tissue antigens should be expressed in quantitative terms. Table 1 illustrates the possible outcomes of such a purified antiserum test procedure. When the antiserum after the adsorption with B still reacts with this component (Table 1, possibility 1), the adsorption apparently was not carried out properly. When, on the other hand, the adsorbed antiserum no longer reacts with component B (Table 1, possibilities 2, 3, and 4) the outcome of the antiserum test procedure may show a discrepancy between the results of the model test system and the tissue section (Table 1, possibility 2). According to the model test the adsorbed antiserum should contain antibodies against A, but in the tissue section (known to contain A) no reaction is observed; the apparent conclusion is that all antigenic determinants on component A in the tissue section are lost or masked (e.g. due to the tissue fixation procedure) and that thus probably the tissue processing has to be revaluated.

When after a successful adsorption with B the reactivity with A is unchanged and also the tissue staining remains (Table 1, possibility 3), apparently two different populations of antibodies are present in the antiserum: one directed against A and one directed against B. In this case, the antibodies directed against B are called 'contaminating antibodies' (see Section XI). Such contaminating antibodies may already be present in the serum prior to immunization (Section VI) or can be induced by impurities in the injected antigen, or especially in the case of small haptens by the carrier protein used to prepare the antigen (Steinbusch *et al.*, 1978).

The last possible reaction of the purified antiserum described in Table 1 is that after a successful adsorption with B also the reactivity with A has changed (Table 1, possibility 4). Apparently in this case at least part of the

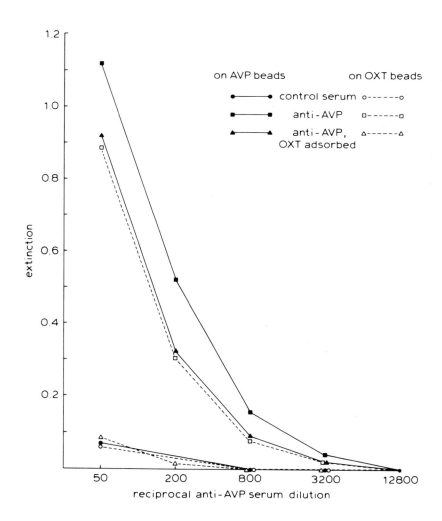

Figure 14 Antiserum dilution curves found after incubation of anti-vasopressin serum (squares), anti-vasopressin serum after adsorption with oxytocin beads (triangles), and control serum (circles) with vasopressin coupled beads (closed symbols) and oxytocin beads (open symbols), followed by a goat anti-rabbit peroxidase conjugate incubation. The immunoreactivity was visualized by a peroxidase reaction using (soluble) OFD as chromogen (see Appendix III). Notice that after the adsorption with oxytocin all (cross)-reactivity of the vasopressin antiserum towards oxytocin has disappeared, while the reactivity towards vasopressin has been reduced.
(Work done in collaboration with Miss A. A. Sluiter)

Table 1   Possible (ICC) reactivities of an adsorbed antiserum determined in
a (model) specificity test and in the tissue section

	Reaction with A (%)	Reaction with B (%)	Reaction on the tissue (%)
Non-adsorbed	100	100	100
Possibility 1	⩾100	⩾100	⩾100
Possibility 2	⩾100	0	0
Possibility 3	100	0	⩾100
Possibility 4	>100	0	>100

An antiserum (raised against A) reacts with two components (A and B) both present in the tissue under study. Since the aim was a specific ICC localization of component A in that tissue, the antiserum was adsorbed with component B.

The final outcome of this adsorption experiment was tested on isolated A and isolated B (for instance with the DASS system) and on tissue sections (the reactivities of the non-adsorbed antiserum were set at 100% in each case).

antibodies against A react also with B. Such antibodies are called cross-reacting antibodies and point to structural similarities between (in our case) A and B (see Section XI). Such cross-reacting antibodies have frequently been observed in ICC studies in the brain, as for example the cross-reactivity of anti-ACTH with alpha-MSH or anti-AVP with oxytocin (Figure 14). In some cases two antigens may be structurally so similar that with an antiserum raised against one of these compounds 100% cross-reactivity towards the other may be found. For instance, in an attempt to remove the vasopressin (cross-)reacting antibodies from an anti-vasotocin serum, all reactivity of this antiserum towards vasotocin disappeared (Swaab, unpublished observation). This means that using this antiserum no distinction can be made, immunocytochemically, between vasotocin and vasopressin.

IX   SPECIFICITY IN IMMUNOCYTOCHEMISTRY

When an antiserum has been sufficiently purified—which means it only reacts with one tissue compound in the antiserum specificity test (step 4 of the flowchart in Figure 5)—one might conclude that this antiserum consequently allows a monospecific localization of this compound in the tissue under study (see Section XI). However, this presupposes a full predictive value of the specificity test system for the reaction of that antiserum with the tissue section, which has to be proven in each case again for all currently used ICC serum-specificity model systems (step 5 of the flowchart in Figure 5; see also Section VII). The tissue section itself is the only final control in this respect, since the consequences of the inevitably different processing of the tissue compounds in the specificity test and in the tissue fixation procedure can never be determined in model specificity tests alone. Theoretically, such a final test on the 'monospecificity' of an immunocytochemical localization procedure must give negative staining (1) in the serum specificity test and on the tissue section after removal of the specific antibodies (adsorption test), and (2) in the same tissue lacking this particular antigen (mutant test).

This pre-adsorption test is different from the commonly used adsorption tests discussed in Sections III and VI to prove the method specificity. At that stage in the flowchart all immunological activity has to be removed, in an attempt to obtain a 'non-immune' serum, however, without any prior knowledge with respect to what components are actually stained immunocytochemically in the tissue. Since the adsorption test mentioned here is not carried out to determine the 'monospecificity of the antiserum reaction' but to test the validity of the specificity of the ICC reaction as determined with the model serum specificity test (step 4 in the flowchart), it also differs fundamentally from that currently mentioned in a great number of ICC papers to prove a 'monospecific' ICC localization (e.g. Petrusz *et al.*, 1977; Section III).

The most direct and probably also the only correct way to obtain an antigen that can be used in the final adsorption test is to isolate it from the tissue itself by using the same separation technique as used in the antiserum specificity test (see Section VII). For instance, after SDS gel electrophoresis, as used in GEDELISA and SGIP, the antigen can be eluted from the gel and coupled to CNBr-activated sepharose beads and subsequently processed in the adsorption procedure (Section VIII; Pool, 1980). Of course, if an antigen preparation is available that in the test systems behaves identically to the remaining single immunoreactive compound from the tissue, this preparation may also be used.

As stated above, the second possibility to prove the validity of the antiserum specificity test used involved an incubation of the purified antiserum with tissue lacking the antigen to be localized. It assumes either the presence of a mutant deficient for that antigen, or the possibility of removing this component specifically from the tissue under study. Unfortunately, both are only available for a very limited number of antigens. The example *par excellence* of such a mutant is the diabetes insipidus Brattleboro rat which is unable to synthesize the peptide arginine vasopressin. In fact, the neural lobe of the pituitary of this animal has been used to demonstrate the specific ICC vasopressin localization both at LM (Swaab and Pool, 1975) and EM level (van Leeuwen and Swaab, 1977). When, either in the adsorption or in the 'mutant test', positive reactions are found, the monospecificity of the immunocytochemical staining procedure—as was suggested on the basis of the single immunoreactive tissue compound in the serum specificity test—must be questioned. In practically all cases this erroneously assumed monospecificity will be caused by limitations of the test system. For instance, the test may not allow the detection of tissue amounts of antigen. An antigen present in high concentrations localized in few elements within the tissue (a few densely stained cells (µm range)) may cover a larger area in the test situation (mm range) (for instance in the SGIP procedure), and may therefore not be 'seen'. Also the antigen immobilization may be less efficient in the test or the preservation of immunoreactivity may be reduced. Such situations may lead to the necessity of processing larger amounts of tissue or more sensitive techniques to detect the immunostaining in the test.

X SPECIFICITY IN IMMUNOCYTOCHEMISTRY (SOME CONCLUDING REMARKS)

Starting from the idea that one of the conditions for specificity in immunocytochemistry is the proof that the component of interest is indeed the only immunoreactive compound present in the tissue under investigation, it will be clear that a positive identification of all immuno(cytochemical)reactive components in the tissue section should be an intrinsic part of an ICC specificity test procedure. In contrast to this 'defined antigen specificity' it has been shown in Section III that the currently used ICC specificity tests (e.g. the adsorption test) will ultimately yield a (possibly very good) characterization of the antibodies that are responsible for the ICC reactivity but fail to give this insight into the binding capacities to unknown compounds in the tissue section. The type of specificity obtained in this 'classical' way can therefore best be termed 'defined antibody specificity'.

The 'defined antigen specificity' as ultimately found using the sequence of control experiments as described in Sections III–IX and schematically visualized in Figure 5 will mainly be dependent on the procedures used for the identification of the immunoreactive tissue components. It is therefore not surprising that in all currently used ICC serum specificity tests the tissue components are separated by an SDS electrophoresis (see Section VII). But at the same time this means that the limitations of these ICC serum specificity tests will be set by the resolution of this type of electrophoresis. For instance, two tissue antigens with (approximately) the same molecular weight will never be recognized as such. In this respect the approach based on a two-dimensional electrophoresis (isoelectric focussing in one direction and SDS electrophoresis in the second dimension) to separate the tissue antigens will definitely be an improvement

A second point which has to be taken into account in every ICC specificity study is that the finally found 'specific ICC reactivity' will always be a procedure-dependent 'specific ICC reactivity'. This is, e.g., illustrated by the second antibody-dependent ICC reactivity with the oxytocin antiserum as given in Figure 7. An example of the role of the first antiserum incubation conditions on the outcome of an ICC staining procedure may be illustrated by the 'first antiserum dilution-dependent specificity' as described by, for example, Keefer *et al.* (1976), van Leeuwen and Swaab (1977), and Petrusz *et al.* (1980), while an illustration of a tissue-dependent ICC reactivity has been given by Vandesande during the EMBO course on Immunocytochemistry in 1980. In hypothalamic preparations from normal rat they found a maximal staining of the vasopressin-containing cells, with an anti-vasopressin serum applied in a PAP procedure at a dilution of 1/200. However, using the same ICC staining procedure for a study in rats from which the hypothalamic magnocellular neurosecretory system had been activated by dehydration combined with a blocking of the axonal transport by colchicine, no 'vasopressin' reaction in the hypothalamus of these animals was observed. Starting with an ICC procedure which has proven to allow the specific ICC localization of vasopressin an apparent conclusion may be that the hypothalamic magnocellular neurons from dehydrated colchicin-treated rats do not contain vasopressin. However, after using a different dilution (1/1000) of the (same) vasopressin antiserum an intense reaction was observed in the vasopressin cells in these rats. The maximal staining intensity that could be obtained after a renewed optimalization of the ICC staining procedure even turned out to be much higher in the experimental (dehydrated, colchicine-treated) animal than in the normal rats.

These three examples all illustrate the procedure-dependent ICC reactivity: a change in one of the components (the tissue, the antisera) or conditions (tissue fixation, antiserum incubation) used to define the specificity of a given ICC localization means that the specificity of the ICC staining procedure has to be revaluated.

Finally, there is the question whether the application of monoclonal antibodies provides an answer to the specificity problems in immunocytochemistry. It will be clear that indeed this type of antibody will abolish all specificity problems caused by the presence of contaminating antibodies (see Sections VIII, XI, and Chapter 9), but beforehand cross-reactivity of a monoclonal antibody (see Sections VIII, XI and Section IX of Chapter 9) cannot be excluded and moreover, if present, it will involve the entire antibody population and a purification as described in Section VIII will be irrelevant.

Theoretically, a clone can be selected that produces an antibody that does react in an ICC staining procedure with no other component in the tissue under study than the antigen of interest. However, practically this implies that a test on the possibility of fulfilling this condition should be an intrinsic part of the clone selection procedures. Since this type of selection procedure will and probably can never be applied, the same series of ICC specificity tests as described in this chapter for polyclonal antibodies will be necessary to prove a 'defined antigen-specific' immunocytochemical localization with a monoclonal antibody.

ACKNOWLEDGEMENTS

The authors wish to thank P. van Nieuwkoop, Dr H. L. Walg, and Dr P. C. Diegenbach for their kind assistance during the preparation of the manuscript, and H. Stoffels and A. T. Potjer for making the drawings and the photographs. We are also greatly indebted to the (other) members of our project group on neuroendocrinology for their valuable suggestions.

XI   GLOSSARY

Method specificity
The absence of staining in an immunocytochemical localization procedure by mechanisms other than an immunological interaction between antibodies from the first antiserum and the tissue.

Serum specificity
The absence of immunological interactions in an immunocytochemical staining procedure between antibodies from the first antiserum with other tissue components than the antigen of interest.

Monospecific immunocytochemical staining procedure
A staining procedure proven to result in the immunocytochemical localization of one defined antigen in a given tissue.

Contaminating antibodies
Antibodies present in the first antiserum which react in an immunocytochemical staining procedure with tissue component(s) which share no antigenic sites with the antigen of interest.

Cross-reacting antibodies
Antibodies present in the first antiserum which react in an immunocytochemical staining procedure with the antigen of interest but also with (an)other tissue component(s).

APPENDIX I
IMMUNOCYTOCHEMICAL STAINING (PAP PROCEDURE) OF VIBRATOME SECTIONS FOR LIGHT AND ELECTRON MICROSCOPY

Buffer for LM: 0.05 M Tris, 0.9% NaCl, 0.5% Triton, pH = 7.6.
Buffer for EM: 0.05 M Tris, 0.9% NaCl, 0.1% Triton, pH = 7.6.

—all antiserum incubations and washings of the sections (20–100 μm) are performed in plastic jars with a diameter of 2.2 cm

—sections of non-perfused fixed brains are pretreated with methanol for at least 15 min to eliminate the pseudo-peroxidase activity in the erythrocytes (only for LM)

—washing of the sections in Tris–NaCl buffer

—incubation with the first antiserum (30–60 min at room temperature followed overnight at 4 °C, shake gently)

—washing three times 30–60 min with the Tris–NaCl buffer depending upon the section thickness (for the following EM incubations use no Triton)

—incubation with the second antibody (60–90 min, room temperature, shake gently)

—wash three times 30–60 min with the Tris–NaCl buffer

—incubation with the PAP complex (60–90 min, room temperature, shake gently)

—wash with Tris buffer (0.05 M Tris; pH = 7.6), (LM), for EM 0.05 M Tris, 0.9% NaCl, pH = 7.6

—enzyme–cytochemical peroxidase reaction (5 mg diaminobenzidine, 0.1 ml 1% H_2O_2 in 9.9 ml 0.05 M Tris buffer; pH = 7.6) (for EM add 0.9% NaCl to this mixture) for 5–20 min at room temperature

—wash in buffer

—(LM) the sections are brought onto a glass slide and stretched with a paint brush and allowed to dry in the air

—dehydration in graded alcohol followed by embedding in malinol

—(EM) incubation in 1% osmium tetroxide in 0.1 M cacodylate buffer (pH = 7.2) for 30 min

—wash in 0.1 M cacodylate buffer

—dehydration in graded alcohol and embedding in Epon 812.

APPENDIX II
IMMUNOELECTRON MICROSCOPIC PROCEDURE FOR POST-EMBEDDING STAINING

—small tissue blocks are fixed, dehydrated in alcohol and embedded in Epon 812

—ultrathin (or semithin) sections are collected on nickel grids

—etching of the sections for 3 min in a droplet of 5% hydrogen peroxide

—wash in 0.05 M Tris saline (pH = 7.6)

—incubation in a droplet normal swine serum (diluted 1:30 in Tris saline) for 10 min

—incubation with the first antiserum for 10 min at room temperature or 24–48 h at 4 °C

—wash in Tris saline and incubation in a droplet swine serum

—incubation for 10 min with the second antibody

—wash in Tris saline and incubation in a droplet swine serum

—incubation with the PAP complex diluted in 1% swine serum in Tris saline (10 min)
—wash in 0.05 M Tris (pH = 7.6)
—incubation with the hydrogen peroxide/DAB mixture (see Appendix I)
—wash (several times) in distilled water
—fixation in 4% osmium tetroxide for 15 min
—wash in distilled water
—dry on filter paper

Alternatively, the second antibody may be labelled with peroxidase or colloidal gold or may be replaced by a protein A–gold incubation (see Chapter 11).

APPENDIX III
DEFINED ANTIGEN SUBSTRATE SPHERE (DASS) SYSTEM
(Modified after Capel (1974) and Streefkerk *et al.* (1975)

(a) Preparation of the Antigen-coupled Beads

—coupling of 200 μg peptide to 1 ml CNBr-activated beads overnight at 4 °C under gentle shaking (coupling buffer 0.1 M borate 0.5 M NaCl (pH = 8.5)
—washing of the beads in the coupling buffer
—inactivation of the residual reactive groups with 1 M ethanolamine (pH = 8.5)
—removal of the non-covalently bound antigen by repeated washings at pH 4.0 (0.1 M acetate buffer, 0.5 M NaCl) and pH 8.5 (coupling buffer)
—storage of the beads at 4 °C in physiological buffered saline containing 0.01% Na-azide.

(b) Immunocytochemical Staining of the Antigen-coupled Beads

—incubation of 1.25 ml diluted antiserum with 12.5 μl (packed) beads 60 min at room temperature followed overnight at 4 °C under gentle shaking
—four washings of the beads with 'supermix' (0.05 M Tris buffer containing 0.5 M NaCl, 0.5–0.05% Triton X-100 0.25% gelatin)
—incubation with the second (and if necessary third) layer antibodies each followed by a washing procedure with 'supermix'
—in case of an immunoperoxidase method (using a HRP conjugate or the unlabelled PAP technique) 4 μl packed beads are washed (twice) in an 0.05 M Tris buffer (pH 7.6) (1) or an 0.1 M phosphate buffer (pH = 6.0) (2), and are incubated either with
   (1) 1 ml of a freshly prepared hydrogen peroxide/DAB medium (see Appendix I) or
   (2) 0.9 ml of a medium containing 40 mg orthophenylene diamine and 0.01% hydrgen peroxide in 200 ml 0.1 M phosphate buffer (pH = 6.0)

—the OPD reaction is stopped after 1–3 min by adding 0.25 ml 2 M H_2SO_4 to the reaction medium.

—the DAB-reaction is stopped after 1 min by adding an excess of 0.1 M HCl

(c) Determination of the Immunocytochemical Reactivity

(1) Beads incubated according to an immunofluorescent procedure (see also Capel (1974), Swaab and Pool (1975), and Pool (1980)).

—8 µl of the beads suspension is brought onto an object slide covered with a glass coverslip (9 × 9 mm) and sealed with nail polish

—the fluorescence of 5–40 randomly selected individual beads is measured in a microscope fluorometer using epi-illumination.

(2) Beads incubated according to an immunoperoxidase procedure using DAB as chromogen.

—8 µl of the stained beads suspension is brought onto an object slide covered with a glass coverslip and sealed with nail polish

—the staining intensity of individual beads (Streefkerk *et al.*, 1975) or large areas in the bead preparation (Pool, 1980) is measured with a scanning microscope photometer at 420 nm.

(3) Beads incubated according to an immunoperoxidase procedure using OPD as chromogen.

—the supernatant is separated from the beads and the staining intensity is measured spectrophotometrically at 492 nm.

APPENDIX IV
IMMUNOCYTOCHEMICAL DETECTION OF OLIGOPEPTIDES AFTER ISOELECTRIC FOCUSSING (IEF) IN POLYACRYLAMIDE GELS
(van der Sluis *et al.*, submitted)

—IEF in flat bed apparatus in 200 µm thick polyacrylamide gel slabs (I = 4; C = 3)

—immobilization of the focussed peptides by pressing a sheet of Whatman 540 paper wetted with a 25% glutaraldehyde solution, onto the gel between two Plexiglas plates; by this procedure the gel is firmly attached to the paper, and this gel–paper combination can be used in the following steps

—washing of about 20 min in distilled water in order to remove the gel–paper combination from the lower Plexiglas plate and the non-bound glutaraldehyde

—inactivation of remaining free aldehyde groups by incubation in 0.5 M Tris–HCl, pH 7.4 for 1 h at room temperature, followed by incubation in rinsing buffer (50 mM Tris–HCl, pH 7.4, 150 mM NaCl, 0.25% gelatin and 0.05% Triton X-100) also for 1 h

—PAP procedure as described in Appendix I except for the duration of the washings after each serum incubation (2 h).

REFERENCES AND FURTHER READING

Aarli, J. A., Aparico, S. R., Lumsden, C. E., and Tonder, O. (1975). 'Binding of normal human IgG to myelin sheaths, glia and neurons.' *Immunology*, **28**, 171–185.

Bargmann, W. (1949). 'Über die neurosekretorische Verknopfung von Hypothalamus und Neurohypophyse.' *Z. Zellforsch.*, **34**, 610–634.

Beauvillain, J. C., Tramu, G., and Dubois, M. P. (1975). 'Characterization by different techniques of adrenocorticotropin and gonadotropin producing cells in the rat pituitary.' *Cell Tiss. Res.*, **158**, 301–317.

Bigbee, J.·W., Kosek, J. C., and Eng, L. F. (1977). 'Effects of primary antiserum dilution on staining of "antigen-rich" tissues with the peroxidase anti-peroxidase technique.' *J. Histochem. Cytochem.*, **25**, 443–447.

Boer, G. J. (1979). 'Development of a specificity test for immunocytochemical of neuropeptides using high voltage electrofocussing in polyacrylamide micro slab gels.' *J. Endocr.*, **80**, 54P.

Boorsma, D. M., Streefkerk, D. F., and Kors, N. (1976). 'Peroxidase and fluorescein isothiocyanate as antibody markers. A quantitative comparison of two peroxidase conjugates prepared with glutaraldehyde or periodate and a fluorescein conjugate.' *J. Histochem. Cytochem.*, **24**, 1017–1025.

De Brabander, M., de Mey, J., Joniau, M., and Gevens, G. (1979). 'Immunoelectron microscopic localization of subcellular fibrillar elements using the unlabeled antibody enzyme method.' *Ultramicroscopy*, **4**, 124–128.

Buijs, R. M. (1978). 'Intra- and extrahypothalamic vasopressin and oxytocin pathways in the rat. Pathways to the limbic system, medulla oblongata and spinal cord.' *Cell Tiss. Res.*, **192**, 423–435.

Buijs, R. M. and Swaab, D. F. (1979). 'Immunoelectronmicroscopical demonstration of vasopressin and oxytocin synapses in the limbic system of the rat.' *Cell Tiss. Res.*, **204**, 355–365.

Buijs, R. M., Swaab, D. F., Dogterom, J., and van Leeuwen, F. W. (1978). 'Intra- and extrahypothalamic vasopressin and oxytocin pathways in the rat.' *Cell Tiss. Res.*, **186**, 423–433.

Buijs, R. M. (1982). 'Ultrastructural localization of amines, aminoacids and peptides in the brain.' In Buijs R. M. *et al.* (eds), *Progress in Brain Research*, Vol 55, Elsevier, Amsterdam, pp 167–183.

Capel, P. J. A. (1974). 'A quantitative immunofluorescent method based on the covalent coupling of protein to Sepharose beads.' *J. Immunol. Methods*, **5**, 165–178.

Capel, P. J. A. (1975). 'The defined Antigen Substrate Spheres (DASS) system and some of its applications.' *Ann. N.Y. Acad. Sci.*, **254**, 108–118.

Chan-Palay, V. and Palay, S. L. (1977). 'Ultrastructural identification of substance P cells and their processes in rat sensory ganglia and their terminals in the spinal cord by immunocytochemistry.' *Proc. Natl. Acad. Sci. U.S.A.*, **74**, 4050–4054.

Cowan, W. M., Gottlieb, D. I., Hendrickson, A. E., Price, J. L., and Woolsey, T. A. (1972). 'The autoradiographic demonstration of axonal connections in the central nervous system.' *Brain Res.*, **37**, 25–51.

Cumming, R. (1980). 'Selection of antibodies for the immunofluorescent localization of cyclic GMP in the central nervous system.' *J. Immunol. Meth.*, **37**, 301–309.

Dacheux, F. (1981). 'Ultrastructural localization of corticotropin, beta-lipotropin and alpha- and beta-endorphin in the porcine anterior pituitary.' *Cell Tiss. Res.*, **215**, 87–101.

Dale, H. (1935). 'Pharmacology and nerve-endings.' *Proc. R. Soc. Med.*, **28**, 319–332.

Deelder, A. M. and Ploem, J. S. (1975). 'An immunofluorescence reaction for *Schistosoma mansonii* using the Defined Antigen Substrate Spheres (DASS) system.' *J. Immunol Methods*, **4**, 239–251.

Dogterom, J., van Wimersma Greidanus, Tj. B., and Swaab, D. F. (1977). 'Evidence for the release of vasopressin and oxytocin into cerebrospinal fluid: measurements in plasma and CSF of intact and hypophysectomized rats.' *Neuroendocrinology*, **24**, 108–118.

Eccles, J. C., Fatt, P., and Koketsu, K. (1954). 'Cholinergic and inhibitory synapses in a pathway from motor–axon collaterals to motoneurones.' *J. Physiol.*, **126**, 524–562.

Engvall, E. and Perlmann, P. (1971). 'Enzyme linked immunosorbent assay (ELISA). III. Quantitative assay of immunoglobulin G.' *Immunochemistry*, **8**, 871–880.

Engvall, E. (1980). 'Enzyme immunoassay ELISA and EMIT.' In Van Vunakis, H. and Langore, J. J. (eds), *Methods in Enzymology*, vol. 70. Academic Press, New York, pp. 418–439.

Falck, B., Hillarp, N. A., Thieme, G., and Torp, A. (1962). 'Fluorescence of catecholamines and related compounds condensed with formaldehyde.' *J. Histochem. Cytochem.*, **10**, 348–354.

Fink, R. P. and Heimer, L. (1967). 'Two methods for selective silver impregnation of degenerating axons and their synaptic endings in the central nervous system.' *Brain Res.*, **4**, 369–374.

Geuze, J. J., Slot, J. W., and Tokuyasu, K. T. (1979). 'Immunocytochemical localization of amylase and chymotrypsin in the exocrine cell with special attention to the Golgi complex.' *J. Cell Biol.*, **82**, 697–707.

Geyer, G. (ed.) (1973). *Ultrahistochemie*. Gustav Fisher Verlag, Stuttgart.

Golgi, C. (1879). 'Di una mova reasione apparentamente nera delle cellule nervose cerebrali ottenuta col bichloruro di mercurio.' *Arch. Sci. Med.*, **3**, 1–7.

Gordon, W. E., Bushnell, A., and Burridge, K. (1978). 'Characterization of the intermediate (10 nm) filaments of cultured cells using autoimmune rabbit serum.' *Cell*, **13**, 249–261.

Graftstein, B. (1967). 'Transport of protein by goldfish optic nerve fibres.' *Science*, **157**, 196–198.

Grouselle, D., Favre Bauman, A., and Tixier-Vidal, A. 'A radio-immuno assay for thyroliberin.' Comparison with TRH radio receptor assay.' *Neurosci. Lett.*, **7**, 7–15.

Grube, D. (1980). 'Immunoreactivities of gastrin (G-) cells. II. Non-specific binding of immunoglobulins to G-cells by ionic interactions.' *Histochemistry*, **66**, 149–167.

Gu, J., de Mey, J., Moeremans, M., and Polak, J. M. (1981). 'Sequential use of the PAP and immunogold staining methods for the light microscopical double staining of tissue antigens.' *Peptides*, **1**, 365–374.

Hebert, G. A., Pittman, B., and Cherry, W. B. (1967). 'Factors affecting the degree of non-specific staining given by fluorescein isothiocyanate labeled globulins.' *J. Immunol.*, **98**, 1204–1212.

Hunt, S. P., Kelly, J. S., and Emson, P. C. (1980). 'The electron microscopic localization of methionine enkephalin within the superficial layers (I and II) of the spinal cord.' *Neuroscience*, **5**, 1871–1890.

Jockusch, B. M., Kelley, K. H., Meijer, R. K., and Burger, M. (1978). 'An efficient method to produce specific anti-actin.' *Histochemistry*, **55**, 177–185.

Keefer, D. A., Stumpf, W. E., and Petrusz, P. (1976). 'Quantitative autoradiographic assessment of ^{3}H-estradiol uptake in immunocytochemically characterized pituitary cells.' *Cell Tiss. Res.*, **166**, 25–32.

Kraehenbuhl, J. P. and Jamieson, J. D. (1974). 'Localization of intracellular antigens by immunoelectron microscopy.' *Int. Rev. Exper. Pathol.*, **13**, 1–53.

Kurki, P., Linder, E., Virtanen, I., and Stenman, S. (1977). 'Human smooth muscle auto antibodies reacting with intermediate 100 A filaments.' *Nature*, **268**, 240–241.

Lazarides, E. (1976). 'Actin, alpha-actinin and tropomyosin interaction in the structural organization of actin filaments in non-muscle cells.' *J. Cell. Biol.*, **68**, 202–218.

Li, J. Y., Dubois, M. P., and Dubois, P. M. (1977). 'Somatotrophs in the human fetal anterior pituitary. An electron microscopic immunocytochemical study.' *Cell Tiss. Res.*, **181**, 545–552.

Lillie, R. D. and Pizzolato, P. (1972). 'Histochemical use of borohydrides as aldehyde blocking reagents.' *Stain. Technol.*, **47**, 13–16.

Livett, B. G. (1978). 'Immunohistochemical localization of nervous system specific proteins and peptides.' *Int. Rev. Cytol.*, Suppl. 7.

Lutz, H., Higgins, J., Pederson, N. C., and Theilen, G. H. (1979). 'The demonstration of antibody specificity by a new technique.' *J. Histochem. Cytochem.*, **27**, 1216–1220.

McLaughlin, B. J., Barber, R., Saiko, K., Roberts, E., and Wu, J. Y. (1975). 'Immunocytochemical localization of glutamate decarboxylase in rat spinal cord.' *J. Comp. Neurol.*, **164**, 308–322.

Nakane, P. K. and Hartman, A. L. (1980). 'Immunocytochemical localization of intracellular antigens with SEM.' *Histochem. J.*, **12**, 435–447.

O'Beirne, A. J. and Cooper, H. R. (1979). 'Heterogeneous enzyme immunoassay.' *J. Histochem. Cytochem.*, **27**, 1148–1162.

Ong, S. L. and Steiner, A. L. (1977). 'Localization of cyclic GMP and cyclic AMP in cardiac and skeletal muscle: immunocytochemical demonstration.' *Science*, **195**, 183–185.

Petrusz, P., Sar, M., Ordronneau, P., and DiMeo, P. (1976). 'Specificity in immunocytochemical staining.' *J. Histochem. Cytochem.*, **24**, 1110–1115.

Petrusz, P., Sar, M., Ordronneau, P., and DiMeo, P. (1977). 'Reply to the letter of Swaab *et al.*, Can specificity ever be proved in immunocytochemical staining?' *J. Histochem. Cytochem.*, **25**, 390–391.

Petrusz, P., Ordronneau, P., and Finley, J. C. W. (1980). 'Criteria for reliability for light microscopic immunocytochemical staining.' *Histochem. J.*, **12**, 333–348.

Pickel, V. M., Joh, T. H., and Reis, D. J. (1976). 'Monoamine synthesizing enzymes in central dopaminergic, noradrenergic and serotonergic neurons. Immunocytochemical localization by light- and electron-microscopy.' *J. Histochem. Cytochem.*, **24**, 792–806.

Pool, Chr. W. (1980). 'An immune- and enzymehistochemical determination of striated muscle fibre characteristics.' Thesis, University of Amsterdam.

Pool, Chr. W., Buijs, R. M., Swaab, D. F., Boer, G. J. and van Leeuwen, F. W. (1982). 'Specificity in immunocytochemistry.' In van Leeuwen, F. W. *et al.* (eds), *ICC and its Application in Brain Research*. Manual of Second EMBO practical course, Amsterdam, pp. 93–128.

van Raamsdonk, W., Pool, Chr. W., and Heyting, C. (1977). 'Detection of antigens and antibodies by an immunoperoxidase method applied on thin longitudinal sections of SDS polyacrylamide gels.' *J. Immunol. Methods*, **17**, 337–348.

Renart, J., Reiser, J., and Stark, G. R. (1979). 'Transfer of proteins from gels to diazobenzyl oxymethyl paper and detection with antisera: a method for studying antibody specificity and antigen structure.' *PNAS USA*, **76**, 3116–3120.

Skowsky, W. R. and Fisher, D. A. (1972). 'The use of thyroglobulin to induce antigenicity to small molecules.' *J. Lab. Clin. Med.*, **80**, 134–146.

van der Sluis, P., Boer, G. J., and Pool, Chr. W. (1983). 'The immunocytochemical detection of oligopeptides immobilized by glutaraldehyde after gel isoelectric focussing.' (In preparation.)

Smith, K. O. and Gehle, W. D. (1980). 'Semiautomation of immunoassays by use of magnetic transfer devices.' In Van Vunakis, H. and Langone, J. J. (eds), *Methods in Enzymology*, vol. 70, pp. 388–416.

Sofroniew, M. V. and Glassmann, W. (1981). 'Golgi-like im immunoperoxidase staining of hypothalamic magnocellular neurons that contain vasopressin, oxytocin or neurophysin in the rat.' *Neuroscience*, **6**, 619–643.

Sofroniew, M. V. and Weindl, A. (1978). 'Extrahypothalamic neurophysin containing perikarya, fiber pathways and fiber clusters in the rat brain.' *Endocrinology*, **102**, 334–337.

Steinbusch, H. W. M., Verhofstad, A. A. J., and Joosten, H. W. J. (1978). 'Localization of serotonin in the central nervous system by immunohistochemistry. Description of a specific and sensitive technique and some applications.' *Neuroscience*, **3**, 811–819.

Sternberger, L. (1979). *Immunocytochemistry*, 2nd edn. John Wiley & Sons, New York, Chichester, Brisbane, Toronto.

Strauss, W. (1971). 'Inhibition of peroxidase by methanol-nitroferricyanide for use in immunoperoxidase procedures.' *J. Histochem. Cytochem.*, **19**, 682–688.

Streefkerk, J. G. (1972). 'Inhibition of erythrocyte pseudoperoxidase activity by treatment with hydrogen peroxide following methanol.' *J. Histochem. Cytochem.*, **20**, 829–831.

Streefkerk, J. G., van der Ploeg, M., and van Duijn, P. (1975). 'Agarose beads as matrices for proteins in cytospectrophotometric investigations of immunohisto-peroxidase procedures.' *J. Histochem. Cytochem.*, **23**, 243–250.

Stumph, W. E., Elgin, S. C. R., and Hood, L. (1974). 'Antibodies to proteins dissolved in sodium dodecyl sulphate.' *J. Immunol.*, **113**, 1752–1756.

Swaab, D. F. (1982). 'Comments on the validity of immunocytochemical methods.' In Palay, S. L. and Chan-Palay, V. (eds), *Cytochemical Methods in Neuroanatomy*. Alan Liss, New York.' pp. 423–440.

Swaab, D. F. and Pool, Chr. W. (1975). 'Specificity of oxytocin and vasopressin immunofluorescence.' *J. Endocr.*, **66**, 263–272.

Swaab, D. F., Pool, C. W., and Nijveldt, F. (1975). 'Immunofluorescence of vasopressin and oxytocin in the rat hypothalamo-neurohypophyseal system.' *J. Neural Transm.*, **36**, 195–215.

Swaab, D. F., Pool, Chr. W., and van Leeuwen, F. W. (1977). 'Can specificity ever be proved in immunocytochemical staining.' *J. Histochem. Cytochem.*, **25**, 388–391.

Towbin, H., Staehelin, T., and Gordon, J. (1979). 'Electrophoretic transfer of proteins for polyacrylamide gels to nitrocellulose sheets: Procedure and some applications.' *Proc. Natl. Acad. Sci. USA*, **76**, 4350–4354.

Trenchev, J. and Holborrow, D. I. (1976). 'The specificity of anti-actin serum.' *Immunology*, **32**, 509–512.

van der Sluis, P. J., Boer, G. J. and Pool, Chr. W. 'Fixation and immunoperoxidase staining of oligopeptides after isoelectric focusing in thin polyacrylamide slabgels (submitted).

Vandesande, F. (1979). 'A critical review of immunocytochemical methods for light microscopy.' *J. Neurosci. Meth.*, **1**, 3–23.

Vandesande, F. and Dierickx, K. (1979). 'The activated hypothalamic magnocellular neurosecretory system and the one neuron–one neurohypophyseal hormone concept.' *Cell Tiss. Res.*, **200**, 29–33.

van Leeuwen, F. W. (1981). 'An introduction to the immunocytochemical localization of neuropeptides and neurotransmitters.' *Acta Histochemica*, Suppl. Bd. **XXIV**, 49–77.

van Leeuwen, F. W. (1982). 'Monospecific localization of neuropeptides: a utopian goal?' In Bullock, G. R. and Petrusz, P. (eds), *Techniques in Immunocytochemistry*, vol. 1. Academic Press, London, New York, pp. 283–299.

van Leeuwen, F. W. and Swaab, D. F. (1977). 'Specific immunoelectronmicroscopic localization of vasopressin and oxytocin in the neurohypophysis of the rat.' *Cell Tiss. Res.*, **177**, 493–501.

van Leeuwen, F. W., Pool, Chr. W. and Sluiter, A. A. (1983). 'Enkephalin immunoreactivity in synaptoid elements on glial cells in the rat neural lobe.' *Neuroscience*, **8**, 229–241.

Van Vunakis, H. and Langone, J. J. (eds) (1980). *Methods in Enzymology*, vol. 70. *Immunochemical Methods*. Academic Press, New York, London, Toronto, Sydney, San Francisco.

Vivien-Roels, B., Pevet, P., Dubois, M. P., Arendt, J., and Brown, G. M. (1981). 'Immunohistochemical evidence for the presence of melatonin in the pineal gland, the retina and the Harderian gland.' *Cell Tiss. Res.*, **217**, 105–115.

Immunohistochemistry
Edited by A. C. Cuello
© 1983 IBRO

CHAPTER 2

Labelling of Proteins with Fluorescent Dyes: Quantitative Aspects of Immunofluorescence Microscopy

J. J. HAAIJMAN

Institute for Experimental Gerontology TNO, PO Box 5815, 2280 HV Rijswijk, The Netherlands

I INTRODUCTION

Coons *et al.* (1941) were the first to use a conjugate of an antibody with a fluorescent dye for the localization of an antigen in a tissue section. Since its introduction, the technique of immunofluorescence has gained an enormous momentum and is used both in clinical diagnosis and research. In this chapter the technique will be evaluated first from the point of view of labelling proteins with fluorochromes. Second, quantitation in immunofluorescence microscopy will be discussed as a tool to arrive at further standardization of the technique. The influence of the microscope equipment on fluorescence yield and image contrast is described. An introduction is given regarding the aspects in which quantitative immunofluorescence microscopy may contribute to the testing of reagent quality and the efficacy of various immunochemical procedures.

II LABELLING OF ANTIBODIES WITH FLUOROCHROMES

In the original report of 1941 Coons and collaborators used β-anthracene for the labelling of anti-pneumococcal antibody. This fluorochrome emits blue light after excitation with near-UV wavelengths. β-Anthracene had several disadvantages: (a) the human eye is relatively insensitive to the blue emission; (b) the excitation of tissues with near-UV light causes autofluorescence, resulting in a rather poor image contrast; and (c) the dye decomposes quickly under excitation. Table 1 lists the requirements for a fluorochrome to be used successfully in immunofluorescence procedures. In 1942, Coons *et al.* introduced fluorescein in immunofluorescence microscopy. Fluorescein emits green to yellow-green light after blue excitation. The maximum emission wavelength corresponds roughly to the maximum in the wavelength sensitivity curve of the human eye. Fluorescein was originally coupled to protein via the isocyanate intermediate. The isocyanate derivative was, however, highly susceptible to hydrolysis and could not be stored for a prolonged period of time. A big improvement was the introduction of fluorescein isothiocyanate (FITC) by Riggs *et al.* (1958). It was prepared by reacting aminofluorescein with thiophosgene. FITC can be stored desiccated at −20 °C for at least 2 years before losing its activity.

Under weakly alkaline conditions it will react with protonated amino groups which will generally be the ε amino groups of lysine residues in proteins. In aqueous solutions FITC will also hydrolyse. Therefore, FITC-protein condensation and FITC hydrolysis will always compete during a labelling. The protein to fluorochrome concentration determines which process will dominate (see below). It is essential to remove non-reacted and hydrolysed dye from the reaction mixture because these may cause non-specific reactions after applying the preparation to a biological substrate. The removal can be accomplished conveniently by dialysis or molecular sieving.

Although FITC is by far the most commonly used fluorochrome in the immunofluorescence technique a brief review will be given here of some of the alternatives.

Table 1   Requirements of a fluorescent dye to be used in IF microscopy

1. The dye should interfere minimally with the antigen–antibody interaction.
2. The emission maximum of the dye should be within the spectral sensitivity of the human eye.
3. The maximum of the excitation spectrum should preferably be above 360 nm.
4. The excitation and emission spectra should be far enough apart on the wavelength scale that they can be separated from each other.
5. Photodecomposition during excitation should be minimal.
6. The dye should be stable upon storage and available in a highly purified form.

(a) Treatment of aminofluorescein with cyanuric chloride results in the formation of dichlorotriazinylaminofluorescein (DTAF—Blakeslee and Baines, 1976; Blakeslee, 1977). This compound was used successfully in the conjugation of protein, and may be applied also to the labelling of polysaccharides.

(b) TRITC. Selective filtering of excitation and emission enables the use of more than one tracer in the same preparation. Clearly, the excitation and/or emission spectra should not overlap with each other. The emission spectra maxima should be separated by at least 50 nm for unambiguous interpretation in visual work, to be appreciated as two distinct colours. Lissamine rhodamine B (RB 200), fluorescing red with green excitation, was the first dye to be combined with fluorescein (Chadwick *et al.*, 1958). The dye was coupled to protein via its sulphonyl chloride derivative. Its use has been superseded by other rhodamines which can be obtained in chemically more purified form. The best known of these is tetramethyl rhodamine which was first used in its isocyanate form (Hiramoto *et al.*, 1958) to be replaced by the more stable isothiocyanate (Riggs *et al.*, 1958). The excitation and emission spectra of FITC and tetramethyl rhodamine isothiocyanate (TRITC) are shown in Figure 1.

The combination of FITC and TRITC is still not ideal for certain applications because the emission of FITC overlaps that of TRITC to a small extent. Other rhodamine derivatives have been studied, of which the XRITC has to be mentioned. This dye emits maximally in the 630 nm region and does not overlap with FITC.

TRITC can be obtained from several commercial sources. The quality of the different batches may vary considerably. Unfortunately, very little is known about the production process nor about the eventual composition and/or purity of the end product. Thin-layer chromatography shows

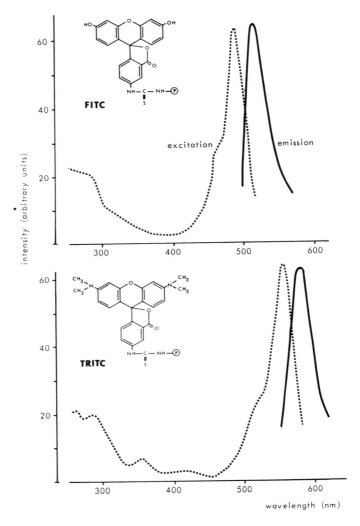

Figure 1 Structural formula, excitation and emission spectra (redrawn from Hansen, 1964) of fluorescein isothiocyanate (FITC) and tetramethyl rhodamine isothiocyanate (TRITC) conjugated to protein ('P' in formula)

a variety of compounds in all of the tested batches (J. J. Haaijman and J. P. R. van Dalen, unpublished observations). Most of these compounds will absorb green light but only a few will fluoresce. No identification of the several components has been attempted yet. Research is urgently needed in this area, aimed at the production of well-characterized and standardized material for protein conjugation. Too often valuable anti-bodies are lost because of unsatisfactory labelling with faultly TRITC preparations. It may be advisable to elaborate on the work of Brandtzaeg (1973, 1975) who tested several rhodamine derivatives other than TRITC and XRITC for their performance in antibody labelling.

(c) SITS (stilbene isothiocyanate). A third tracer is badly needed in some areas of immunology for combination with fluorescein and rhodamine. Extensive research has been devoted to this subject. A blue light-emitting fluorochrome is the only practical choice for visual interpretation, because yellow cannot be distinguished with enough certainty from the green of FITC and the red of TRITC. Rothbart *et al.* (1978) used the SITS which was introduced by Sinsheimer *et al.* (1968). Conjugation of protein with SITS requires very careful monitoring of the pH, in contrast to FITC and TRITC which are less sensitive to pH variations during the conjugation step. SITS conjugates have not been employed routinely, mainly because the dye decomposes very rapidly during excitation (so-called fading).

(d) MDPF (2-methoxy-2,4-diphenyl-3(H)furanone) and Fluram (Udenfriend *et al.*, 1972; marketed by Hoffman-La Roche A. G. Diagnostica, Basel, Switzerland) have been suggested (Weigele *et al.*, 1973; Handschin and Ritschard, 1976) as third fluorochromes. The practical use of these compounds is again forfeited by their rapid fading. In conclusion, we feel that no completely satisfactory third fluorochrome has been developed yet.

III LABELLING OF PROTEINS WITH FITC AND TRITC; PRACTICAL CONSIDERATIONS

The aim of a fluorochrome labelling is the even distribution of a given number of fluorochrome molecules over a given number of protein mole-cules. The conditions should be chosen to reduce the possibility of the generation of strongly over-conjugated as well as strongly under-conjugated molecules since this will complicate the interpretation of the results after-wards. This condition holds even more true if the conjugate is to be used in quantitative work. Taken together, the labelling of proteins should be done in a reaction mixture which is as homogeneous as possible. Therefore we discourage the use of the original Cebra and Goldstein (1965) method in which solid FITC or TRITC is added to the antibody solution. Because these dyes dissolve rather slowly in aqueous solutions this will result in high local concentrations of dye with the risk of over-conjugation of a part of the protein molecules. Hijmans *et al.* (1969) advocated the dropwise addition of FITC and TRITC dissolved in the conjugation buffer. This method (especially for FITC) combines convenience and the possibility of a limited time interval between dissolving FITC and mixing it with protein. The latter is important because of the hydrolysis of FITC in solution. This factor played a significant role in the method in which a dialysis bag containing the protein solution was placed in a beaker of FITC solution (Clark and Shepard, 1963). The last method, however, ensures a very gentle conjugation which is easily controlled. TRITC is difficult to dissolve in water. Dissolving TRITC first in a small volume of dimethylsulphoxide was introduced by Bergquist and Nilsson (1974). This procedure is now generally adopted for the conjugation of most isothiocyanate and succinimide derivatives of fluorochromes and haptens (see Goding, 1976; and Appendix I for a detailed description of procedure). The DMSO will not interfere with the antigen binding of antibodies if used below a final concentration of 50% (v/v) in the conjugation mixture.

IV   THE DETERMINATION OF FLUOROCHROME TO PROTEIN RATIO

Measurement of the average number of fluorochrome molecules per molecule of antibody (molar F/P ratio) is necessary to evaluate the efficiency of the labelling procedure. F/P determinations are done spectrophotometrically using 280 nm for maximum protein absorbance and 495 and 550 nm for maximum fluorescein and rhodamine absorbance, respectively. Both FITC and TRITC absorb also significantly at 280 nm, so a correction based on the 495 and 550 nm absorbance is used to determine the true protein concentration (see Appendix II, for formulas). Alternatively, the nomogram constructed by Wells *et al.*, 1966, can be employed. It should be recognized that an F/P ratio gives only an impression of the average protein substitution. If conjugates are fractioned by ion-exchange chromatography it becomes apparent that the range of F/P ratios is extensive within one preparation (Thé, 1970a,b). The usefulness of the F/P determination in the routine laboratory is questionable, because of the following considerations:

(a) Very little is known about the efficiency of labelling of various serum proteins (see White, 1970). This means that the F/P ratio will only be indicative for the relevant portion of the protein if purified antibody preparations are used for labelling.
(b) The F/P ratio is related to performance of the conjugates in biological systems, only in a very non-linear way: highly over-conjugated molecules tend to give high non-specific staining and severely under-conjugated molecules tend to give no signal at all. Between these two extremes no clear-cut relationship exists between F/P ratio and conjugate quality. Too much appears to depend on the properties of different antisera.
(c) The determination of rhodamine F/P ratios is still a rather controversial subject. The molecular extinction coefficient of TRITC bound to polyacrylamide films was determined by van Dalen and Haaijman (1974).

It appears, however, that different batches of TRITC may cause different absorption spectra (Brandtzaeg, 1975) depending on the F/P ratio. Notably, a second absorption peak between 515 and 520 nm is evident in conjugates with more extensive fluorochrome substitution. The nature of this 520 nm absorbing material is not known. It is clear, however, that absorption at 520 nm does not cause fluorescence.

Differences in absorption spectra depending on the F/P ratio of course make a reliable estimation of the F/P ratio impossible. Quite a few investigators, therefore, present only the ratio between the optical density at 280 and 550 nm as an indication of the degree of labelling of a TRITC conjugate.

(d) Stabilizing proteins are often added to fluorescent conjugates. This is true for purified antibody preparations which will degrade more rapidly if stored at too low a concentration and most likely for commercial conjugates which are diluted to give a certain acceptable strength. In both cases, the F/P ratio of the labelled proteins is impossible to check.

It may be concluded that determination of the F/P ratio is only of importance in quality-control situations in which batches of the same antiserum have to be labelled frequently.

Implicit to the appreciation of F/P determination is the notion that too high substitution ratios will cause damage to the antibody molecules. Reports on this phenomenon are surprisingly scarce. Klugerman (1966) showed that the electrical charge of FITC-labelled gamma globulins is proportional to the F/P ratio, as is understandable since FITC is negatively charged. Arnold and Mayersbach (1972) studied the changes in solubility of IgG preparations after FITC labelling. In Figure 2 Sepharose beads conjugated with ovalbumin were used to measure the binding efficiency of rabbit-anti-ovalbumin antibodies conjugated to various F/P values. Beads coupled with human IgG were used to estimate the non-specific binding of the preparations (see Section VI of this chapter for a more extensive description of this model system). Specific and non-specific binding increases linearly up to an F/P ratio of approximately 10. Above an F/P of 10 the specific binding was not increased whereas the non-specific binding was considerably higher, resulting in a lower specific to non-specific contrast.

The performance measurement of conjugates, as shown in Figure 2, is only of limited validity since:

(a) the non-specific staining properties in a model system are often not comparable to non-specific staining on biological substrates;
(b) no distinction is made between the destruction of antigen-binding sites, resulting in less fluorescence of beads incubated with conjugates with high F/P ratio, and possible effects of self-quenching. The quench phenomenon was demonstrated for instance by Bergquist and Nilsson

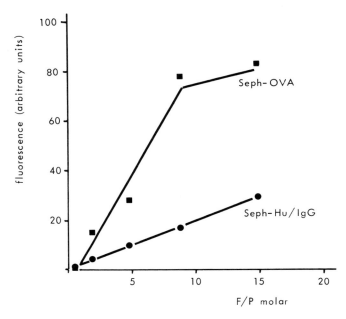

Figure 2 The influence of F/P ratio in the Sepharose bead immunofluorescence system. Rabbit antibodies directed against ovalbumin (OVA) were purified using affinity chromatography. These antibodies were conjugated with TRITC to different F/P ratios which were determined spectrophotometrically. Sepharose beads coupled with OVA and human IgG were incubated with the different anti-ovalbumin conjugates. After 60 min of incubation the beads were washed and the fluorescence of individual beads was measured microfluorometrically. Each point is the average fluorescence intensity of at least 10 individual beads. The fluorescence of Seph-OVA and Seph-Hu/IgG incubated with a conjugate with an F/P ratio of 0.5 was taken as 1.0, arbitrarily

(1975) who found with their model system (glutaraldehyde polymerized immunoglobulin) a lower fluorescence intensity with a conjugate with an F/P ratio of 5.3 than with a conjugate with F/P of 1.2. If the interpretation of the authors is correct, quenching should occur between fluorochrome molecules of different antibody molecules and not between fluorochrome molecules on the same molecule. In the Sepharose model system (Figure 2) the antigen densities are never high enough to allow the approximation of two antibody molecules to such a small distance that quenching can occur.

A more definitive method is illustrated in Figure 3 for the measurement of the influence of fluorochrome or hapten substitution on protein molecules. A monoclonal antibody directed against an allotype determinant on mouse

IgG$_{2a}$ was conjugated with biotin succinimide. Biotin-conjugated antibodies may be used together with fluoresceinated avidin in a so-called hapten-sandwich method (Wofsy *et al.*, 1974; Bayer and Wilchek, 1974; Heitzmann and Richards, 1974). To determine the damage to the anti-mouse/IgG$_{2a}$ caused by the biotin conjugation, a solid-phase competition radioimmuno-assay (Oi and Herzenberg, 1979) was used.

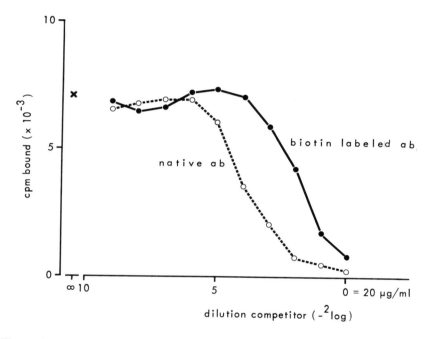

Figure 3 Estimation of the damage caused by hapten substitution. A monoclonal mouse antibody directed atainst the 'b' allotypic determinant on mouse IgG$_{2a}$ (kindly provided by Dr V. T. Oi, Stanford University, Stanford, Cal., USA) was conjugated with biotin succinimide. Microtitration plates (flexible, polyvinyl) were coated for 60 min with 30 μl of 100 μg/ml mouse/IgG$_{2a}$ ('b' allotype) in PBS. Non-occupied adsorption sites were blocked by washing with 1% bovine serum albumin in PBS (PBS–BSA). Individual wells were then incubated with a mixture of ^{125}I-labelled anti-IgG$_{2a}$ (20 kcpm) and various concentrations of biotin-labelled anti-IgG$_{2a}$ and native (unconjugated) anti-IgG$_{2a}$, respectively. Excess antibody was washed away with PBS–BSA and the amount of (^{125}I) anti-IgG$_{2a}$ bound to the individual wells was determined with a gamma-counter

Flexible polyvinyl 96-well microtitration plates were coated with purified mouse/IgG$_{2a}$ (passive adsorption). Non-occupied adsorption sites were saturated with 1% bovine serum albumin (BSA) in phosphate buffered saline (PBS). Various concentrations of native anti-IgG$_{2a}$ and biotin-conjugated anti-IgG$_{2a}$ were added to individual wells of the microtitration plate, followed immediately by 20 kcpm of ^{125}I-labelled anti-IgG$_{2a}$. The mixture of radio-active and non-radioactive antibodies was incubated for 60 min. After rinsing the plates with BSA–PBS the number of cpm bound to the wells was determined by γ-counting.

Evidently, the biotin conjugate in Figure 3 was about 75% less efficient in the competition assay than the native antibody. Using this assay it was established (Dr V. T. Oi, personal communication) that F/P ratios of FITC and TRITC up to about 4 will not change the antigen-binding efficiency of antibodies, although labelling in itself destroys a significant proportion of the antibody molecules.

V   QUANTITATION IN IMMUNOFLUORESCENCE MICROSCOPY

V.1   Introduction

Immunofluorescence (IF) microscopy as a tool in clinical diagnosis and research is beset by a large number of variables influencing the eventual quality of the slides for visual examination. Three main variables in IF microscopy are apparent: the IF equipment, the antisera, and the preparative procedures. Several approaches have been taken to arrive at what was tentatively called 'defined immunofluorescent staining' (Beutner, 1971a). It should be clear that consistency of diagnoses is of utmost importance for the application of IF to clinical immunology. Interlaboratory trials, involving the distribution of reference test samples, were initiated in the late 1960s (Anderson *et al.*, 1971; Cherry and Reimer, 1973). In this approach, only the final scoring of the test preparations counts. With the different microscope set-ups, the different substrates, the different ways of preparing the slides, and the inherent subjectivity of visual screening, it was not surprising that the progress in the interlaboratory trials was slow. In more recent years the World Health Organization has started to provide reference fluorescent conjugates and very detailed protocols for the most commonly performed tests. Together with the introduction of epi-illumination microscopes (see below) this has led to a much improved status of clinical IF microscopy. Another approach to the tangles of routine IF microscopy has been the introduction of very elaborate specifications of the chemical composition of antisera and conjugates. This method has been advocated by Beutner (1971b) and Wick (1972). The staining of conjugates was related to specific antibody content and F/P ratio. Beutner (1971b) assumes that the desired specific staining (DSS) is directly related to the antibody content and that the non-specific staining (NSS) is related to the F/P ratio. The degree of DSS and NSS was estimated in this system using checkboard titrations (anti-immuno-globulin technique). Quantitation of IF results, in terms of the number of conjugate molecules bound to a given substrate, is an alternative way of arriving at data which can be compared between different laboratories. In quantitation several levels can be recognized:

—measurement of fluorescence intensities *per se*;
—the influence of microscope equipment on the observed fluorescence intensity;
—the influence of the reagents on the eventual test result;
—the efficacy of various IF procedures.

These four aspects of IF quantitation will be dealt with in the subsequent sections of this chapter.

V.2 The Measurement of Fluorescence Intensity in IF Microscopy

Fluorescence is a self-lighting phenomenon, that is, under ideal circumstances the excitation light is shut from the eye or photomultiplier and the fluorescence is observed or measured against a completely dark background. This implies that in IF quantitation there does not exist a meaningful 'blank value' as in absorption photometry. For this reason, fluorescence can only be measured relative to a fluorescent standard sample. Several such standards have been described in the literature. They may be divided into two main categories: (a) macro or conus standards, (b) standard objects of microscopical dimensions.

The first macro standard for the IF microscopy was suggested by Rigler (1966) in the form of a uranyl glass (GG17 of Schott and Gen., Mainz, West-Germany). Ploem (1970a,b) and Ruch (1970) used the same uranyl glass as a conus standard: the objective was rested against the glass and the fluorescence is measured from a conus determined by the focal length and numerical aperture of the objective. Jongsma *et al.* (1971) gave a description of the uranyl standard together with its limitations: first, all readings are influenced by the position of the collector lens in the lamp housing and the diameter of the excitation diaphragm, and, second, the spectral properties of uranyl are not the same as those of fluorescein. Ploem (1970b) introduced the standard of microscopical dimensions in the form of microdroplets of fluorochrome solution suspended in mineral oil. Because the size of the droplets permits them to be measured *in toto* and because the fluorochrome content of individual droplets can be measured accurately, the microdroplets provide an absolute standard which will calibrate also for collector lens position and excitation diaphragm width. However, only a stable reference solution is known for FITC (free fluorescein generated by quantitative hydrolysis of fluorescein diacetate) and not for TRITC. Moreover, the microdroplet preparations could not be stored and were rather tedious to work with. The same holds true for the microcapillaries filled with

Table 2   Requirements for a standard in immunofluorescence microscopy

1. Microscopical dimension.
2. Applicable for TRITC and FITC.
3. Excitation and emission spectra the same as those of cell-bound conjugate.
4. Incorporability in an immunofluorescence slide.
5. Stable upon storage.
6. Easy to handle and suitable for routine application.

fluorochrome solutions as introduced by Sernetz and Thaer (1970, 1972). A more theoretical disadvantage of these standards was the unknown quantum efficiency of the conjugated form of fluorescein and rhodamine compared to free fluorescein and rhodamine. In Table 2 the requirements for a standard in IF microscopy are summarized.

Because of the limitations of already existing standards, the Sephadex conjugated FITC and TRITC standard was developed (Haaijman and van Dalen, 1974). In brief, Sephadex G25 beads are provided with amino groups which can then be derivatized with regular FITC and TRITC (Appendix III). It was proven that the fluorochrome is distributed throughout the whole volume of the beads. The influence of several variables in the bead preparation on the fluorescence/volume was investigated; notably, amination time, staining time, and concentration of dye during staining. The amount of fluorochrome per individual bead, a parameter essential to the use as a standard, was measured originally by absorption photometry of individual beads. More recently, radioactive FITC (Haaijman, 1977) and measurements of FITC conjugated beads in suspension (Visser *et al.*, 1978) have been used. The fluorescent Sephadex beads fulfill most of the requirements for a proper IF standard, except for the fact that the quantum efficiency of Sephadex-bound FITC is not necessarily identical to that of protein-bound FITC.

V.3   Evaluation of Fluorescence Microscope Components with Fluorescent Microspheres

Figure 4 shows a simplified diagram of a modern fluorescence microscope equipped with epi-illumination according to Ploem (1967) and a photometer attachment. The measurements presented below were performed using either a Leitz Orthoplan microscope or a Leitz Diavert inverted microscope (Leitz GmbH, Wetzlar, W. Germany) with MPV 1 measuring devices (Weber, 1965) (MPV 2 and 3 have recently been introduced by Leitz). Operations necessary for controlling the different light paths during measurements were provided electromechanically, pneumatically, or electronically (Haaijman and Wijnants, 1975; Haaijman, 1977). Recently, also, a microprocessor-controlled version of the Diavert microscope has become available commercially. Only one standardization example will be dealt with here in more

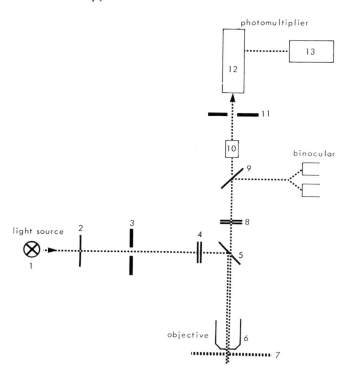

Figure 4 Simplified diagram of a fluorescence microscope equipped with epi-illumination and microfluorometry. 1 = light source; 2 = collector lens; 3 = excitation diaphragm; 4 = excitation filters; 5 = interference dividing plate; 6 = objective; 7 = object; 8 = emission filters; 9 = mirror; 10 = measuring eye piece; 11 = measuring diaphragm; 12 = photomultiplier; and 13 = power supply of photomultiplier

detail, namely the influence of excitation and measuring diaphragm diameters on the fluorescence of the standard beads. The fluorescence per picolitre value was determined (Figure 5) of one particular TRITC-conjugated Sephadex batch using either of two methods: (a) keeping the measuring diaphragm constant and changing the diameter of the excitation diaphragm only; and (b) changing the diameter of the measuring diaphragm, keeping the excitation diaphragm 20 μm larger than the measuring diaphragm. Evidently, the diameter of either of the two diaphragms is not critical. The measured background fluorescence, of course, depends on the diameter of the measuring diaphragm (Figure 6), and although to a lesser extent, on the diameter of the excitation diaphragm. Consequently, in practice one will opt for measuring diaphragms with a diameter as small as possible, so as to reduce the contribution of background fluorescence.

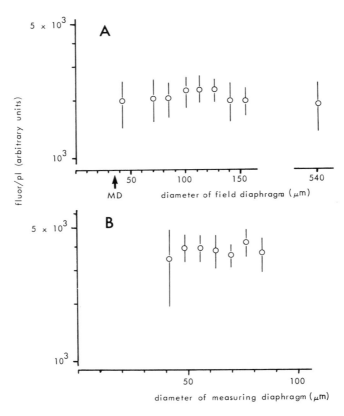

Figure 5   The influence of the diameter of the excitation (= field) diaphragm (A) and measuring diaphragm (B) on the fluorescence per picolitre of amino-ethyl Sephadex beads stained with TRITC. The diameter of the measuring diaphragm was held constant (arrow) in A. In B the excitation diaphragm was always 20 μm larger than the measuring diaphragm. Each point is the average of at least 15 individual bead measurements. Bars indicate standard deviation

The following microscope components are of importance in determining the overall fluorescence yield.

V.3.a   *Light source*

The performance of several types of light sources has been measured using the Sephadex microbeads (Haaijman, 1977). Optimal results were obtained with 100 W high-pressure mercury arcs, whereas the 50 W mercury and 200 W mercury arcs scored second best. The 100 W variety has the disadvantage that it has to be operated on a DC power supply but this source is also, for this

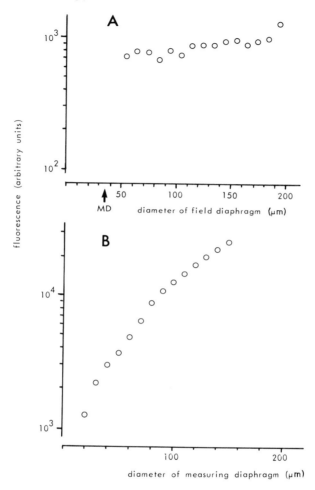

Figure 6 The influence of the diameter of excitation (field) diaphragm (A) and measuring diaphragm (B) on the fluorescence reading from an empty part of the preparation used in Figure 5. Each point is the average of 15 separate readings

reason, indispensable for quantitative work. If a choice has to be made between the 200 W and 50 W mercury AC arcs, the latter is advisable for its small dimensions and relative low cost.

The output spectrum of mercury arcs has a strong line at 546 nm, and this makes them eminently suitable for TRITC excitation. No strong emission line is available with mercury, however, in the wavelength region of maximum absorption of FITC. Xenon arcs emit almost a flat spectrum between 400 and 800 nm, and their output power in the 470–490 nm range is larger than of mercury arcs. In our measurements the expected better performance of Xenon arcs over mercury arcs could not be confirmed for FITC fluorescence. Also because of the inconvenience of switching light sources in evaluating double-stained preparations, we suggest the use of mercury arcs for routine purposes. It should be indicated, however, that performance measurement of light sources is a hazardous undertaking since, first, there appears to exist a considerable variation between different specimens of the same manufacturer and, second, because the collector design in the different brands of micro-scopes may influence the results.

V.3.b   *Filters for fluorescence microscopy*

The excitation or primary filters are chosen to transmit the wavelength band corresponding to the excitation maximum of the fluorescent dyes under study. The emission, secondary, or barrier filters ought to transmit all fluorescence emission and block all excitation light. In an epi-illumination system (Figure 4) the dichroic mirror serves as an additional filter: it will reflect largely excitation light and transmit largely emission light. Additional filter requirements are posed by two-colour fluorescence microscopy: not only should the emission of one fluorochrome be transmitted, but the emission of the second fluorochrome should be blocked. Selectivity in visualizing two different dyes is of course a result of the combination of excitation and emission filtering. At present the excitation and emission windows are constructed by combinations of long-pass (LP filters, alternative-ly called K filters) and short-pass (SP filters, alternatively called KP) filters. The first are constructed of coloured glass, the second of dielectric layers, deposited on a glass base. Generally, additional 'old-fashioned' glass filters are needed to alleviate the shortcomings of the LP and SP filters. Several filter sets commonly in use have been tested for their efficiency (Table 3) using FITC and TRITC stained Sephadex beads. AL and SAL filters in Table 3 stand for small-band interference filters. These are constructed by glueing together dielectric filters and coloured glass filters. The small-band filters have largely been replaced now by combinations of LP and SP filters. In brief, a high fluorescence yield is always accompanied by a rather small contrast between FITC and TRITC (the F/T and T/F ratios in Table 3). In other words: high selectivity is paid for by low fluorescence yield. The following filter combinations for FITC and TRITC have proven to be a useful compromise between yield and selectivity:

FITC
   excitation
      Long-pass: 2 mm GG450 or GG475 (note 1)
      Short-pass: 2 × KP490

Table 3 The influence of different filter combinations on the fluorescence of FITC and TRITC

No.	Excitation filter(s)	Mirror	Emission filter(s)	FITC fluor/pl	TRITC fluor/pl	F/T
1	2 × 2 mm UG 1	TK 430	K 430	361	375	1.0
2	3 mm BG 3 + S 405	TK 455	K 460	114	133	0.9
3	AL 481	TK 510	SAL 525	134	10	13.4
4	AL 481	TK 510	SAL 525 + K 515	82	4	20.5
5	AL 481	TK 510	KP 560 + K 515	294	8	38.7
6	2 × KP 490	TK 510	SAL 525 + K 515	557	171	3.3
7	2 × KP 490 + BG 38	TK 510	SAL 525 + K 515	391	104	3.7
8	2 × KP 490 + BG 38 + GG 455	TK 510	SAL 525 + K 515	241	51	4.7
9	2 × KP 490	TK 510	KP 560 + K 515	1812	902	2.0
10	2 × KP 490 + BG 38	TK 510	KP 560 + K 515	1524	673	2.3
11	2 × KP 490 + BG 38 + GG 455	TK 510	KP 560 + K 515	970	259	3.7
12	2 × KP 490	TK 510	K 515	1042	94	11.1
						T/F
13	1 mm BG 36 + S 546	TK 580	K 580	9	320	34.7
14	1 mm BG 36 + KP 560 + K 515	TK 580	K 580	38	456	12.1
15	KP 560 + K 515	TK 580	K 580	78	634	8.1

Aminoethyl-Sephadex beads were stained with FITC or TRITC. The fluorescence per picolitre (fluor/pl) of both preparations was measured with different filter combinations. Each fluor/pl value is the average of 15 individual bead measurements. For each filter combination, the excitation diaphragm was focussed optimally in the object plane. F/T and T/F stand for ratios between, respectively, FITC and TRITC and TRITC and FITC fluorescence. Objective: 25×/0.60W; eyepiece: 6.3×.

Additional: 2–4 mm BG38 (note 2)
interference dividing plate (dichroic mirror): TK490
emission
    Long-pass: LP520
    Short-pass: KP560 (note 3)

TRITC
    excitation
        Long-pass: LP520
        Short-pass: KP560
        Additional: 1–2 mm BG36 (note 4)
    interference dividing plate: TK580
    emission
        Long-pass: LP580

Notes

(1) The choice between the GG450 or GG475 depends largely on the type of substrate under investigation. The combination with GG450 will cause more autofluorescence than with GG475. This may be advantageous if some orientation is needed, for instance in tissue sections. For other applications (suspended cells, etc.) the GG475 may prove optimal. The image contrast is the parameter of prime importance in IF microscopy. It may therefore be that eventually a combination of filters is chosen which does not give the maximum absolute fluorescence intensity but which gives a better contrast between background and specimen fluorescence.

(2) The BG38 filter blocks the leakage of red light through the KP490 filters.

(3) The short-pass filter in the emission pathway is only obligatory in two-colour IF applications. The combination LP520 + KP560 is sometimes referred to as BP (broad pass) 525.

(4) The BG36 filter reduces the unwanted excitation leaked by the KP560 filters. Mostly, the 1 mm filter will be sufficient; however, sometimes 2 mm gives a better image contrast. These differences appear to be related to the specification of the individual KP560 specimens.

(5) In most modern microscopes the excitation and emission are combined together with an interference dividing plate in interchangeable modules and the lamp-housing is provided with non-exchangeable heat-absorbing filters (KG1). It is advisable to test the performance of a number of modules using one's own system before deciding on what combination suits the purpose best.

   The modular design of the filter combinations enables the rapid switching between different combinations which is indispensable in two-colour work, since visual memory for spatial relationships is relatively poor.

V.3.c *Microscope Objectives*

In an epi-illumination system the intensity of excitation is proportional to the square of the numerical aperture (NA) of the objective. Also the collecting power of the objective for emission varies with the second power of the NA. Therefore, in an epi-illumination fluorescence microscope the fluorescence intensity is proportional to the 4th power of the NA. Recently, objectives have been constructed especially for fluorescence microscopy which combine a high NA with only moderate magnifications (for instance objectives with 40× and 63× magnification and an NA of 1.30). These objectives always require oil-immersion. If only objectives of low magnifications are suited for the experiments it may be questionable whether epi-illumination is optimal. In that case diaillumination with a high aperture dark-field condensor of the Tiyoda type with toric lens will be advisable. It should be added, however, that rapid switching of filter combinations is hardly possible with diaillumination and that quantitation is an almost impossible task because of the uncertainty in the focussing of the condensor.*

V.3.d *Microscope Eye Pieces*

Evidently, high-magnifying eye pieces collect the emission energy in a microscope from a smaller part of the image plane of the objective than do low-magnifying eye pieces. The fluorescent standard was used to establish the quantitative relationship between fluorescence intensity and eye piece magnification. It appeared (Haaijman and Slingerland-Teunissen, 1978) that for flat objects the intensity is proportional to $1/M^2$ in which M stands for the eye piece magnification. It follows then that for maximum fluorescence yield as low as possible magnifying eye pieces should be combined with objectives with an NA as high as possible.

VI QUANTITATIVE IMMUNOFLUORESCENCE MICROSCOPY AS APPLIED TO THE TESTING OF REAGENT QUALITY

VI.1 Introduction

Antisera are the pivot on which the whole technique of immunofluorescence microscopy hinges. A superb microscope cannot help to interpret a faulty preparation. Several methods have been used in the past to assess the

---

* *Editor's Note.* For very low magnifications objective (4×, 6×), fluorescence diaillumination is clearly more effective than epi-illumination. This is relevant in neuroanatomical immunohistochemistry when surveying fluorescence of entire brain sections.

quality of reagents for IF microscopy. Notably, performance testing (Hijmans *et al.*, 1971) has been widely accepted, using a test substrate related as closely as possible to the substrate on which the antiserum or conjugate will eventually be used. Performance testing requires prior knowledge about the composition of the substrate and the availability of a reference set of monospecific reagents.

VI.2 The Sepharose Bead Immunofluorescence System

Purified immunoglobulin preparations coupled covalently to Sepharose beads were used as the substrate for the immunofluorescence procedure. The coupling procedure ensuring homogeneous distribution of the protein over the bead surface is described in Appendix IV.

Van Dalen *et al.* (1973) were the first to employ Sepharose conjugated immunoglobulins to test conjugated antisera against human immunoglobulins. These authors used an activation procedure which yielded homogeneous distribution of immunoglobulin throughout the whole bead volume. This condition made it necessary to measure the fluorescence/volume values for different bead preparations. Capel (1974) introduced an activation procedure for conjugate testing purposes at a much higher pH (pH 10.5 instead of 8.0) with which the antigens are bound primarily in the direct vicinity of the surface (Figure 7). It thus became possible to measure only a fixed area of the bead surface (plug method) after incubation of these beads with fluorescent antisera. Understandably, the plug measurements are far less time-consuming than fluorescence + diameter readings. We have employed the plug method for all our experiments.

Deelder *et al.* (1978, 1980) introduced another approach for the measurement of Sepharose-associated fluorescence. These authors used relatively low magnifying objectives and determined the total emission from the excitation cone. The volume of the measured bead mass is determined by the focal length and NA of the objective. This method enables the automatic scanning of large numbers of samples and was successfully employed for the evaluation of anti-*Schistosoma mansoni* antibodies.

Still another approach was used by Phillips *et al.* (1980). These authors describe an assay in which antigens (human immunoglobulins) are coupled to polystyrene beads. After incubation with fluorescent antisera the bead-bound fluorescence is measured with a macrofluorometer on beads kept in suspension.

An even distribution of antigens over the Sepharose bead surface and, even more important, only a small variation in antigen density between individual beads from one preparation, is a *sine qua non* for successful application of the conjugate test system, using single bead measurements. Most commercial preparations of pre-activated Sepharose will not fulfil this requirement: with

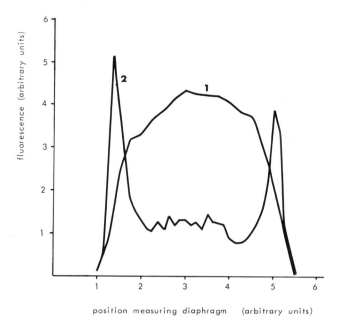

position measuring diaphragm   (arbitrary units)

Figure 7 Surface and volume staining in the Sepharose bead immunofluorescence system. Bead preparation 1 was activated according to van Dalen *et al.* (1973) using pH 8.0. Bead preparation 2 was activated according to Capel (1974). Both kinds of beads were coupled with human IgG and incubated with a TRITC-conjugated rabbit antiserum directed against human IgG. The profiles were obtained by scanning manually the bead fluorescence with a small measuring and excitation diaphragm. Curve 1 indicates that Hu/IgG is distributed throughout the whole volume of the bead; curve 2 suggests that the Hu/IgG is present only in the direct vicinity of the surface of the bead

those preparations often a large range between under- and over-substituted beads is observed.

VI.3   Titration of Antisera with Antigen-coupled Sepharose Beads

In the testing of conjugates or antisera with the Sepharose bead immunofluorescence assay four reactions can be distinguished (see also Beutner, 1971b and flowchart in Chapter 1):

(a) The desired specific staining (DSS)—this is the staining an antiserum is meant to perform.
(b) The undesired specific staining (USS). The observed reaction is caused by a specific immunological reaction, but is not desired. The USS may be

divided into two types: USS caused by antibodies also responsible for the DSS, and USS caused by antibodies contaminating the antiserum.

(c) Cross-reactive specific staining (XSS). The reaction is caused by the presence of the same or similar epitopes on molecules other than the antigen used for raising the antiserum or conjugate.

(d) Non-specific staining (NSS). This category of staining is caused by non-immunological reactions between the Sepharose beads (coupled with antigens or not) and the test antiserum or conjugate.

An ideal conjugate should exhibit only DSS. However, in addition to the DSS, antisera always show NSS and sometimes USS and XSS. In the Sepharose bead system, the antisera are incubated in different dilutions with a variety of bead specimens to ascertain the relationship between these different antiserum reactivities. Idealized titration curves of an antiserum with different beads are shown in Figure 8. The logarithm of the average bead

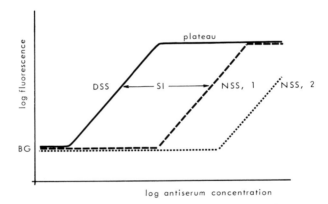

Figure 8 Idealized titration curves of antisera reacting with antigens bound to Sepharose beads. Beads coupled with the homologous antigen serve to estimate the degree of DSS. Beads with heterologous antigens yield data for NSS, USS, or XSS. The antiserum is incubated with the different bead species in a number of dilutions. NSS, 1 and NSS, 2 refer to two hypothetical antisera sharing the same DSS. BG = background; SI = specificity interval. Ordinate = logarithm of the average bead fluorescence in arbitrary units; abscissa; logarithm of antiserum concentration

fluorescence is plotted against the logarithm of the antiserum dilution. Up to a certain dilution no specific reaction is measured. The SS (specific staining) equals the background (BG) fluorescence. Above this dilution the logarithm of the fluorescence is linearly related to the logarithm of the antiserum concentration up to a concentration which saturates all available antigen sites on the beads. A similar result is obtained for both the DSS and USS or NSS. The difference in concentration for which the same DSS and USS/NSS fluorescence values are obtained constitutes the specificity interval (SI). Two hypothetical antisera are shown in Figure 8. Both antisera have the same DSS but one shows appreciable NSS (NSS-1) and the other has a much lower NSS (NSS-2). It has been shown to be an essential point that the USS/NSS curves are parallel to the DSS curve, only that they are shifted to higher concentrations. The level of the plateau in Figure 8 is determined by the available binding sites on the Sepharose beads. The effect of changing the antigen density on the beads is shown schematically in Figure 9. The slope of the curve will not change, only the plateau and consequently the length of the plateau. Haaijman *et al.* (1975) presented experimental evidence for this model.

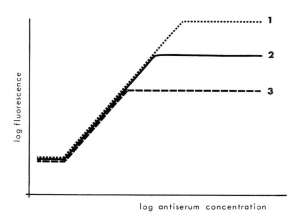

Figure 9 The influence of the amount of antigen coupled to Sepharose on the titration curve with an antiserum. The numbers 1–3 refer to decreasing amounts of antigen (1 is the highest amount of antigen). Only the height of the plateau is influenced and not the slope of the curve in the concentration-dependent range. Ordinate and abscissa as in Figure 8

VI.4 Antiserum and Conjugate Evaluation with Antigens Bound to Sepharose Beads

Figure 10 shows a typical example of an antiserum test. A commercial rabbit antiserum directed against mouse/IgM was incubated in different dilutions with Sepharose beads coupled with highly purified IgM, IgG$_{2a}$ and ovalbumin, respectively. After washing, the antibodies bound to the beads were revealed with a fluorescent horse antiserum directed against rabbit immunoglobulins. Following the second incubation the beads were washed and the individual bead fluorescences were measured microfluorometrically. The average fluorescence of 10 individual beads is shown in Figure 10.

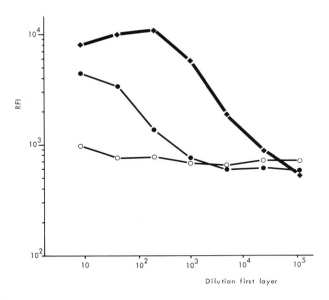

Figure 10   Specificity test for a rabbit antiserum directed against mouse/IgM. The antiserum was incubated in different dilutions with Sepharose-coupled mouse/IgM (◆), mouse/IgG$_{2a}$ (●—●), and ovalbumin (○—○), respectively. After removing the excess antiserum by washing, the beads were incubated with a fluorescent horse anti-rabbit/IgG. Individual bead fluorescences were determined microfluorometrically. Plotted values represent the average of at least ten individual beads. Ordinate: relative fluorescence intensity (RFI) in arbitrary units; abscissa: dilution of the rabbit anti-mouse/IgM

The antiserum reacts clearly most strongly with the homologous beads, but in lower dilutions also appreciably with the IgG$_{2a}$ beads. The ovalbumin serves as a control for NSS and it is assumed that the reaction with these beads is non-immunological. To evaluate the results obtained with the model system, it was necessary to 'calibrate' the results of the model system on the results obtained with the same antisera in a biological test system. Knapp *et al.* (1975) compared the behaviour of six conjugates in the Sepharose bead system and the monoclonal bone marrow system of Hijmans *et al.* (1969). The aim of this study was to express the relative reactivities observed in the bead system in the quality of a given conjugate. For the visual interpretation of IF slides the image contrast is of paramount importance: an antiserum giving a strong DSS can be allowed to give more NSS (or USS for that matter) than a weak antiserum. Because the DSS is a more or less fixed parameter of the antiserum, a lot of effort has been spent on the reduction of NSS. The influence on NSS of fixation, embedding, and washing technique was investigated by von Mayersbach (1972) and Arnold *et al.* (1975). Free fluorochrome remaining in the protein solute after conjugation may enhance NSS (Nisengard and Beutner, 1972) as can antibodies with too high an F/P ratio (Thé, 1967; Herbert *et al.*, 1971; Calcagno *et al.*, 1973). USS phenomena are the major concern in the specificity testing of antibodies. The means of removing USS, if not stronger than the DSS, are dilution (cf. Figure 10) or further purification. The technique of affinity chromatography has been of great importance in IF microscopy for the removal of antibodies to known impurities. The logical next step, namely to purify antibody on antigen columns, has not been employed routinely. Several facts may account for this:

(a) The stability of purified antibodies appears to be less than of, for instance, IgG fractions. Therefore, stabilizing proteins often have to be added and the preparations should be stored at $-70\,°C$ or below.
(b) Elution of antibodies from antigen columns invariably results in some denaturation. From a practical point of view the eluting buffer should be removed as soon as possible from the eluate. This is most easily accomplished by joining the immunoadsorbent column tandem-wise with a Sephadex-G50 column.
(c) Preparation of antigen columns of sufficient purity and capacity is often difficult or even impossible.
(d) The financial costs involved in the preparation of immunoadsorbent-eluted antibodies prohibits the use of these antibodies on such a large scale as in clinical immunology.
(e) Factors other than the chemical purity of the antibody will determine the quality of a given antibody for research, using biological substrates (see below).

In conclusion, most investigators and commercial sources will reserve the preparation of antigen-column-eluted antibodies for special cases only, and conjugates prepared from IgG fractions of antisera and absorbed for impurities on solid immunoadsorbents appear to be suitable for most systems.

Solid-phase adsorption is the only good choice because: conjugates can be mixed without the risk of precipitation of the material intended for absorption, antibody or antigen excess is avoided, and a properly treated solid immunoadsorbent can be re-used almost indefinitely.

Two aspects should be taken into account when comparing the results obtained with the Sepharose bead system and those obtained with biological substrates:

(a) the concentration relationship differs between the antigen on beads and the antigen in cells on the one hand, and the conjugate molecules on the other hand;
(b) in the model system only those contaminants can be detected which are directed against the antigens bound to the beads.

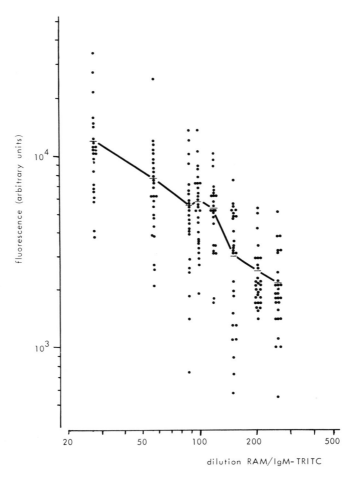

Figure 11 Quantitation of antiserum bound intracellularly. Cytocentrifuge slides were prepared of a cell suspension of spleens from 13-week-old CBA mice. The cells were treated with acid ethanol, washed and incubated with various dilutions of a rabbit antiserum specific for the Fc part of IgM. Individual fluorescent plasma cells were located with a 100 W halogen lamp and the fluorescence was measured using a 100 W mercury arc. The procedure was adopted to avoid fading of fluorescence prior to the measurement. Individual fluorescence values are indicated together with the averages

The working dilution of a conjugate for visual work is determined by scoring the fluorescence intensity of preparations treated with different dilutions of conjugate. The highest dilution is first found, which still gives a '++' reading. The working dilution is then taken to be 1 step less. The concentration difference covered by 1 step is determined by the concentration range, e.g., the working dilution of a conjugate whose last '++' dilution is 1/60 should be used at 1/40 and one which can be diluted 1/16 will be used at 1/12. We have tried to quantitate the visual plateau in Figure 11. The fluorescence of individual plasma cells spreaded on cytocentrifuge slides was measured after incubation of the slides with different dilutions of a rhodamine-labelled rabbit antiserum directed against mouse IgM. The working dilution of this conjugate was determined previously as 1:60. No plateau is observed in Figure 11. It must be concluded that quantitation of the fluorescence of cells does not give an indication with regard to the working dilution for visual work. It then follows that a single dilution cannot be selected for testing the conjugate specificity and/or quality in a model system. The parameter independent of dilution in the bead system in the specificity interval (SI) indicated in Figure 8. Determination of the SI for a number of conjugates may prove to be difficult; first, because it requires a lot of conjugate and, second, because good strong conjugates appear to have a low NSS and USS, even in undiluted form. Unexpected results may be obtained in the comparison of the behaviour of conjugates with beads and cells if the antigen coupled to the beads contains impurities not normally present in the biological test system. As an example, IgG preparations may contain trace amounts of fibrinogen, and antisera may contain anti-fibrinogen antibodies. These antisera will prove to be highly non-specific in the model system but may be very adequate for tracing IgG-containing cells. Alternatively, antisera may contain antibodies against, e.g., cell surface proteins which cannot be obtained in sufficient quantities to couple to beads. These antiserum contaminants may make a conjugate completely unsuited for biological work but will go unnoticed in the model system.

In conclusion, the Sepharose bead immunofluorescence system is very useful to determine the extent of contamination of a given antiserum by antibodies to known antigens. However, it has not been possible to find conditions, yet, for predicting the quality of a conjugate in biological systems from data obtained with model systems alone.

The above discussion was tailored to the use and testing of conventional reagents. With monoclonal antibodies derived by somatic cell fusion (Köhler and Milstein, 1975; see also Chapter 9) several aspects have to be reconsidered. A monoclonal antibody recognizes, by definition, only one epitope. The 'specificity' of a monoclonal reagent is then only determined by the distribution of that epitope in tissues, or on cells within a given tissue. Monoclonal antibodies have primarily been used, to date, in fluorescence and radioimmunoassay applications.

VII   QUANTITATION OF SERUM ANTIBODIES BY MICRO-FLUOROMETRY ON ANTIGEN-COUPLED SEPHAROSE BEADS

Microfluorometry can be applied to the determination of antibody concentration using the same system as outlined in the previous section. Figure 12 shows the results of an experiment in which the antibody response of CBA mice was measured, following intravenous injection with 200 μg of soluble chicken gamma-globulin (CGG). CGG-coupled beads were incubated with a fixed dilution of mouse serum and then with fluorescent conjugates directed specifically to the Fc part of mouse IgM, IgG_1, IgG_2, IgG_{2b}, IgG_3, and IgA. The dilution of the sera was chosen in the antibody-dependent concentration range, as determined in pilot experiments. The fluorescence of the individual beads was measured using the automated inverted microfluorometer, described earlier (Haaijman, 1977). To normalize the curves all fluorescence data were calculated relative to the values obtained with preimmune serum, resulting in a measure called 'contrast'. The first antibodies to appear in serum upon intravenous injection of antigen are of the IgM class. These can

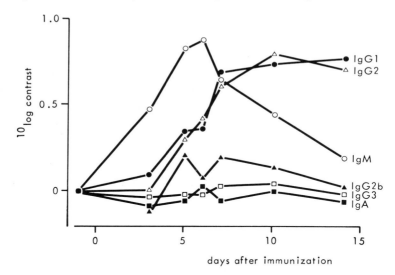

Figure 12   Quantitation of the antibody response using the Sepharose bead immunofluorescence assay. 12-week-old CBA mice received 200 μg chicken gamma-globulin (CGG), intravenously. Ten to twenty μl of serum was obtained from the tail vein at indicated days. Sepharose beads coupled with CGG were first incubated with 1 : 100 diluted serum samples and then with fluorescent antisera specific for IgM, IgG_1, IgG_2, IgG_{2b}, IgG_3, and IgA, respectively. The fluorescence of at least five individual beads was determined microfluorometrically, after washing. Plotted was the ratio between the average fluorescence at any given day and the fluorescence observed with preimmune serum ('contrast'). The contrast was calculated for each conjugate separately

be detected at least 3 days after immunization. The concentration of IgM anti-CGG is maximal at day 6 and declines thereafter, to be replaced by antibodies of the IgG class, notably IgG_1 and IgG_{2a} (although no anti-IgG_{2a} antibody was used, this conclusion can be inferred from the appearance of IgG_2 antibodies and the undetectability of IgG_{2b} antibodies).

VIII   TESTING THE EFFICACY OF VARIOUS IMMUNOFLUORESCENCE PROCEDURES WITH THE SEPHAROSE BEAD SYSTEM

A large number of different techniques are available for demonstrating the binding of antibodies to antigens, using immunofluorescence. The most well known of these are the direct technique and the anti-immunoglobulin technique. Quite a few discussions have been devoted to the various merits of these two methods (see Nairn, 1976). The Sepharose bead system was used to evaluate both specificity and sensitivity using a rabbit anti-ovalbumin antiserum. Beads coupled with human/IgM served as controls for NSS activity. For Figure 13 ovalbumin and IgM coupled beads were incubated with different dilutions of either fluorescein-conjugated rabbit anti-ovalbumin (direct technique) or with unlabelled antiserum followed by fluorescent goat anti-rabbit/Ig (anti-Ig technique). The antibody content was the same in the labelled and unlabelled anti-ovalbumin preparations. The specificity interval for the direct technique was about 2 log units larger than for the indirect technique in this experiment. On the other hand, the anti-Ig technique proved to be about four times as sensitive as the direct technique. A large number of different antigen–antibody combinations would have to be tested to draw general conclusions. This remains to be done. Several indirect techniques other than the anti-Ig technique were compared by Haaijman and Slingerland-Teunissen (1978) following the procedures outlined above. By and large the anti-Ig technique proved to be superior to the other multi-layer techniques with regard to general applicability, simplicity, sensitivity, and specificity.

IX   CONCLUDING REMARKS

The technique of immunofluorescence has been improved tremendously over the past years. This has been due to a number of simultaneous developments in the fields of fluorochrome characterization, microscope design, and the purification of antisera.

This chapter deals with the method of fluorochrome conjugation, being usually the first step in the application of an immunofluorescence technique. Fluorescein isothiocyanate has now been purified and characterized to such an extent that it could be added to the list of certified drugs in the USA. The

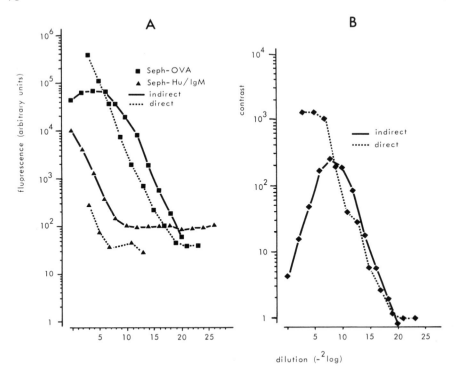

Figure 13   Comparison of the direct technique and anti-Ig method with the Sepharose bead immunofluorescence system. A = titration curves; B = contrast curves (specific/non-specific fluorescence). For details of the procedure see text

situation with tetramethyl rhodamine isothiocyanate is so far not that good: at the moment no reliable (commercial) source is available and research on the synthesis of this compound is urgently needed. The different reaction products and isomeric forms have to be characterized and tested for their conjugation and fluorescence properties. In addition to fluorescein and rhodamine new fluorochromes have to be developed which can be used in combination with the other two, for applications using three or more colours.

A first breakthrough for fluorescence microscopes was the application of the epi-illumination system. This system increased the fluorescence yield remarkably, especially when using moderate- to high-magnifying objectives. Objectives were later constructed which combined a high numerical aperture with medium magnification, because the numerical aperture largely determines this yield of fluorescence, thus exploiting the assets of epi-illumination to the utmost. Along the same line of reasoning eye pieces with an extra-low magnification factor were made especially for fluorescence work. Unfortunately, the special eye pieces will only fit the larger research microscopes and have not yet been adapted to the routine microscopes. Originally, the light sources for fluorescence excitation were attached to the general-purpose (research) microscope, resulting in an awkwardly long light path. The collector lens design, moreover, was not optimal for filling out the back entrance pupil of the various objectives. More recently, special-purpose fluorescence microscopes have been marketed with a shorter light path and better collectors. Improvements, however, are still needed to adapt the collector system to applications in which different objectives are used within a large range of magnifications. Zoom-optics may be one of the promising solutions to this. Modern microscopes often feature rapidly interchangeable filter arrangements, and this is of importance in two-colour fluorescence applications. The filters themselves have also been improved. It is now possible to obtain dielectric short-pass filters covering the whole range of visible wavelengths, enabling the investigator to construct his own filter 'window' by combining these short-pass filters with the already available long-pass filters. In this chapter methods were introduced to quantitate the fluorescence intensity and to compare the efficiency in this respect of various microscope designs. The quality of antisera is the most important factor in determining success or failure of an immunofluorescence technique. A large part of this chapter is devoted to the evaluation of antiserum specificity and potency. The Sepharose bead immunofluorescence system was introduced, in which the reaction of antisera or conjugates with antigens bound to Sepharose beads is measured by microfluorometry. This system proved helpful for making an inventory of the specificities against known antigens within a single antiserum, but was not able to furnish conclusive data on the quality and thus applicability of that antiserum in biological work. The same holds true for any system in which the assay depends on the use of purified or semi-purified antigens. The best evaluation of the quality of an antiserum is still the testing of performance on a number of biological substrates with restricted antigenic composition (see Chapter 1). Prior knowledge about substrate specificity is often only to be obtained by testing with immunological means, e.g. monospecific antisera. It then follows that the reasoning implicit to performance testing is circular. The circle can now be broken after the recent introduction of monoclonal antibodies in immunofluorescence (see Chapter 3). Provided all necessary controls are taken into consideration the presence or absence (given a certain lower detection limit) of an antigenic determinant can be demonstrated unequivocally. The specificity of a monoclonal antibody is no longer in doubt, and only the cellular or organ distribution of the recognized determinants is of importance. It should also be understood that monoclonal antibodies may be found to react with more than one determinant. Mostly, however, the reactions with different determinants will have vastly different affinity constants.

Although it is to be expected that monoclonal antibody preparations will gradually replace a large number of the conventional reagents, there are several reasons for caution. First of all the fluorescence obtained with a good conventional antiserum or conjugate is often substantially brighter than with a monoclonal preparation. It may prove necessary to use a combination of several monoclonal antibodies directed against different determinants on the same molecule to boost the signal over noise sufficiently for visual examination and appreciation. It is evident that the financial consequences of such a method will weigh heavily, and may restrict the widespread application of such preparations. Another point of concern is the general applicability of monoclonal preparations: one antibody may be optimal for fluorescence, the other for cytotoxicity, and still another for precipitation assays. If more than one monoclonal antibody preparation is used in different assays, it has to be proven that the recognized determinants are identical. Conventional antisera will probably still be used for a long time, and these antisera will have to be tested for specificity in the systems for which they are intended. The guarantee of specificity can be obtained only by the individual investigator using his own assay.

ACKNOWLEDGEMENT

The help of Marion Roggenkamp with the preparation of this manuscript is gratefully acknowledged.

APPENDIX I
THE CONJUGATION OF PROTEIN WITH FLUOROCHROMES

Materials
Protein solution (between 1 and 10 mg/ml).
0.1 M $NaHCO_3$, pH 9.0.
FITC, fluorescein isothiocyanate (Nordic Immunological Laboratories, Tilburg, The Netherlands).
Dimethylsulphoxide.
PD-10 column (Pharmacia Fine Chemicals, Uppsala, Sweden).
Phosphate buffered saline (PBS).
PBS with 1% bovine albumin and 0.1% NaN_3 (PBS–BSA).

Procedure
The protein solution is dialysed against 0.1 M $NaHCO_3$ for at least 4 h. If the protein concentration is above 5 mg/ml the solution can be diluted, e.g., with an equal volume of 10% $NaHCO_3$. FITC is dissolved in DMSO at 1 mg/ml. The relative amount of FITC to be added for optimal conjugation depends on

the protein concentration. The following amounts can only be taken as a rough indication.

Protein concentration (mg/ml)	μg FITC added per mg protein
10	10
5	25
2	50
1	100

The indicated amount of FITC in DMSO is added in small aliquots (e.g. 10 μl) to the protein under continuous stirring, using either a magnetic bar stirrer or a Vortex mixer. The protein–FITC mixture is left for 3 h at room temperature or 8 h at 4 °C. A PD-10 column is washed with 25 ml of PBS–BSA; 2 ml of the conjugation mixture is applied per column and the drop-through is discarded. The conjugate is eluted from the column with 3 ml of PBS–BSA. If an F/P ratio is to be measured then elution can be performed with PBS. It is advisable to add BSA and NaN_3 later.

APPENDIX II
CALCULATION OF THE F/P RATIO OF IgG CONJUGATES FROM THE OD_{280} AND OD_{495}

OD_{280} and OD_{495} are measured in 1 cm cuvettes.

$$\text{Molar concentration of protein P} = \frac{OD_{280} - 0.35\ OD_{495}}{2.24 \times 10^5}$$

2.24×10^5 is the molar absorption coefficient of IgG at 280 nm.

$$\text{Molar concentration of fluorescein F} = \frac{OD_{495}}{0.7 \times 10^5}$$

0.7×10^5 is the molar absorption coefficient of bound FITC at pH 7.8. The molar F/P ratio is found by dividing F by P.

APPENDIX III
PREPARATION OF FLUORESCENT MICROBEADS

Materials
Sephadex G25 SF (Pharmacia Fine Chemicals, Uppsala, Sweden).
Aminoethylsulphuric acid (Fluka AG, Buchs, Switzerland).
2 M NaOH.
0.05 M sodium carbonate, pH 9.5.

FITC, fluorescein isothiocyanate (Nordic Immunological Laboratories, Tilburg, The Netherlands).
Phosphate buffered saline (PBS).
Glycerol p.a. (Merck AG, Darmstadt, West Germany).

Procedure
The Sephadex beads are suspended in the NaOH solution and swollen for at least 3 h. The suspension is centrifuged in a graded tube for 1 min at 3000 g. The supernatant is discarded and the volume of the packed beads is measured. Four times this volume is added of 100 mg aminoethylsulphuric acid/ml 2 M NaOH. The suspension is heated to 85 °C for 2 h, preferably in a large Petri dish. The beads are washed extensively after the reaction, with 2 M NaOH followed by a large volume of distilled water. The aminoethyl– Sephadex beads can now be stored either in suspension or as a dry powder after substitution of the water by acetone, and evaporation to dryness. For conjugation with FITC, aminoethyl–Sephadex beads are suspended in, or washed with, 0.05 M sodium carbonate pH 9.5; 1 mg of FITC is dissolved in 100 ml carbonate buffer; 10 ml of the freshly prepared fluorochrome solution is incubated with 1 ml of sedimented aminoethyl–Sephadex beads for 3 h under continuous rotation on a roller bank. The beads are then washed, first with the carbonate buffer (three changes of 15 ml per ml of beads) and subsequently with PBS (three changes plus one wash overnight under rotation). One volume of a suitably diluted bead suspension is mixed with nine volumes of glycerol for the preparation of standard slides.

APPENDIX IV
THE PREPARATION OF ANTIGEN-COUPLED SEPHAROSE BEADS FOR QUANTITATIVE IMMUNOFLUORESCENCE

Materials
Sepharose 4B (Pharmacia Fine Chemicals, Uppsala, Sweden).
2 M sodium carbonate.
CNBR, cyanogen bromide (Fluka AG, Buchs, Switzerland).
Acetonitrile.
Washing solutions:
    (A) 0.1 M sodium bicarbonate pH 9.5
    (B) Distilled water
    (C) 0.2 M sodium bicarbonate pH 9.5
    (D) 0.1 M sodium acetate pH 4.0   with 0.65 M NaCl
    (E) 2 M urea   with 0.65 M NaCl
    (F) 0.1 M sodium bicarbonate pH 9.5   with 0.65 M NaCl
0.5 M ethanolamine (solution should be colourless; discard if yellowish due to polymers).

Procedure according to March *et al.* (1974).

The Sepharose is washed with a large volume of distilled water to remove the preservative added by the manufacturer. A volume of *a* ml of Sepharose suspension consisting of equal parts of packed Sepharose and distilled water is mixed with *a* ml of 2 M sodium bicarbonate. The suspension is slowly stirred on a magnetic stirrer and 0.05 *a* ml of CNBR in acetonitrile (2 g/ml) is added. During the addition the rate of stirring is momentarily increased. The mixture is allowed to react for 1–2 min. The now activated gel is then washed on a coarse-sintered glass funnel with 5–10 *a* volumes of wash solutions A, B, and C. After the last wash the gel is sucked almost dry and transferred to a tube containing *a* ml of 0.2 M sodium bicarbonate and *a* ml of protein solution (usually in PBS). Routinely, 1–2 mg of protein is mixed with 1 ml of packed beads. The coupling takes place under continuous agitation on a roller bank for 8–12 h at 4 °C. Residual active groups on the Sepharose are blocked by incubation of the beads overnight in 0.5 M ethanolamine, also under agitation. Finally, the beads are washed with 20 *a* volumes of the solutions D, E, and F and are stored in PBS containing 0.1% NaN_3.

Note: The continuous mixing of the Sepharose bead suspension during the activation, coupling, and deactivation is essential in the above procedure. This procedure ensures an even distribution of the antigens over the beads.

REFERENCES

Anderson, S. G., Addison, I. E., and Dixon, H. G. (1971). 'An international collaborative study of the proposed research standard 66/223.' *Ann. N.Y. Acad. Sci.*, **177**, 337–345.

Arnold, W., Kalden, J. R., and Mayersbach, H. von (1975). 'Influence of different histological preparation methods on preservation of tissue antigens in the immunofluorescent antibody technique.' *Ann. N.Y. Acad. Sci.*, **254**, 227–234.

Arnold, W. and Mayersbach, H. von (1972). 'Changes in the solubility of immunoglobulins after fluorescent labeling and its influence on immunofluorescent techniques.' *J. Histochem. Cytochem.*, **20**, 975–985.

Bayer, E. A. and Wilchek, M. (1974). 'Insolubilized biotin for the purification of avidin.' *Methods in Enzymol.*, **34**, 265–267.

Bergquist, N. R. and Nilsson, P. (1974). 'The conjugation of immunoglobulins with tetramethyl rhodamine isothiocyanate by utilization of dimethylsulfoxide (DMSO) as a solvent.' *J. Immunol. Methods*, **5**, 189–198.

Bergquist, N. R. and Nilsson, P. (1975). 'Laser excitation of fluorescent copolymerized immunoglobulin beads.' *Ann. N.Y. Acad. Sci.*, **254**, 157–162.

Beutner, E. H. (1971a). 'Field trials by ten laboratories of six commercial conjugates prepared from antisera to human IgG.' *Ann. N.Y. Acad. Sci.*, **177**, 361–404.

Beutner, E. H. (1971b). 'Defined immunofluorescent staining: past progress, present status and future prospects for defined conjugates.' *Ann. N.Y. Acad. Sci.*, **177**, 506–526.

Blakeslee, D. (1977). 'Immunofluorescence using dichlorotriazinylaminofluorescein (DTAF). II. Preparation, purity and stability of the compound.' *J. Immunol. Methods*, **17**, 361–364.

Blakeslee, D. and Baines, M. G. (1976). 'Immunofluorescence using dichlorotriazinylaminofluorescein (DTAF). I. Preparation and fractionation of labelled IgG.' *J. Immunol. Methods*, **13**, 305–320.

Brandtzaeg, P. (1973). 'Conjugates of immunoglobulin G with different fluorochromes. I. Characterization by anionic exchange chromatography.' *Scand. J. Immunol.*, **2**, 273–290.

Brandtzaeg, P. (1975). 'Rhodamine conjugates: specific and non-specific binding properties in immunohistochemistry.' *Ann. N.Y. Acad. Sci.*, **254**, 35–54.

Calcagno, J. V., Sweeny, M. J., and Oels, H. C. (1973). 'Rapid batch method for the preparation of fluorescein isothiocyanate-conjugated antibody.' *Infect. Immun.*, **7**, 336–369.

Capel, P. J. A. (1974). 'A quantitative immunofluorescent method based on the covalent coupling of protein to Sepharose beads.' *J. Immunol. Methods*, **5**, 165–178.

Cebra, J. J. and Goldstein, G. (1965). 'Chromatographic purification of tetramethyl rhodamine–immune globulin conjugates and their use in the cellular localization of rabbit γ-globulin polypeptide chains.' *J. Immunol.*, **95**, 230–245.

Chadwick, C. S., McEntegart, M. G., and Nairn, R. C. (1958). 'Fluorescent protein tracers: a trial of new fluorochromes and the development of an alternative to fluorescein.' *Immunology*, **1**, 315–327.

Cherry, W. B. and Reimer, C. B. (1973). 'The standardization of diagnostic immunofluorescence.' *Bull. World Health Org.*, **48**, 737–746.

Clark, H. F. and Shepard, C. G. (1963). 'A dialysis technique for preparing fluorescent antibody.' *Virology*, **20**, 642–644.

Coons, A. H., Creech, H. J., and Jones, R. N. (1941). 'Immunological properties of an antibody containing a fluorescent group.' *Proc. Soc. Exp. Biol. Med.*, **47**, 200–202.

Coons, A. H., Creech, H. J., Jones, R. N., and Berliner, E. (1942). 'The demonstration of pneumococcal antigen in tissues by the use of fluorescent antibody.' *J. Immunol.*, **45**, 150–170.

Dalen, J. P. R. van, and Haaijman, J. J. (1974). 'The determination of the molar absorbance coefficient of tetramethyl rhodamine isothiocyanate relative to fluorescein isothiocyanate.' *J. Immunol. Methods*, **5**, 103–106.

Dalen, J. P. R. van, Knapp, W., and Ploem, J. S. (1973). 'Microfluorometry on antigen–antibody interactions in immunofluorescence using antigens covalently bound to agarose beads.' *J. Immunol. Methods*, **2**, 383–392.

Deelder, A. M., Tanke, H. J., and Ploem, J. S. (1978). 'Automated quantitative immunofluorescence using the aperture defined microvolume (ADM) method.' In Knapp, W., Holubar, K., and Wick, G. (eds), *Immunofluorescence and Related Staining Techniques*, pp 31–44. Elsevier/North-Holland, Amsterdam/New York.

Deelder, A. M., Koper, G., de Water, R., Tanke, H. J., Rotmans, J. P., and Ploem, J. S. (1980). 'Automated measurement of immunogalactosidase reactions with a fluorogenic substrate by the aperture defined microvolume measurement method and its potential application to *Schistosoma mansoni* immunodiagnosis.' *J. Immunol. Methods*, **36**, 269–283.

Goding, J. W. (1976). 'Conjugation of antibodies with fluorochromes: modification to the standard methods.' *J. Immunol. Methods*, **13**, 215–226.

Haaijman, J. J. (1977). 'Quantitative Immunofluorescence Microscopy. Methods and Applications.' PhD thesis, University of Leiden, The Netherlands.

Haaijman, J. J., Bloemmen, F. J., and Ham, C. M. (1975). 'Microfluorometric immunoassays with antigens bound to Sepharose beads.' *Ann. N.Y. Acad. Sci.*, **254**, 137–150.

Haaijman, J. J. and Dalen, J. P. R. van (1974). 'Quantitation in immunofluorescence microscopy. A new standard for fluorescein and rhodamine emission measurements.' *J. Immunol. Methods*, **5**, 359–374.

Haaijman, J. J. and Slingerland-Teunissen, J. (1978). 'Equipment and preparative procedures in immunofluorescence microscopy: quantitative studies.' In Knapp, W., Holubar, K., and Wick, G. (eds), *Immunofluorescence and Related Staining Techniques*, pp. 11–29. Elsevier/North-Holland, Amsterdam/New York.

Haaijman, J. J. and Wijnants, F. A. C. (1975). 'Inexpensive automation of the Leitz Orthoplan microfluorometer using pneumatic microcomponents.' *J. Immunol. Methods*, **7**, 255–270.

Handschin, U. E. and Ritschard, W. J. (1976). 'Spectrophotometric determination of fluorophor, protein, and fluorophor/protein ratios in fluorescamine and MDPF fluorescent antibody conjugates.' *Anal. Biochem.*, **71**, 143–155.

Hansen, P. A. (1964). 'Fluorescent compounds used in protein tracing. Absorption and emission data.' Report Dept. Health, NIH, Bethesda, Md., USA.

Hebert, G. A., Pittman, B., and Cherry, W. B. (1971). 'The definition and application of evaluation techniques as a guide for the improvement of fluorescent antibody reagents.' *Ann. N.Y. Acad. Sci.*, **177**, 54–69.

Heitzmann, H. and Richards, F. M. (1974). 'Use of the avidin–biotin complex for specific staining of biological membranes in electron microscopy.' *Proc. Natl. Acad. Sci.*, **71**, 3537–3541.

Hijmans, W., Schuit, H. R. E., and Hulsing-Hesselink, E. (1971). 'An immunofluorescence study on intracellular immunoglobulins.' *Ann. N.Y. Acad. Sci.*, **177**, 290–305.

Hijmans, W., Schuit, H. R. E., and Klein, F. (1969). 'An immunofluorescence procedure for the detection of intracellular immunoglobulins.' *Clin. Exp. Immunol.*, **4**, 457–472.

Hiramoto, R. N., Engel, K., and Pressman, D. (1958). 'Tetramethyl rhodamine as an immunochemical fluorescent label in the study of chronic thyroiditis.' *Proc. Soc. Exp. Biol. Med.*, **97**, 611–614.

Jongsma, A. P. M., Hijmans, W., and Ploem, J. S. (1971). 'Quantitative immunofluorescence. Standardization and calibration in microfluorometry.' *Histochemie*, **25**, 329–343.

Klugerman, M. R. (1966). 'Chemical and physical variables affecting the properties of fluorescein isothiocyanate and its protein conjugates.' *J. Immunol.*, **95**, 1165–1173.

Knapp, W., Haaijman, J. J., Schuit, H. R. E., Berg, P. van den, Ploem, J. S., and Hijmans, W. (1975). 'Microfluorometric evaluation of conjugate specificity with the Defined Antigen Substrate Spheres (DASS) system.' *Ann. N.Y. Acad. Sci.*, **254**, 94–107.

Köhler, G. and Milstein, C. (1975). 'Continuous cultures of fused cells secreting antibody of predefined specificity.' *Nature*, **256**, 495–497.

March, S. C., Parikh, I., and Cuatrecasas, P. (1974). 'A simplified method for cyanogen bromide activation of agarose for affinity chromatography.' *Anal. Biochem.*, **60**, 149–152.

Mayersbach, H. von (1972). 'Quantitatieve Aussagemöglichkeiten der Immunofluoreszenz', *Acta Histochem.* Suppl. **XII**, 87–95.

Nairn, R. C. (1976). *Fluorescent Protein Tracing*, 4th edn. Churchill Livingstone, London.

Nisengard, R. and Beutner, E. H. (1972). 'Quantitative studies of immunofluorescent staining. IV. Nonspecific staining by free fluorescein and labeled protein.' *Int. Arch. Allergy Appl. Immunol.*, **43**, 383–389.

Oi, V. T. and Herzenberg, L. A. (1979). 'Localization of murine Ig-1b and Ig-1a (IgG$_{2a}$) allotypic determinants detected with monoclonal antibodies.' *Molec. Immunol.*, **16**, 1005–1017.

Phillips, D. J., Reimer, C. B., Wells, T. W., and Black, C. M. (1980). 'Quantitative characterization of specificity and potency of conjugated antibody with solid-phase, antigen bead standards.' *J. Immunol. Methods*, **34**, 315–327.

Ploem, J. S. (1967). 'The use of a vertical illuminator with interchangeable dichroic mirrors for fluorescence microscopy with incident light.' *Z. Wiss. Mikroskopie*, **68**, 129–142.

Ploem, J. S. (1970a). 'Quantitative immunofluorescence.' In Holborow, E. J. (ed.), *Standardization in Immunofluorescence*, pp. 63–73. Blackwell Scientific Publications, Oxford.

Ploem, J. S. (1970b). 'Standards for fluorescence microscopy.' In Holborow, E. J. (ed.), *Standardization in Immunofluorescence*, pp. 137–154. Blackwell Scientific Publications, Oxford.

Riggs, J. L., Seiwald, R. J., Burckhalter, J. H., Downs, C. M., and Metcalf, T. G. (1958). 'Isothiocyanate compounds as fluorescent labeling agents for immune serum.' *Am. J. Pathol.*, **34**, 1081–1097.

Rigler, R. (1966). 'Microfluorometric characterization of intracellular nucleic acids and nucleoproteins by acridine orange.' *Acta Physiol. Scand.*, **67**, Suppl. 267.

Rothbarth, Ph. H., Tanke, H. J., Mul, N. A. J., Ploem, J. S., Vliegenthart, J. F. G., and Ballieux, R. E. (1978). 'Immunofluorescence studies with 4-acetamido-4'-isothiocyanate stilbene-2,2'-disulphonic acid (SITS).' *J. Immunol. Methods*, **19**, 101–109.

Ruch, F. (1970). 'Principles and some applications of cytofluorometry.' In Wied, G. L., and Bahr, G. F. (eds), *Quantitative Cytochemistry*, vol II, pp. 431–450. Academic Press, New York.

Sernetz, M. and Thaer, A. A. (1970). 'A capillary fluorescence standard for microfluorometry.' *J. Microscopy*, **91**, 43–52.

Sernetz, M. and Thaer, A. A. (1972). 'Microfluorometric binding studies of fluorescein-albumin conjugates in single fibroblasts.' *Anal. Biochem.*, **50**, 98–109.

Sinsheimer, J. E., Stewart, J. F., and Burckhalter, J. H. (1968). 'Stilbene isothiocyanates as potential fluorescent tagging agents.' *J. Pharm. Sci.*, **57**, 1938–1944.

Thé, T. H. (1967). 'Conjugatie van fluoresceine isothiocyanaat aan antistoffen.' Thesis, University of Amsterdam.

Thé, T. H. (1970a). 'Conjugation of fluorescein isothiocyanate to antibodies. I. Experiments on the conditions of conjugation.' *Immunology*, **18**, 865–873.

Thé, T. H. (1970b). 'Conjugation of fluorescein isothiocyanate to antibodies. II. A reproducible method.' *Immunology*, **18**, 875–881.

Udenfriend, S., Stein, S., Böhlen, P., Dairman, W., Leimgruber, W., and Weigele, M. (1972). 'Fluorescamine: a reagent for assay of amino acids, peptides, proteins and primary amines in the picomole range.' *Science*, **178**, 871–872.

Visser, J., Haaijman, J. J., and Trask, B. (1978). 'Quantitative immunofluorescence in flow cytometry.' In Knapp, W., Holubar, K., and Wick, G. (eds), *Immunofluorescence and Related Staining Techniques*, pp. 147–160. Elsevier/North-Holland, Amsterdam/New York.

Weber, K. (1965). 'Leitz-Mikroskop-Photometer MPV mit variabeler Messblende.' *Leitz Mitt. Wiss. Techn.*, **3**, 103–107.

Weigele, M., DeBernardo, S., Leimgruber, W., Cleeland, R., and Grunberg, E. (1973). 'Fluorescent labeling of proteins. A new methodology.' *Biochem. Biophys. Res. Comm.*, **54**, 899–906.

Wells, A. F., Miller, C. E., and Nadel, M. K. (1966). 'Rapid fluorescein and protein assay method for fluorescent antibody conjugates.' *Appl. Microbiol.*, **14**, 271–275.

White, R. G. (1970). 'Fluorochromes and labelling.' In Holborow, E. J. (ed.), *Standardization in Immunofluorescence*, pp. 49–53. Blackwell, Scientific Publications, Oxford.

Wick, G. (1972). 'Immunofluoreszenz-Versuche zur Standardisierung.' *Wiener Klin. Wochenschr.*, **84**, 2–18.

Wofsy, L., Baker, P. C., Thompson, K., Goodman, J., Kimura, J., and Henry, C. (1974). 'Hapten-sandwich labeling. I. A general procedure for simultaneous labeling of multiple cell surface antigens for fluorescence and electronmicroscopy.' *J. Exp. Med.*, **140**, 523–537.

Immunohistochemistry
Edited by A. C. Cuello
© 1983 IBRO

CHAPTER 3

Preparation of HRP-labelled Antibodies

D. M. BOORSMA

Department of Dermatology, Academic Hospital Free University, De Boelelaan 1117, 1081 HV Amsterdam, The Netherlands

I INTRODUCTION

In 1966 Nakane and Pierce introduced a breakthrough in immunocyto-chemistry when they succeeded in the application of enzymes as markers of antibodies. In the same year Graham and Karnovsky described a method for the histochemical demonstration of the enzyme horseradish peroxidase (HRP) at ultrastructural level. This method could also be used for visualization of HRP by light microscopy. From that year on, methods that make use of the enzyme HRP as marker for the demonstration of antibodies were called *immunoperoxidase* methods. Since then, immunoperoxidase methods have successfully been applied for the localization of antigens both at light and electron microscopic level. Peroxidase-labelled antibodies, frequently called HRP conjugates, have a broad field of application in immunohisto-chemistry and immunocytochemistry. Furthermore these HRP conjugates find application in the rapidly expanding field of enzyme immunoassay and to a lesser extent in that of immunochemistry.

Immunoperoxidase methods do not always depend on the use of HRP conjugates. Another important technique makes use of the soluble immune complex HRP–anti HRP, called PAP (Sternberger, 1979; see also Chapter 4).

In this chapter attention will be focussed on the preparation, purification, analysis, and application of HRP conjugates. Moreover the properties of differently prepared HRP conjugates will be compared.

HRP conjugates are prepared by the coupling of HRP and antibody by means of a suitable agent (Avrameas *et al.*, 1978). This coupling agent has the possibility of reacting via the active groups with both the enzyme and the antibody, thus bridging the two molecules.

Some requirements which must be fulfilled by the coupling agent are: it must produce an irreversible bond between HRP and antibody; it must act in such a way that the biological activity of both the HRP and the antibody will be preserved as much as possible in the HRP conjugate; it must not induce properties of the HRP conjugate, e.g. altered charge through polymerization, which might cause non-specific attachment to tissue components.

The complexity of the coupling reaction in fact always leads to a reaction mixture that, after the reaction, consists of a mixture of reactants, the HRP conjugate being one of them. The appearance of dimers and even polymers of both HRP and antibody is a common feature, while the HRP conjugate formed is seldom of homogeneous composition. The extent to which the HRP conjugate is formed considerably differs from method to method. This means that after the conjugation uncoupled starting reactants (HRP and/or antibody) will be found in the final reaction mixture.

II METHODS OF COUPLING

Until now there have been described two types of methods of coupling: one-step methods and two-step methods. In the one-step methods antibody, HRP, and the coupling agent are mixed. The reaction is allowed to proceed for a certain period and thereafter it is stopped by an agent or it stops spontaneously. In the two-step methods the first step consists of activation of HRP or antibody with the coupling agent. Subsequently the activated protein, after removal of the excess coupling agent, is added to the other reactant and again the reaction proceeds for a certain period. In general these coupling agents should possess at least two active groups, of which one couples to the first protein, while the other active groups remain available for coupling to the second reactant. Two-step reactions are more controlled and provide in most cases a more homogeneous HRP conjugate than the one-step reactions.

III COUPLING AGENTS

Several agents have been used for preparation of HRP conjugates since their introduction in 1966.

(1) *p,p'*-Difluoro-*m,m'*-dinitrodiphenyl sulphon (FNPS). This reagent was the first one which had successfully been applied in the preparation of HRP conjugate (Nakane and Pierce, 1966). The method used was a one-step method. The HRP conjugate obtained was heterogeneous and polymeric of structure, while the yield of the reaction was low.

(2) Cyanuric chloride (Avrameas and Lespinats, 1967). On the HRP conjugate obtained using this agent the same comment is applicable as for the FNPS.

(3) Carbodi-imides (Clyne *et al.*, 1973). HRP conjugate prepared with this agent proved to be unstable, and lost its biological activity after a few days.

(4) Toluene di-isocyanate (Clyne *et al.*, 1973). This agent has been used in a two-step method. However, it has not found wide application.

(5) Glutaraldehyde (Avrameas, 1969; Avrameas and Ternynck, 1971). This dialdehyde has gained a very wide popularity as coupling agent. With this agent not only the enzyme HRP, but also many other enzymes, can be coupled to antibodies. Glutaraldehyde can be used in a one-step method as well as in a two-step method. The action of glutaraldehyde is based on the following assumption: of the two aldehyde groups one reacts with an epsilon-amino group in the first protein and the second aldehyde group reacts with an amino-group in the other protein.

Using glutaraldehyde in a one-step method (Avrameas, 1969) the HRP conjugate is of heterogeneous composition, polymeric of structure, and contains relatively few HRP molecules per antibody molecule (Boorsma and Kalsbeek, 1975). When glutaraldehyde is used in a two-step method (Avrameas and Ternynck, 1971), firstly HRP is allowed to react with an excess of this agent. The activated HRP, after removal of excess glutaraldehyde, is added in excess to antibody. A homogeneous HRP conjugate is then formed, though in a low yield. This HRP conjugate has a high biological activity because of the mild method of preparation. The superior quality of this HRP conjugate makes this method of preparation very popular.

(6) Sodium periodate (Nakane and Kawaoi, 1974; Wilson and Nakane, 1978). This chemical is not an authentic coupling agent because it does not itself act as the bridge between HRP and antibody. The mechanism of action of this method is ingenious. Until now the method has almost only been applied for HRP conjugation. The protein HRP has a considerable polysaccharide shell. The sugar moieties in this shell can be oxidized by periodate in such a way that aldehyde groups are introduced. The HRP aldehyde obtained reacts subsequently in a second step with the amino groups of the antibody and the HRP conjugate will be formed.

This method for preparation of HRP conjugate is also very popular especially because of the simplicity and the high yield of the reaction.

(7) *p*-Benzoquinone (Ternynck and Avrameas, 1976; 1977). This agent is used in two-step methods for coupling HRP or other enzymes and antibody. The first step may be the activation of either HRP or antibody with *p*-benzoquinone. Subsequently the other reactant is coupled to the activated one in a second step. This relatively recent method has not been commonly applied till now, though it is said to give good results (Avrameas, personal communication, 1980).

(8) *N*-Succinimidyl 3-(2-pyridyldithio)propionate (Carlsson *et al.*, 1978). This agent must be used in a two-step method. Both HRP and antibody must be activated separately. Coupling is accomplished by introducing S–S bonds between the proteins. This method for preparing HRP conjugate is as yet in a stage of development.

IV   REVIEW OF THE MOST COMMONLY USED METHODS

The two-step method using glutaraldehyde, and the periodate method, are by far the most often applied methods for the preparation of HRP conjugate. Therefore these methods will be considered in more detail. The analysis of the reaction product and purification of HRP conjugate from contaminating constituents, like starting reactants and by-products will be discussed for these two procedures.

IV.1   Two-step Glutaraldehyde Method

The two-step glutaraldehyde method starts with the activation of HRP by means of excess glutaraldehyde. This HRP must be of very high quality. The RZ (this parameter is the ratio of the optical density at 403 nm and 280 nm) must be about 3, in any case not below 2.8. Since this HRP contains only few free amino groups available for reaction with glutaraldehyde, it remains for the major part in monomeric form. Dimerization occurs, dependent on the batch, in maximally 30% (Boorsma and Streefkerk, 1976a). Figure 1 shows a gel chromatography pattern of activated HRP where dimerization is obvious. In addition it can be concluded that polymerization with HRP of RZ 3 hardly occurs. HRP of RZ lower than 2.8 has considerably more free amino groups that can react with glutaraldehyde. Therefore the lower the RZ of HRP the more polymerization takes place during glutaraldehyde activation. The polymers are probably very reactive but have a very low enzyme activity, thus causing large polymeric conjugates of insufficient and low sensitivity.

After the activation step with glutaraldehyde, the excess of this reagent has to be removed. This is usually done by column chromatography, e.g. with Sephadex G25 fine. The choice of a different gel (e.g. Ultrogel AcA-44) for column chromatography additionally provides separation of the monomeric and dimeric HRP. After having obtained the activated HRP the antibody is

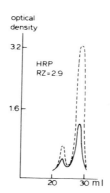

Figure 1   Gel chromatography on Ultrogel AcA–44 (55 × 1 cm, flow rate 7 ml/cm²/
h) of glutaraldehyde-activated HRP. ——— OD_{280nm}; – – – – OD_{403nm}

added. The former must be present in large excess, since the reaction
proceeds only partially. Afterwards about 5% of the originally added HRP
and about 30% of the antibody is found in the HRP conjugate; the rest of the
starting proteins has not reacted. This is clear from Figure 2 (left), where an
elution pattern of a column chromatography of an HRP conjugate is shown.
In the first peak both antibody and HRP were found, in the second peak only
antibody was found, and in the last large peak only HRP. From the elution
volume of the HRP conjugate in this chromatography pattern it could be
concluded that this conjugate had a molecular weight of about 200,000

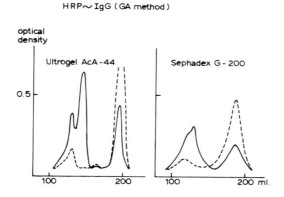

Figure 2   Gel chromatography on Ultrogel AcA–44 (left) and Sephadex G–200
(right) of HRP conjugate prepared by the two-step glutaraldehyde method. Column:
100 × 2 cm, flow rate 3.2 ml/cm²/h. Reproduced by permission of the Histochemical
Society Inc.

daltons. From the optical density ratio of 403 to 280 nm it could be calculated that the molar ratio of antibody to HRP was 1:1. This means that the HRP conjugate was composed of one molecule antibody to which one molecule HRP has been coupled. It is obvious that the HRP conjugate was of defined and homogeneous composition. Extensive studies (Boorsma *et al.*, 1976) have shown that both the antibody activity and the enzyme activity of HRP in the conjugate were well preserved.

IV.2   The Periodate Method

The periodate method starts with a mild oxidation of HRP by means of sodium periodate. This type of oxidation is a well-known reaction in carbohydrate chemistry: glycol groups in sugars can be oxidized by periodate to aldehyde groups. Also in this method the HRP must be of very high quality (RZ ± 3). HRP of lower RZ lacks the extensive carbohydrate shell and has more free amino groups. Oxidation of this lower RZ HRP results either in non-activated HRP or self-coupling by polymerization. The oxidation reaction usually takes place in bicarbonate solution (Nakane and Kawaoi, 1975) or, more recently proposed, in distilled water (Wilson and Nakane, 1978). The introduction of aldehyde groups in HRP does under these circumstances lead to only minor amounts of dimeric activated HRP (Boorsma and Streefkerk, 1976a) and not to polymeric moieties, as can be seen from Figure 3. The prevention from self-coupling can be explained from the well-documented paucity of accessible amino groups in HRP. The excess periodate in the reaction mixture can be removed by dialysis (Wilson and Nakane, 1978) or neutralized with excess glycol followed by column chromatography (Boorsma and Streefkerk, 1979). Subsequently this HRP aldehyde is reacted with antibody. The reaction is very efficient; almost all HRP and antibody react to HRP conjugate (Boorsma and Streefkerk, 1976b, 1979). By

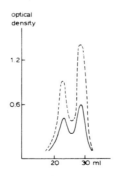

Figure 3   Gel chromatography on Ultrogel AcA–44 (55 × 1 cm, flow rate 7 ml/cm^2/ h) of HRP-aldehyde activated with periodate

varying the ratio HRP to antibody in the reaction mixture it is possible to obtain HRP conjugate with different HRP antibody ratios. The optimal ratio is usually considered to be about 2.2 moles HRP per antibody. This results in the HRP conjugate in a molar ratio of two HRP to one antibody. In Figure 4 (left) an elution pattern is shown from a chromatography of a HRP conjugate

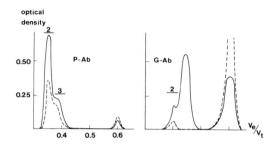

Figure 4 Gel chromatography on Ultrogel AcA–44 after conjugation of HRP to antibodies (Ab) by the periodate (P) and the two-step glutaraldehyde (G) methods. Left: P conjugation; right: G conjugation. The numbers P–Ab–2, P–Ab–3 refer to pools of fractions (conjugates) studied (number 1 refers to the non-chromatographed, 'crude' reaction mixtures)

prepared with the periodate method. From that pattern it can be concluded that the molecular dimensions of the major part of this HRP conjugate are of considerable molecular weight, over 400,000 daltons (Boorsma and Streef-kerk, 1976b). A minor fraction had a lower molecular weight (between 200,000 and 400,000 daltons). A small amount of HRP did not react and no unreacted antibody was detected. Other studies have revealed that this HRP conjugate is a heterogeneous mixture with molecular weights ranging from 200,000 to several million daltons. The HRP conjugate should retain both antibody activity and enzyme activity (Boorsma *et al.*, 1976; Boorsma and Streefkerk, 1979), though to a lesser extent than conjugates prepared with the two-step glutaraldehyde method.

V PURIFICATION OF HRP ANTIBODY CONJUGATES

From the above discussions and analyses it is clear that after coupling HRP and antibody there always results a mixture of reactants from which the HRP conjugate is one component. Since other products, present in the reaction mixture, may interfere when HRP conjugate is applied, it is in most cases useful to isolate HRP conjugate as much as possible from by-products and/or starting proteins.

Some methods of purification which can be applied:

(a) Ammonium sulphate precipitation (Avrameas, 1969; Boorsma and Kals-
    beek, 1975). This method is used to separate uncoupled HRP from the
    other components. It is unsuitable for isolation of HRP conjugate from
    uncoupled antibody.
(b) Gel chromatography. In most cases the following gels have been applied:
    Sephadex G200 (Avrameas, 1969; Boorsma and Kalsbeek, 1975; Boors-
    ma and Streefkerk, 1976b), Ultrogel AcA-44 (Boorsma and Streefkerk,
    1976b, 1979), Ultrogel AcA-34; Sephacryl S200 (Wilson and Nakane,
    1978). This gel chromatography method is not only suitable for analysis
    of HRP conjugates but also purification can be achieved in this way. The
    gels produce different results, as can be seen in Figure 2. It is clear that,
    under optimal circumstances Ultrogel is much more efficient than a
    comparable Sephadex, in separating HRP conjugate (Boorsma and
    Streefkerk, 1976b). However, these methods are only applicable at
    small-scale level.
(c) Affinity chromatography. This method is as yet little known and there-
    fore hardly applied in purification of HRP conjugate. However, it is
    possible to use a combination of protein A–Sepharose and Concanavalin
    A–Sepharose (Boorsma and Streefkerk, 1978). Protein A has affinity for
    antibody (IgG, coupled with HRP or uncoupled) and not for HRP.
    Concanavalin A has affinity for HRP (also when coupled with antibody)
    but not for antibody. A separation scheme can thus be devised:

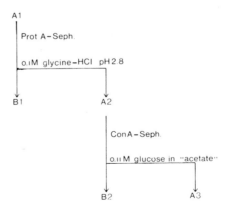

SEPARATION SCHEME

A1

Prot A–Seph.

o.ıM glycine–HCl pH 2.8

B1   A2

ConA–Seph.

o.ıı M glucose in "acetate"

B2   A3

An HRP conjugate prepared by the two-step glutaraldehyde method (A1)
is applied on protein A–Sepharose. The unbound fraction B1 is collected
and the bound fraction eluted (A2) and applied on the Concanavalin

A–Sepharose. The unbound fraction B2 is collected and the bound fraction (A3) is eluted. Elution patterns thus obtained are shown in Figure 5. The respective fractions A1, 2, B1, 2, 3 analysed on Ultrogel

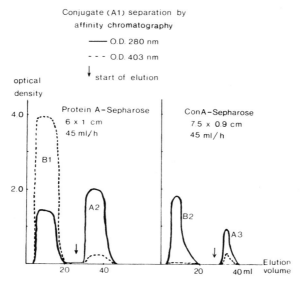

Figure 5 Affinity chromatography elution pattern of HRP conjugate prepared by the two-step glutaraldehyde method. Elution is performed with (left) 0.1 M glycine–HCl pH 2.8 and (right) glucose in acetate buffer

chromatography gave results as depicted in the elution patterns of Figure 6. It is clear from these results that it is possible to obtain in this way an almost pure HRP conjugate. Fraction B1 consists of uncoupled HRP, fraction B2 of uncoupled antibody. Fraction A3 represents an HRP conjugate which possibly is only slightly contaminated with uncoupled antibody. This HRP conjugate compares favourably with those isolated by gel chromatography (Boorsma and Streefkerk, 1978).

This method of purification allows separation of products on a large scale. The separation capacity of this method is about 600 times that of gel chromatography. In addition, it is faster; a complete sequence can be performed in just 4 h.

It must be noted that the method has limitations. The first limitation of this method lies in the fact that protein A does not have affinity for immunoglobulins of all species, e.g. from sheep globulins a considerable fraction is not bound*. These problems can be circumvented by using as a first step a gel

---

* *Editor's Note:* The same lack of affinity of protein A has been observed with some monoclonal antibodies.

Immunohistochemistry

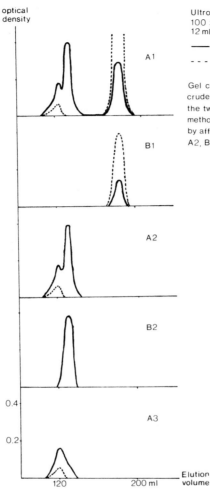

Figure 6

chromatography that gives separation of the unbound HRP, instead of affinity chromatography with protein A. The second limitation lies in the high affinity of Concanavalin A for HRP, which results in some irreversible adherence and therefore loss of HRP conjugate. Maximally loading of Concanavalin A diminishes these effects.

VI APPLICATION OF DIFFERENT HRP CONJUGATES

It has been shown (Boorsma *et al.*, 1976; Boorsma and Streefkerk, 1979) that both types of HRP conjugate are suitable in immunocytochemistry and other fields. However it is generally accepted that there exist some differences as to the degree of suitability of these preparations in different fields.

In general two techniques can be distinguished: (a) the direct technique, and (b) an indirect (sandwich) technique in which the first antibody is unlabelled and developed with a labelled second antibody. Both techniques (direct and indirect) can be used for detection of antigen in unfixed, cryostat-sectioned tissue, on cell surfaces, in formalin-fixed, paraffin-embedded tissue, and in ELISA techniques. Results of comparative studies (Boorsma and Streefkerk, 1979) for the suitability of periodate prepared and two-step glutaraldehyde prepared HRP conjugates are represented in Figure 7. It is clear that in the direct technique for detection of antigen in unfixed cryostat sections the two-step glutaraldehyde HRP conjugate is superior to the periodate HRP conjugate, while in ELISA techniques the reverse is true. Both types of HRP conjugates were about equally efficient for the detection of surface immunoglobulins of lymphocytes. The same holds true for the

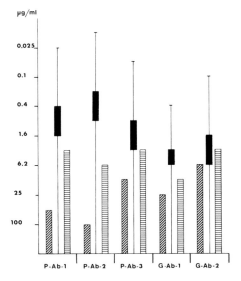

Figure 7 Diagrammatic representation of test results with the different HRP conjugates. For nomenclature of conjugates see legend of Figure 4. Vertical axis: concentration of conjugates in μg/ml. For each conjugate the concentration giving positive reactions is shown as follows: left bar, tissue immunohistochemistry (skin of LE patients); straight line and black bar, direct and indirect ELISA (reaction of human IgG and detection of anti-penicillin antibodies, respectively); right bar, surface antigen detection (Ig on human lymphocytes)

detection of intracytoplasmic immunoglobulins in plasma cells of mouse spleen (Boorsma, unpublished observations).

VII HRP CONJUGATES AND PAP

No proper comparisons between the efficiency of HRP conjugate and PAP have been reported. In some comparative studies good PAP and a bad HRP conjugate have been compared. Of the presumed higher sensitivity and lower background of PAP over HRP conjugate, only the slightly higher sensitivity of PAP survives when it is compared with an optimally prepared HRP conjugate (Tougard *et al.*, 1979; van Leeuwen and Boorsma, unpublished observations). This higher sensitivity probably must be attributed to the multiplication effect of the three-step method.

In conclusion optimally prepared HRP conjugate is a very suitable and sensitive reagent in immunocytochemistry and in other immunological methods. In addition, new possible applications of these conjugates are expected with the advancement of monoclonal antibodies, such as the revival of the direct immunoperoxidase technique (Boorsma *et al.*, 1982).

APPENDIX 1

Two-step glutaraldehyde conjugation procedure (Avrameas and Ternynck, 1971):

(1) Dissolve 10 mg HRP (RZ = 3) in 0.2 ml of a 0.1 M phosphate buffer, pH 6.8, containing 1.25% glutaraldehyde.
(2) After 18 h at room temperature this solution is filtrated on a Sephadex G25 fine column, equilibrated with 0.15 M NaCl, to remove the excess glutaraldehyde.
(3) The fractions containing the activated (brown) HRP are pooled and concentrated to ± 10 mg/ml; subsequently 5 mg/ml antibody in 0.15 M NaCl is added.
(4) The pH is raised to 9.0–9.5 with sodium carbonate–bicarbonate buffer (pH 9.5).
(5) After 24 h at 4 °C 0.1 ml of a 0.2 M lysine–HCl solution is added.
(6) After 2 h at 4 °C the solution is dialysed against PBS (pH 7.2).

Notes
(a) Instead of step (2) it is possible to isolate the monomeric activated HRP fractions by column chromatography on Ultrogel AcA-44 and to pool the fractions with monomeric activated HRP. In this way activated dimers of HRP are excluded from the conjugation reaction.
(b) A possible step (7) could be the removal of uncoupled antibody and HRP by, e.g. gel chromatography.

APPENDIX 2

Periodate conjugation procedure (Wilson and Nakane, 1978)

(1) Dissolve 4 mg HRP (RZ = 3) in distilled water.
(2) Add 0.2 ml freshly prepared solution of 0.1 M $NaIO_4$ and mix gently for 20 min. The colour should turn from brown to dark green.
(3) The solution is subsequently dialysed against 0.001 M sodium acetate buffer pH 4.4, at 4 °C for 20 h.
(4) The pH of the HRP solution is then raised to 9.5 by the addition of 20 µl 0.2 M sodium carbonate–bicarbonate buffer (pH 9.5) and immediately 8 mg antibody is added in 1 ml 0.01 M sodium carbonate–bicarbonate buffer (pH 9.5). Mix gently and let the reaction proceed for 2 h at room temperature.
(5) Subsequently add 0.1 ml of a freshly prepared solution of sodium borohydride (4 mg/ml distilled water). Let this mixture stand for 2 h at 4 °C.
(6) The HRP conjugate is thereafter chromatographed (on e.g. Ultrogel or Sephacryl) or dialysed against PBS.

Note: For minor modifications see Boorsma and Streefkerk, 1979.

REFERENCES

Avrameas, S. (1969). 'Coupling of enzymes to proteins with glutaraldehyde. Use of the conjugates for the detection of antigens and antibodies.' *Immunochemistry*, **6**, 43–52.

Avrameas, S. and Lespinats, G. (1967). 'Enzymes couplées aux protéines; leur utilisation pour la détection des antigènes et des anticorps.' *C.R. Acad. Sci. Paris*, **265**, 1149–1153.

Avrameas, S. and Ternynck, T. (1971). 'Peroxidase labelled antibody and Fab conjugates with enhanced intracellular penetration.' *Immunochemistry*, **8**, 1175–1179.

Avrameas, S., Ternynck, T., and Guesdon, J. L. (1978). 'Coupling of enzymes to antibodies and antigens.' *Scand. J. Immunol.*, **8**, Suppl. 7, 7–23.

Boorsma, D. M. and Kalsbeek, G. L. (1975). 'A comparative study of horseradish peroxidase conjugates prepared with a one-step and a two-step method.' *J. Histochem. Cytochem.*, **23**, 200–207.

Boorsma, D. M. and Streefkerk, J. G. (1976a). 'Some aspects of the preparation, analysis and use of peroxidase-antibody conjugates in immunohistochemistry.' *Protides Biol. Fluids*, **24**, 795–802.

Boorsma, D. M. and Streefkerk, J. G. (1976b). 'Peroxidase–conjugate chromatography. Isolation of conjugates prepared with glutaraldehyde or periodate using polyacrylamide-agarose gel.' *J. Histochem. Cytochem.*, **24**, 481–486.

Boorsma, D. M. and Streefkerk, J. G. (1978). 'Improved method for separation of peroxidase conjugates.' In Knapp, W., Holubar, K., and Wick, G. (eds), *Immunofluorescence and Related Staining Techniques*, pp. 225–235. Elsevier/North Holland Biomedical Press, Amsterdam.

Boorsma, D. M. and Streefkerk, J. G. (1979). 'Periodate or glutaraldehyde for preparing peroxidase conjugates?' *J. Immunol. Methods*, **30**, 245–255.
Boorsma, D. M., Streefkerk, J. G., and Kors, N. (1976). 'A quantitative comparison of two peroxidase conjugates prepared with glutaraldehyde or periodate and a fluorescein conjugate.' *J. Histochem. Cytochem.*, **24**, 1017–1025.
Boorsma, D. M., Cuello, A. C., and van Leeuwen, F. W. (1982). 'Direct immunocytochemistry with a horseradish peroxidase conjugated monoclonal antibody against substance P.' *J. Histochem. Cytochem.*, **30**, 1211–1216.
Carlsson, J., Drevin, H., and Axén, R. (1978). 'Protein thiolation and reversible protein–protein conjugation.' *Biochem. J.*, **173**, 723–737.
Clyne, D. H., Norris, S. H., Modesto, R. R., Pesce, A. J., and Pollak, V. E. (1973). 'Antibody enzyme conjugates. The preparation of intermolecular conjugates of horseradish peroxidase and antibody and their use in immunohistology of renal cortex.' *J. Histochem. Cytochem.*, **21**, 233–240.
Graham, R. C. and Karnovsky, M. J. (1966). 'The early stages of absorption of injected horseradish peroxidase in the proximal tubules of mouse kidney: ultrastructural cytochemistry by a new technique.' *J. Histochem. Cytochem.*, **14**, 291–302.
Nakane, P. K. and Kawaoi, A. (1974). 'Peroxidase-labeled antibody. A new method of conjugation.' *J. Histochem. Cytochem.*, **22**, 1084–1091.
Nakane, P. K. and Pierce, G. B. (1966). 'Enzyme-labeled antibodies: preparation and application for the localization of antigens.' *J. Histochem. Cytochem.*, **14**, 929–931.
Sternberger, L. A. (1979). *Immunocytochemistry*. 2nd edn. John Wiley, New York.
Ternynck, T. and Avrameas, S. (1976). 'A new method using *p*-benzoquinone for coupling antigens and antibodies to marker substances.' *Ann. Immunol. (Inst. Pasteur)*, **127C**, 197–208.
Ternynck, T. and Avrameas, S. (1977). 'Conjugation of *p*-benzoquinone treated enzymes with antibodies and Fab fragments.' *Immunochemistry*, **14**, 767–775.
Tougard, C., Tixier-Vidal, A., and Avrameas, S. (1979). 'Comparison between peroxidase-conjugated antigen or antibody and peroxidase–anti-peroxidase complex in a postembedding procedure.' *J. Histochem. Cytochem.*, **27**, 1630–1633.
Wilson, M. B. and Nakane, P. K. (1978). 'Recent developments in the periodate method of conjugating horseradish peroxidase (HRPO) to antibodies.' In Knapp, W., Holubar, K., and Wick, G. (eds), *Immunofluorescence and Related Staining Techniques*, pp. 215–224. Elsevier/North Holland Biomedical Press, Amsterdam.

Immunohistochemistry
Edited by A. C. Cuello
© 1983 IBRO

CHAPTER 4

Peroxidase–antiperoxidase Techniques

F. VANDESANDE

Zoölogical Institute, K. U. Leuven, Louvain, Belgium

I INTRODUCTION

Many of the shortcomings of the enzyme-labelled antibody methods are due to the conjugation procedure itself. The circumstances in which the covalent binding between the antibody and the peroxidase molecule is formed, partly destroy the antibody activity and give rise to a mixture of conjugated and non-conjugated antibody, which is very difficult to purify. Recently, however, an ingenious purification method has been developed by Boorsma and Streefkerk (1978) (see Chapter 3).

To overcome the problems due to conjugation procedures Mason *et al.* and Sternberger and Cuculis simultaneously developed the unlabelled antibody enzyme method and showed that the immunohistochemical localization of antigen can be enzymatically visualized without the use of conjugated antibodies (Mason *et al.*, 1969a,b; Sternberger, 1969; Sternberger and Cuculis, 1969).

All unlabelled antibody enzyme methods have one point in common: for detection of the primary antibody bound to the tissue antigen, only immunological reactions are used.

The unlabelled antibody enzyme methods may be divided into two groups:

(a) the original unlabelled antibody enzyme and related methods;
(2) the PAP and related methods.

This contribution will deal only with the original unlabelled antibody method and the PAP method. As it is almost impossible to cover all the literature the reader is referred to the excellent monograph *Immunocytochemistry* by Sternberger (1979).

II THE ORIGINAL UNLABELLED ANTIBODY ENZYME METHOD

II.1 Principle

The principle of the original unlabelled antibody enzyme method is depicted in Figure 1. The method consists of five sequential steps.

In the first step the tissue section is incubated with a specific primary antiserum produced in species A and directed against the tissue antigen under investigation. This primary antiserum is usually used at high dilutions, so that the antibody will bind with both antigen binding sites.

In a second step the tissue section is incubated with an antiserum produced in species B and directed against IgG of species A. It is important to use this antiserum in excess, in order to leave one antigen binding site free after reaction with the primary antibody.

In a third step the tissue section is incubated with an antiserum produced in the same species as the primary antiserum, but now directed against

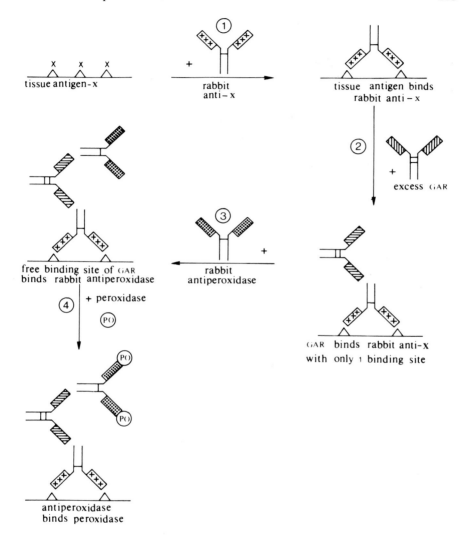

Figure 1 Staining sequence in the original unlabelled antibody enzyme method. GAR, goat anti-rabbit immunoglobulin; PO, horseradish peroxidase. Reproduced by permission of Elsevier/North Holland from *Journal of Neuroscience Methods,* 1979, **1**, 3–23

horseradish peroxidase. The free binding site of the anti-IgG, applied in the second step, now binds the antiperoxidase antibodies. As the anti-IgG used in the second step contains mainly antibodies directed against the Fc fragments of IgG molecules of species A, usually both, but in any event at least one, of the specific peroxidase binding sites of the antiperoxidase antibodies remains free.

In a fourth step the section is incubated with horseradish peroxidase that will react with the free binding sites of the antiperoxidase antibodies applied during the third step.

In a last step the section is incubated with hydrogen peroxide and 3,3'-diaminobenzidine tetrahydrochloride (DAB) as substrates for peroxidase.

This incubation results in the formation of a brown, insoluble polymeric oxidation product of DAB over the antigenic sites in the tissue section.

II.2 Discussion

In the original unlabelled antibody enzyme method all problems concerned with conjugation procedures are eliminated. The method suffers, however, from major shortcomings. A first problem concerns the antiperoxidase antiserum used in the third step. A normal antiperoxidase antiserum contains not only antiperoxidase antibodies but also many other IgG molecules not directed against peroxidase. In the third step these IgG molecules, not directed against peroxidase, will also be bound by the free antigen binding sites of the secondary antibodies. This markedly decreases the efficiency of the staining, as IgG of specificities other than peroxidase will not bind peroxidase in the fourth step. Therefore it is extremely important to use purified antiperoxidase antiserum in the third step. Antiperoxidase antisera can only be purified by affinity chromatography on a specific immunoadsorbent such as for example a Sepharose-4B–peroxidase complex.

Affinity chromatography is a very good method for the purification of antibodies directed against most proteins.

Unfortunately with some other proteins and peptides this method gives very bad results. This is caused by the strong binding of some proteins and peptides to their antibodies so that pH changes, or the use of chaotropic agents are not able to dissociate the antigen–antibody binding. This is the case for the peroxidase–antiperoxidase binding.

After affinity chromatography with an immunoadsorbent only those antiperoxidase antibodies with the lowest affinities are recovered, and the antibodies with higher affinities remain bound to the column. Low-affinity antibodies are easily lost by dissociation during washing and this again markedly decreases the efficiency of the staining.

In immunocytochemistry an excess of antibody is usually applied to the antigen present in the tissue preparation. This results in a preferential binding of the antibodies with the highest affinities, while the low-affinity antibodies remain in solution. Dissociation during washing is thereby minimized. In the third step of the unlabelled antibody enzyme method, however, antiperoxidase has the role of antigen that will be bound by the free binding site of the secondary antibody. This binding depends on the affinity of the secondary antibody for IgG, and not on the affinity of antiperoxidase for peroxidase. Consequently, antiperoxidase with low affinity, as well as antiperoxidase with high affinity, will be bound by the secondary antibody. Weakly bound peroxidase will be lost during washing after the fourth step, resulting again in a decrease of staining efficiency. According to Sternberger, 75% of the peroxidase is lost during washing after the fourth step. These major short-comings have been overcome in an ingenious and elegant manner, thanks to the development of the PAP technique by Sternberger *et al.* (1970).

III THE PAP METHOD

III.1 Principle

The principle of the PAP method is the same as for the original unlabelled antibody enzyme method except that steps (3) and (4) of the original method are replaced by a single incubation with PAP complex. PAP is a soluble complex of peroxidase with antiperoxidase and is prepared *in vitro*. The principle of the PAP method is illustrated in Figure 2. In the third step of the staining sequence, PAP possesses a dual function: it has enzymatic activity and is an antigen for the secondary antibody attached to the tissue section during the second step. This secondary antibody is also called link antibody (Rickert *et al.*, 1976).

III.2 Preparation and Properties of PAP

PAP is prepared *in vitro* by precipitation of antibody from specific rabbit antiserum with horseradish peroxidase at equivalence. The precipitate is washed and solubilized with excess peroxidase at pH 2.3, 1 °C, followed by immediate neutralization and separation of PAP from free peroxidase by half-saturation with ammonium sulphate. The ratio of peroxidase to antiper-oxidase in PAP is 3:2, irrespective of the source of the antiserum. This unexpected ratio of peroxidase to antiperoxidase is presumed to be due to stabilization by a pentagonal ring structure in which three corners are supposed to be peroxidase, while the other two are antibody Fc (constant) fragments.

The amount of free peroxidase necessary to maintain PAP in solution may vary with antibodies from different sera. At times it has been immeasurably small.

The fact that PAP, in contrast to other soluble antigen–antibody complexes, can be maintained in solution with small amounts of free peroxidase, indicates strong binding between peroxidase and antiperoxidase. Sternberger

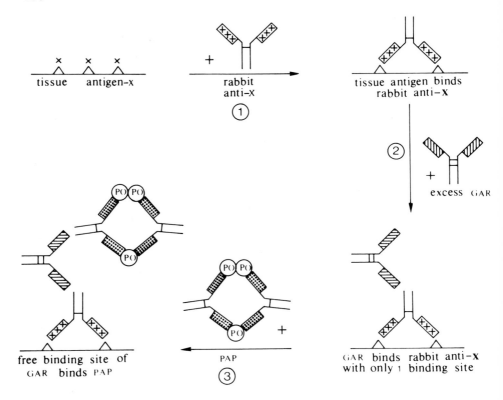

Figure 2 Staining sequence in the PAP method. GAR, goat anti-rabbit immunoglubulin; PO, horseradish peroxidase. Reproduced by permission of Elsevier/North Holland from *Journal of Neuroscience Methods*, 1979, **1**, 3–23

established the association constant of PAP as 10^8. This unusual stability of PAP is, as we shall see, very important for the sensitivity of the immunocytochemical staining. It is also important that peroxidase activity is not destroyed in PAP. According to Sternberger the impairment of peroxidase activity in PAP varies from 2 to 30%. This has no practical influence on the sensitivity of the method.

For more details concerning the preparation of PAP see Section IV.1.3.

III.3   Discussion

III.3.1   Advantages of the PAP method

With the PAP technique all problems concerned with conjugation procedures are eliminated. In contrast to the preparation of enzyme-labelled antibodies, the preparation of PAP is an economical and simple procedure. High-quality PAP preparations are commercially available and some of these preparations can be used at a working dilution of 1:300. The sensitivity of the PAP method is sometimes 20–200 times higher than that of other immuno-cytochemical methods (Sternberger *et al.*, 1970; Moriarty *et al.*, 1973; Petrali *et al.*, 1974; Baker *et al.*, 1975; Burns, 1975; Marucci and Dougherty, 1975). This high sensitivity is due to the high stability of the PAP complex and to the high signal-to-noise ratio of the method.

The low background staining of the PAP method as well as of the original unlabelled antibody enzyme method can partly be explained by the fact that the presence in the link antiserum of antibodies directed against unwanted antigens in the tissue section will not result in method non-specificity (see Chapter 1). In the enzyme-labelled antibody method, however, these un-wanted antibodies are conjugated with peroxidase and will be detected by the histochemical reaction in the last step. Consequently they will show up as background staining and increase method non-specificity. Both situations are illustrated in Figure 3 and 4 (see also Sternberger, 1977).

III.3.2 Shortcomings of the PAP method

For light microscopical purposes the PAP method is, at least for the moment, the best of all existing immunocytochemical techniques.

Investigators using the PAP technique, however, may be misled by false-negative results (see also Bigbee *et al.*, 1977). This phenomenon can best be explained by means of an example. During an investigation of the supraoptic and paraventricular nuclei in normal rats we obtained with one of our antivasopressin antisera an intense immunocytochemical staining of vasopressinergic cells with a primary antiserum dilution 1:200. About 1 year later we used the same antiserum at the same dilution for studies of hypothalamic preparations from experimental rats in which the hypothalamic magnocellular neurosecretory system had been activated by dehydration, and axonal transport blocked by intracisternal injection of colchicine. Since in these circumstances vasopressin accumulates in the vasopressinergic cells of the paraventricular and supraoptic nuclei, we expected a very intense staining. To our great surprise, however, all of the vasopressinergic cells remained unstained. At first we thought that this negative staining result was due to a deterioration of our anti-vasopressin antiserum. However, incuba-tion of hypothalamic preparations from normal rats with this supposedly deteriorated antiserum resulted again in a positive staining. This result proved that our antivasopressin serum was still active and that some other factor had caused the negative staining result in the experimental animals. By running simultaneous staining reactions with increasing dilutions of the primary antiserum we found that in normal rats the staining intensity

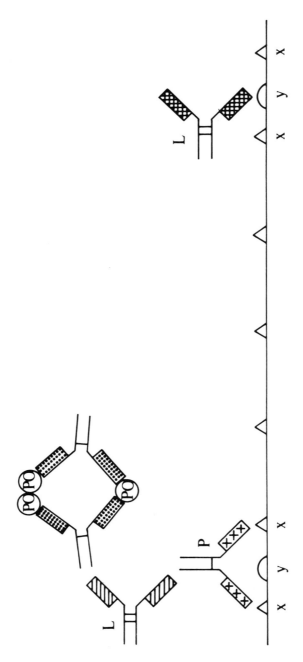

Figure 3 Illustration of possible events during the localization of a tissue antigen X with the PAP technique if the link antiserum contains antibodies directed against an antigen Y also present in the tissue section. The antibodies directed against Y are not directed against rabbit IgG and will not react with PAP. This results in a blocking of the non-specific staining. L, link antibody; P, specific primary antibody. Reproduced by permission of Elsevier/North Holland from *Journal of Neuroscience Methods*, 1979, **1**, 3–23

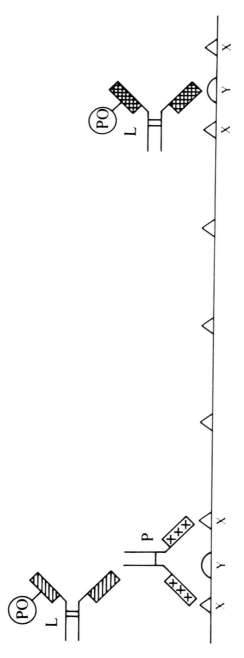

Figure 4 Illustration of possible events during the localization of a tissue antigen X with the indirect enzyme-labelled antibody method, if the link antiserum contains antibodies against antigen Y also present in the tissue section. During conjugation of the link antiserum also, antibodies directed against Y were conjugated. When these antibodies bind to antigen Y in the tissue section they will show up as background staining. L, link antibody; P, specific primary antibody. Reproduced by permission of Elsevier/North Holland from *Journal of Neuroscience Methods*, 1979, **1**, 3–23

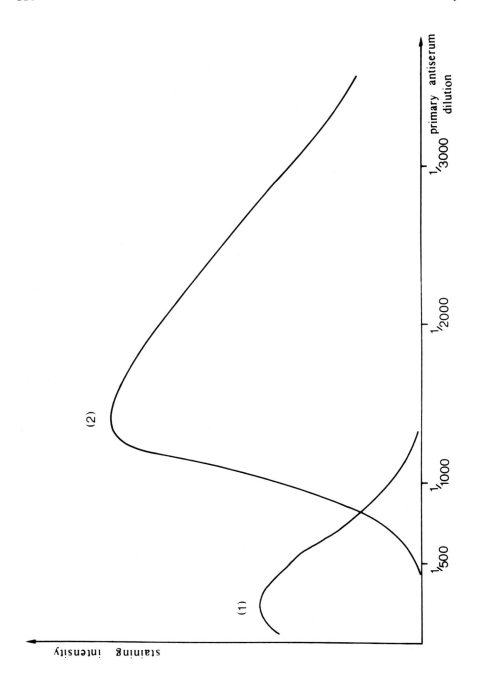

decreased with increasing dilution. In contrast, in dehydrated-colchicine treated rats the staining remained negative until a serum dilution of 1 : 600 was reached. Further dilution of the primary antiserum resulted in an increasing staining intensity to reach an optimal staining at a dilution 1 : 1500. Still further dilution resulted, in these animals also, in a decreasing staining intensity. The maximum staining intensity that could be obtained was much higher in the experimental animals than in the normal animals. These results are summarized in Figure 5. These results can best be explained by suggesting that at high antibody and antigen concentration the primary antibody binds in such a way with the tissue antigen that the distance d between the Fc fragments becomes appropriate to allow a preferential binding of both Fab (antigen-binding) fragments of the link antibody. In such a situation only the unreactive Fc fragments of the link antibody remain uncovered. As staining can only occur if free unreacted Fab is present to pick up the PAP molecules, this will result in a negative staining. This situation is illustrated in Figure 6.

The amount of primary antibody that will bind to tissue antigen during incubation with primary antiserum depends on several parameters. These parameters are: (1) tissue antigen concentration; (2) titre, avidity, and dilution of the primary antiserum; (3) incubation time; (4) incubation temperature; and (5) accessibility of the antigen.

Tissue antigen concentration itself depends on several parameters: (1) physiological condition of the animal; (2) fixation procedure; and (3) embedding procedure. Thus it is clear that it cannot be overemphasized that a serum dilution appropriate for one tissue may not be so for another. From all these facts we may conclude that when applying an untested antiserum to tissue, or a tested serum to unknown tissue, a broad range of primary antisera dilutions should be tried to safeguard against this type of false-negative results.

IV PROTOCOLS

IV.1 Preparation of PAP

The following PAP preparation protocol is a modification of the original protocol of Sternberger. We use it for our own PAP preparations. Starting with a good antiperoxidase antiserum this protocol results in a PAP preparation with a working dilution of $\pm 1 : 1000$.

Figure 5 Staining intensity of vasopressinergic cells in function of primary antiserum dilution. (1): normal rats; (2): dehydrated rats intracisternally injected with colchicine. In both cases the same antivasopressin serum has been used. Reproduced by permission of Elsevier/North Holland from *Journal of Neuroscience Methods*, 1979, **1**, 3–23

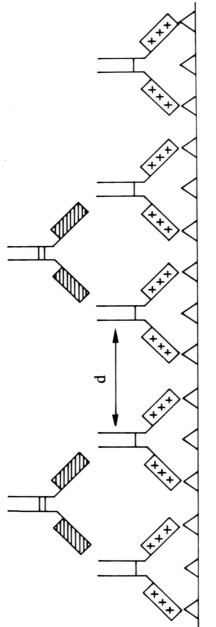

Figure 6 Illustration of the situation in which too much primary antibody had been bound to the antigen in the tissue section as a result of an inappropriate primary antiserum dilution. The distance *d* between the Fc fragments of the primary antibody is appropriate to allow a preferential binding of both Fab fragments of the goat anti-rabbit immunoglobulin (GAR) molecules. As the free Fc fragments of the GAR molecules are unreactive, no PAP will be bound during the third step. Reproduced by permission of Elsevier/North Holland from *Journal of Neuroscience Methods*, 1979, **1**, 3–23

IV.1.1 Production of antiperoxidase antiserum

(a) *Reagents*
—Horseradish peroxidase Sigma type VI.
—Complete Freund's adjuvant.
—0·9% NaCl solution.
—*Bordetella pertussis* suspension.

(b) *Materials*
—Virtis homogenizer.
—Plastic disposable 5 ml syringe.

(c) *Immunization procedure*
Dissolve 1 mg horseradish peroxidase in the closed barrel of a 5 ml plastic disposable syringe containing 0.5 ml 0.9% NaCl solution. Add 0.5 ml complete Freund's adjuvant. Homogenize (in the barrel) with a Virtis homogenizer at 30,000 rpm until a stable emulsion is obtained. Inject a rabbit with this emulsion into the footpads, and also into multiple sites of the back. Give in addition an intramuscular injection of a suspension containing 6×10^9 *Bordetella pertussis*. Give three fortnightly booster injections with the same antigen-complete Freund's adjuvant emulsion. Collect blood from an ear artery 1 week after the third booster injection. Store the blood serum at $-25\,°C$.

IV.1.2 Determination of the antiperoxidase titre of antiperoxidase sera

This determination is based on the fact that when an increasing amount of peroxidase is added to a given amount of antiperoxidase serum all of the peroxidase will take part in the reaction and precipitate until the equivalence point is reached. Beyond this point free peroxidase will remain in solution and can be detected in the supernate by means of an enzymatic reaction for peroxidase.

(a) *Reagents*
—0.9% NaCl solution.
—2.1 ml of a solution containing 0.66 mg/ml horseradish peroxidase Sigma Type VI in 0.9% NaCl.
—21 ml of a 1:10 dilution of antiperoxidase serum in 0.9% NaCl.
—50 ml of a 5% pyrogallol solution in H_2O.
—25 ml 0.15 M H_2O_2.
—100 ml 0.1 M phosphate buffer pH 6.0.
—25 ml 2 N H_2SO_4.

(b) *Materials*
Centrifuge, spectrophotometer, refrigerator 4 °C, water bath with thermostat set at 20 °C, and pH meter.

(c) *Procedure*

Place into a series of 21 test tubes 0, 10, 20 . . . 180, 190, 200 μl of the solution containing 0.66 mg/ml horseradish peroxidase in 0.9% NaCl. Add to these tubes respectively 200, 190, 180 . . . 20, 10, 0 μl 0.9% NaCl solution. The volume of the liquid in each tube is now 200 μl. Add to each tube 1 ml of the 1:10 dilution of antiperoxidase serum in 0.9% NaCl.

Mix well and incubate for 1 h at room temperature and for 48 h in the refrigerator at 4 °C.

Centrifuge and collect 0.5 ml of the supernates into a second set of 21 tubes with thermostat set at 20 °C and containing 2.0 ml of the 5% pyrogallol solution, 1.0 ml 0.15 M H_2O_2, 3.0 ml 0.1 M phosphate buffer pH 6.0 and 10 ml H_2O. Mix very well and add, after 60 s, 1 ml 2 N H_2SO_4 for blocking the enzymatic reaction.

Immediately measure the extinction at 420 nm.

Use a mixture containing 2.0 ml 5% pyrogallol, 1.0 ml 0.15 M H_2O_2, 3.0 ml 0.1 M phosphate buffer pH 6.0, 1 ml 2 N H_2SO_4 and 10 ml H_2O as blank.

Make a diagram of the results and read the equivalence point. See Figure 7.

Suppose that the equivalence point is situated at 110 μl peroxidase (0.66 mg/ml), then (0.66 × 110):1000 = 0.073 mg peroxidase is equivalent to 1 ml of the 1:10 diluted antiperoxidase serum.

This means that for precipitation of 1 ml of antiperoxidase serum in the equivalence zone, 0.73 mg peroxidase are needed.

IV.1.3 *PAP preparation procedure*

(a) *Reagents*
—Horseradish peroxidase Sigma type VI.
—Antiperoxidase serum of known titre.
—1 N and 0.1 N HCl solution.
—1 N and 0.1 N NaOH solution.
—0.9% NaCl solution.
—Ammonium acetate buffer pH 6.9; prepare the buffer by mixing 0.08 N $NaOOCCH_3$ and 0.15 N NH_4OOCCH_3.
—Saturated ammonium sulphate solution.
—50% saturated ammonium sulphate solution.
—Dialysis buffer: 48.6 g NaCl + 30 ml 1.5 N $NaOOCCH_3$ + 30 ml 3 N $(NH_4)_2SO_4$ + 5.941 H_2O.

(b) *Materials*
Refrigerated centrifuge, pH meter, ice bath, refrigerator 4 °C, dialysis tubing, magnetic stirrer.

(c) *Procedure*
Assuming that the antiperoxidase serum has a titre of 0.73 mg peroxidase/

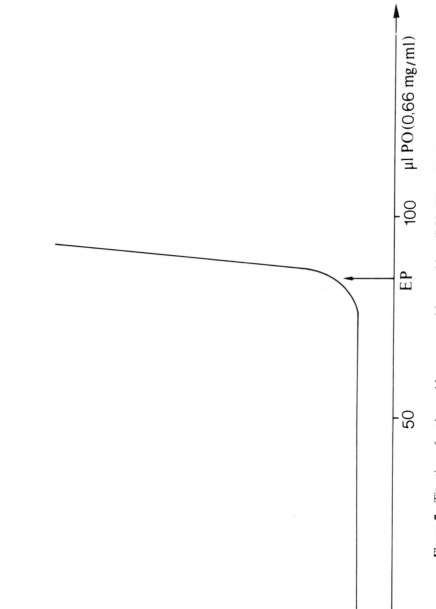

Figure 7 Titration of antiperoxidase serum with peroxidase (PO). EP, equivalence point

ml. Add to 10.5 ml antiperoxidase serum a solution of 7.66 mg peroxidase in 7.66 ml H_2O.

After mixing, incubate for 1 h at room temperature. Isolate the formed precipitate by centrifugation for 15 min at 16,000 g and 4 °C. Resuspend precipitate in a cold 0.9% NaCl solution and centrifuge at 4 °C and 16,000 g for 5 min. Carry out a total of four such washes. Thoroughly resuspend the precipitate at room temperature in a solution of 30.64 mg peroxidase in 15.3 ml H_2O. Under mild stirring bring to pH 2.3 at room temperature with 1.0 N and 0.1 N HCl. Neutralize as quickly as possible to pH 7.2 with 1.0 N and 0.1 N NaOH. Add ±1 ml ammonium acetate buffer to bring the pH to 6.9.

Chill the solution in an ice bath and add slowly, under mild stirring, the same volume of a cold saturated solution of $(NH_4)_2SO_4$. Keep stirring for 45 min at 0 °C and centrifuge for 15 min at 0 °C and 35,000 g. Collect the supernate* and twice wash the precipitate with 50% saturated $(NH_4)_2SO_4$ at 0 °C. Dissolve the precipitate in 10.5 ml H_2O and dialyse at 4 °C against the dialysis buffer.

Eliminate the precipitate formed during dialysis by centrifugation. Re-adjust the volume to 10.5 ml by addition of dialysis buffer.

Aliquot the PAP solution in fractions of 10 µl, freeze in liquid nitrogen and store at −25 °C.

IV.2 PAP Staining for Light Microscopy (for electron microscopy see Chapter 11)

(a) *Reagents*
—Lugol solution: 10 mg/ml KI and 5 mg/ml I_2.
—$NaHSO_3$ solution: 5 g $NaHSO_3$ in 100 ml H_2O.
  Remark: Lugol and $NaHSO_3$ solutions are only needed if the fixative contained sublimate.
—Buffered saline: 0.01 M Tris/HCl pH 7.6 in 0.9% NaCl.
—Pre-immune goat serum diluted 1/5 in buffered saline.
—Specific rabbit primary antisera optimally diluted in buffered saline.
—Goat anti-rabbit IgG serum diluted 1/20 in buffered saline. (for the alternative use of protein A as link reagent see Chapter 7, Section VII.3)
—PAP (peroxidase–antiperoxidase complex) diluted 1/300 (this dilution depends on the batch PAP).
—DAB solution: Dissolve 25 mg 3,3′-diaminobenzidine in 200 ml 0.05 M Tris-HCl buffer. Filter and add 2 ml 0.3% freshly prepared H_2O_2. This

---

* After precipitation of the PAP complex with $(NH_4)_2SO_4$, excess of free peroxidase can easily be recuperated from the collected supernate by affinity chromatography on Concanavalin A–Sepharose.

results in a final DAB concentration of 0.0125% and H_2O_2 concentration of 0.003% (prepare just before use).

(b) *Materials*

Appropriately fixed paraffin sections, paper tissue, rotating shaking apparatus, moist chamber, plain glass trays with removable slide racks.

(c) *Steps for staining procedure*
  (1) Xylene (2×5 min)
  (2) dry ethanol (2×2 min)
  (3) wash by immersion in H_2O
  (4) Lugol solution (2 min) ⎱ only if sublimate was present in the fixative
  (5) $NaHSO_3$ solution (2 min) ⎰
  (6) wash by immersion in H_2O
  (7) wash by immersion in buffered saline
  (8) incubate with pre-immune goat serum 1/5 (moist chamber, 15 min)
  (9) jet-wash with buffered saline
  (10) wash on a rotating–shaking apparatus with buffered saline (5 min) and blot with tissue paper
  (11) incubate overnight in the moist chamber at room temperature with the appropriate dilution of the first primary antiserum (250 μl per slide)
  (12) jet-wash with buffered saline
  (13) wash on the rotating–shaking apparatus (5 min) and blot
  (14) incubate with goat anti-rabbit IgG serum (1/20, moist chamber, 25 min)
  (15) jet-wash with buffered saline
  (16 wash on the rotating–shaking apparatus (5 min) and blot
  (17) incubate with PAP 1/300 (moist chamber, 25 min)
  (18) jet-wash with buffered saline
  (19) wash on the rotating–shaking apparatus with buffered saline (5 min) and blot
  (20) equilibrate the slides in 0.05 M Tris-HCl buffer pH 7.6
  (21) stain for 3–5 min in freshly prepared DAB solution at 20 °C in the rotating–shaking apparatus
  (22) wash with buffered saline
  (23) control the staining under the microscope
  (24) dehydrate in graded ethanol and xylene, mount in fluormount.

V SUPPLIERS

—Goat anti-rabbit IgG serum: Nordic, Immunological Laboratories, Langestraat, 57–61. POB 22, Tilburg, The Netherlands.
—Peroxidase–rabbit antiperoxidase complex (PAP): UCB—Christiaens. Bioproducts–peptide department, Rue Berkendael 68, B-1060 Brussels, Belgium.

—Dealer for Canada: Bio-Ria, 109000 rue Hamon, Montreal, PQ Canada H2M 3A2.

—Dealer for USA: Bio-Ria, 9809 Merioneth Drive, Louisville, Kentucky, USA 40299.

—Rotating-shaking apparatus: Taumler typ 54131, Heidolph-Elektro HG, 0842, Kelheim, Germany.

REFERENCES

Baker, B. L., Dermody, W. C., and Reel, J. R. (1975). 'Distribution of gonadotropin-releasing hormone in the rat brain as observed with immunocytochemistry.' *Endocrinology*, **97**, 125.

Bigbee, J. W., Kosek, J. C., and Eng, L. F. (1977). 'Effects of primary antiserum dilution on staining of "antigen rich" tissues with the peroxidase antiperoxidase technique.' *J. Histochem. Cytochem.*, **25**, 433–447.

Boorsma, D. M. and Streefkerk, J. G. (1978). 'Improved method for separation of peroxidase conjugates.' In Knapp, W., Holubar, K., and Wick, G. (eds), *Immunofluorescence and Related Staining Techniques*, pp. 225–235. Elsevier/North Holland Biomedical Press, Amsterdam.

Burns, J. (1975). 'Background staining and sensitivity of the unlabelled antibody-enzyme (PAP) method. Comparison with the peroxidase labelled antibody sandwich method using formalin fixed paraffin embedded material.' *Histochemistry*, **43**, 291–294.

Marucci, A. A. and Dougherty, R. M. (1975). 'Use of unlabelled antibody immunohistochemical technique for the detection of human antibody.' *J. Histochem. Cytochem.*, **23**, 618–623.

Mason, T. E., Phifer, R. F., Spicer, S. S., Swallow, R. A., and Dreskin, R. B. (1969a). 'New immunochemical technique for localising intracellular tissue antigen.' *J. Histochem. Cytochem.*, **17**, 190.

Mason, T. E., Phifer, R. F., Spicer, S. S., Swallow, R. A., and Dreskin, R. B. (1969b). 'An immunoglobulin-enzyme bridge method for localizing tissue antigens.' *J. Histochem. Cytochem.*, **17**, 563–569.

Moriarty, G. C., Moriarty, C. M., and Sternberger, L. A. (1973). 'Ultrastructural immunocytochemistry with unlabelled antibodies and the peroxidase-antiperoxidase complex. A technique more sensitive than radioimmunoassay.' *J. Histochem. Cytochem.*, **21**, 825–833.

Petrali, J. P., Milton, D. M., Moriarty, G. C., and Sternberger, L. A. (1974). 'The unlabelled antibody enzyme method of immunocytochemistry. Quantitative comparison of sensitivities with and without peroxidase-antiperoxidase complex.' *J. Histochem. Cytochem.*, **22**, 782–801.

Rickert, D. E., Fischer, L. J., Burke, J. P., Redick, J. A., Erlandsen, S. L., Parsons, J. A., and Van Orden, L. S. III (1976). 'Cyproheptadine-induced insulin depletion in rat pancreatic beta cells: demonstration by light and electron microscopic immunocytochemistry.' *Horm. Metabol. Res.*, **8**, 430.

Sternberger, L. A. (1969). 'Some new developments in immunocytochemistry.' *Mikroskopie*, **25**, 346–361.

Sternberger, L. A. (1977). 'Immunocytochemistry of neuropeptides and their receptors.' In Gainer, H. (ed.), *Peptides in Neurobiology*, pp. 61–97. Plenum Press, New York.

Sternberger, L. A. (1979). *'Immunocytochemistry.'* John Wiley, New York, Chichester, Brisbane, Toronto.

Sternberger, L. A. and Cuculis, J. J. (1969). 'Method for enzymatic intensification of the immunocytochemical reaction without use of labelled antibodies.' *J. Histochem. Cytochem.*, **17**, 90.

Sternberger, L. A., Hardy, P. H., Jr., Cuculis, J. J., and Meyer, H. G. (1970). 'The unlabelled antibody-enzyme method of immunohistochemistry. Preparation and properties of soluble antigen-antibody complex (horseradish peroxidase–antihorseradish peroxidase) and its use in the identification of spirochetes.' *J. Histochem. Cytochem.*, **18**, 315–333.

Immunohistochemistry
Edited by A. C. Cuello
© 1983 IBRO

CHAPTER 5

Preparation of Catecholamine-synthesizing Enzymes as Immunogens for Immunohistochemistry

TONG H. JOH and M. ELIZABETH ROSS

Laboratory of Neurobiology, Cornell University Medical College, 1300 York Avenue, New York, N.Y. 10021

I INTRODUCTION

The development of purification methods for catecholamine synthesizing enzymes, tyrosine hydroxylase (TOH), dopamine-β-hydroxylase (DBH), and phenylethanolamine *N*-methyltransferase (PNMT) has made possible the production of specific antibodies to these proteins. A tremendous volume of immunohistochemical literature has been generated on the anatomical local-ization of these enzymes. However, there is a dearth of publications describing the practical details of purifying the catecholaminergic enzymes as immunogens for specific antibody production.

To fill this need, several brief but effective purification schema will be described which can readily be carried out in any biochemistry laboratory. In the interest of simplicity, unnecessary and lengthy citations of alternative methods for enzyme purification will be omitted from the discussion. All of the procedures appearing in this chapter are currently used in the authors' laboratory.

II MATERIALS AND ENZYME ASSAY METHODS

Chromatographic gels for enzyme purification, including phenyl Sepharose CL-4B, Sepharose 4B and Sephadex G100 (Pharmacia), DEAE cellulose (DE52) (Whatman) were prepared. Linear concentration gradients for elution of adsorbed protein from DE52 were produced with a *GM-1 Gradient Mixer* ® (Pharmacia). Bovine pancreatic trypsin (type III, Sigma) was used for partial digestion of tyrosine hydroxylase (TH) and the reaction was stopped with Soybean trypsin inhibitor (type IS, Sigma). Ultrapure sucrose for sucrose density gradient centrifugation was purchased from Schwartz/Mann. Acrylamide and *N-N*-methylene bisacrylamide were purchased from Eastman.

Tyrosine hydroxylase activity was assayed by a modification of the method of Coyle (Coyle, 1972; Reis *et al.*, 1975). Dopamine-β-hydroxylase activity was measured by a modification of the methods of Reis and Molinoff (1972). Phenylethanolamine *N*-methyltransferase activity was assayed using the method of Wurtman *et al.* (Wurtman *et al.*, 1967). Protein was quantitated by the Lowry method (Lowry *et al.*, 1951). During chromatography, protein contents of column fractions were estimated from their optical densities measured at 280 nm.

III   TYROSINE HYDROXYLASE

TH has been purified from a number of different tissues as well as species, including rat brain (Joh *et al.*, 1978), cultured cell lines (Joh *et al.*, 1978; Vulliet *et al.*, 1980), bovine adrenal medulla (Petrack *et al.*, 1968; Shiman *et al.*, 1971; Joh *et al.*, 1969; Joh and Goldstein, 1973) and human phaeochromocytoma (Park and Goldstein, 1976). In the authors' laboratory, all these tissues have been used as sources of TH antigen.

Homologous antibody–antigen systems have frequently been observed to yield the most vigorous and specific immunochemical and immunohistochemical reactions. Consequently, one would expect that antibodies raised against TH from different sources might vary in their affinity to, for example, rat brain TH. Such variation could reflect tissue and species differences in tertiary structure and immunogenicity of the enzyme. However, the fact that immunocytochemical localization of rat TH in both the central and peripheral nervous system is equivalent using antisera raised against a variety of TH species (Pickel *et al.*, 1975a,b,c; Rothman *et al.*, 1981; and Hokfelt *et al.*, 1972) suggests that the physical structure of the molecule is conserved.

Important pragmatic aspects to be considered in designing or selecting a purification method for these antigens include:

(a) how easily and reliably the protocol will isolate highly purified TH which is suitable for immunization;
(b) how economically the antiserum can be produced; and
(c) whether the tissue selected as antigen source will yield antibodies of sufficiently broad species reactivity to be used in several experimental systems.

The most satisfactory TH antibody for immunocytochemical use is produced against the 'trypsin digested' form of bovine adrenal medullary TH (TTH). Numerous laboratories which have received this antiserum from the author have reported that it can be used for labelling TH in brain, adrenal medulla, and ganglia of rodent (Pickel *et al.*, 1975a,b,c), human (Pickel *et al.*, 1981), Chicken (Rothman *et al.*, 1981) and tortoise (Karten, personal communication). Furthermore, TTH is easily purified in relatively large quantities from an economical tissue source, making production of antiserum to this antigen quite practical.

An attractive feature of this method for production of TTH antibody is that another catecholamine synthesizing enzyme, PNMT, can also be purified from the same tissue homogenate. TTH is isolated from the sediment obtained from high-speed centrifugation of adrenal medulla homogenate, while the supernatant can be used for the purification of PNMT.

III.1 Trypsin digested TH (TTH)

A diagrammatic scheme for the purification of TTH appears in Figure 1. In each step the buffer used is potassium phosphate, pH 7.0, of a concentration designated in the text. The isolation method is designed to yield a large quantity of highly purified, but not homogeneous, TH. Approximately 200 g of bovine adrenal medulla are required to obtain enough antigen to inject into three rabbits.

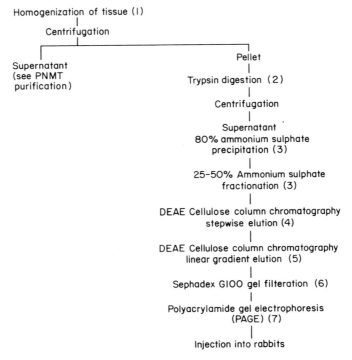

Figure 1   Purification of trypsin digested tyrosine hydroxylase (TTH)

After Sephadex G100 column chromatography the highly purified TTH can be further purified to homogeneity by affinity column chromatography on an antibody-linked Sepharose column. However, the production of specific antiserum does not require this final step. Furthermore, the yield of homogeneously purified enzyme is low and therefore is not practically suited for immunization of rabbits. Following the purification illustrated in Figure 1, TTH is directly subjected to either tube or slab polyacrylamide gel electrophoresis (PAGE) and finally isolated for immunization as detailed later.

III.1.1 *Homogenization of tissue*

Fresh or frozen bovine adrenal glands are cut open and adrenal medulla are dissected out and collected. A 50 g portion of tissue is homogenized in a Waring Blender for 30 s at low speed in 150 ml of 0.25 M sucrose in 5 mM buffer (see procedure for purification of PNMT). The homogenate is passed through several layers of gauze, and filtrate is centrifuged at 105,000 g for 60 min.

III.1.2 *Trypsin digestion*

The supernatant is stored at −80 °C for subsequent purification of PNMT as detailed later. The sediment is homogenized in 20 mM buffer and the final volume is adjusted to 100 ml with the same buffer. To this homogenate is added 5 mg trypsin which is dissolved in 1 ml of 20 mM buffer and the mixture is incubated for 30 min with mild agitation in a 30 °C water bath. Trypsin inhibitor (10 mg dissolved in 2 ml buffer) is then added to the mixture. At this stage the enzyme preparations can be frozen in order to accumulate several batches for further purification.

III.1.3 *Ammonium sulphate fractionation*

The trypsin-treated homogenate is then centrifuged at 105,000 g for 60 min and sediment is discarded. A layer of very loosely packed sediment will overlie the pellet so that only the clear supernatant, which has been removed carefully with a pipette, should be used. The supernatant is subjected either to lyophilization or ammonium sulphate precipitation at 80% saturation.

The lyophilized protein or 80% ammonium sulphate precipitate is dialysed against 20 mM buffer and the protein is fractionated, taking the protein which precipitates between 25 and 50% saturation in ammonium sulphate (see step 3 in purification of total adrenal medullary DBH). This fraction is dialysed against 20 mM buffer, and the total amount of protein is determined.

III.1.4 *DEAE cellulose column chromatography*

A DEAE cellulose (DE52) column is then built and equilibrated with 20 mM buffer. The size of the column is calculated so that 10 ml of bed volume is present for every 100 mg protein chromatographed. The column is layered with the sample and unadsorbed proteins are washed out with 20 mM buffer. Separation of proteins on the column is carried out by stepwise elution with 50, 200, and 300 mM potassium chloride in 20 mM buffer. A majority of TH activity is eluted with 200 mM KCl. The fractions containing the highest specific activity (TH activity per mg protein) are collected, the protein is concentrated by lyophilization, and dialysed against 20 mM buffer.

III.1.5 *Second DEAE cellulose column chromatography*

A second DE52 column is built (100 mg protein/20 ml bed volume) and equilibrated with 20 mM buffer. This time the column elution is carried out with a linear concentration gradient between 50 mM and 200 mM KCl in 20 mM buffer. The total elution buffer volume used is 10 times the bed volume of the column. The peak TH activity generally appears at KCl concentrations around 150 mM. The fractions containing highest specific activity are pooled, the protein is concentrated by lyophilization, and is dialysed against 20 mM buffer.

III.1.6 *Sephadex G100 gel filtration*

The second DE52 eluate is then put on a Sephadex G100 column which is well equilibrated with 20 mM buffer. The optimal protein concentration for this molecular seiving is 10 mg protein per ml. The best protein separation is achieved when 3 ml of a 25–30 mg protein solution is passed over a 450 ml bed volume of Sephadex G100, packed in a 2.6 × 85 cm column.

III.1.7 *Polyacrylamide gel electrophoresis (PAGE)*

When the protein from this purification stage is subjected to polyacrylamide gel electrophoresis (PAGE) at pH 8.2 (see 'Production of Antisera'). One major protein band possessing TH activity and several minor protein bands are detected. The enzyme can be further purified to homogeneity by other column chromatographic procedures such as substrate affinity or antibody-linked affinity chromatography. However, immunization with enzyme finally isolated from PAGE gels has been found to be most satisfactory.

III.2 Purification of Native Form(s) of TH

Native forms of TH can be purified using methods elsewhere described (Joh *et al.*, 1978; Vulliet *et al.*, 1980). Several difficulties are encountered in purifying native forms of the enzyme. First, native TH from bovine adrenal medulla tends to aggregate, making it virtually impossible to purify without partial digestion of the enzyme with trypsin (Petrack *et al.*, 1968) or chrymotrypsin (Shiman *et al.*, 1971). Therefore, native TH must be purified from rat tissues so that each animal sacrificed yields relatively little tissue for purification. Second, the yield of purified enzyme from collected tissues is extremely low, making the expense of such antibody production quite high. Third, the electrophoretic mobility of the native enzyme is much slower than TTH; thus it is rather difficult to separate the TH band from other contaminant protein bands on PAGE gels.

However, in the authors' laboratory, native forms of TH from rat nigrostriatum, rat adrenal glands, cultured cell lines of human neuroblastoma, SK-N-BE2 (Joh *et al.*, 1978), and rat phaeochromocytoma, PC12 (Joh, unpublished; Vulliet *et al.*, 1980) have been purified and some of these are used to produce antibodies. Although there is no advantage in using these antisera when compared with TTH antibodies for immunocytochemical localization, they are better suited for immunochemical uses such as direct immunoprecipitation of native TH from crude tissue preparations or *in vitro* mRNA translation products (Baetge *et al.*, 1981). A schematic view of the procedure appears in Figure 2.

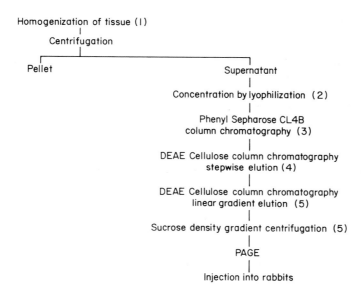

Figure 2   Purification of native forms of tyrosine hydroxylase (TH)

III.2.1   *Homogenization of tissue*

Frozen tissues (rat nigrostriatum, rat adrenal gland, cultured cell lines such as rat phaeochromocytoma (PC12), or human neuroblastoma (SK-N-BE2)) are homogenized with a polytron tissue homogenizer in 10 mM buffer (1 g tissue/20 ml buffer). Homogenate is then centrifuged at 105,000 g for 30 min at 4 °C.

III.2.2 *Concentration of protein*

The supernatant is lyophilized to dryness. The freeze-dried protein is resuspended in water and dialysed first against 10 mM buffer and then 10 mM buffer containing 20% ammonium sulphate (11.4 g ammonium sulphate/ 100 ml). Following dialysis, protein that is insoluble in 20% ammonium sulphate is removed by centrifugation at 15,000 g for 10 min at 4 °C.

III.2.3 *Phenyl sepharose CL-4B column chromatography*

Phenyl Sepharose CL-4B is equilibrated with 10 mM buffer containing ammonium sulphate to 20% saturation and the gel is de-aerated under vacuum. The size of the column is calculated as 10 ml bed volume per 100 mg protein. Care is taken when pouring the column to avoid introducing air into the gel by agitation. Once built, the column is equilibrated in the same de-aerated buffer and after applying the protein, elution is carried out in a stepwise manner with 10 mM buffer containing 5% saturated ammonium sulphate, 5 mM buffer, and finally water. The fractions which contain high specific activity of TH, eluting with 5 mM buffer, are collected and the protein is concentrated by lyophilization. The dry powder is then resuspended in water and dialysed against 10 mM buffer.

III.2.4 *DEAE cellulose column chromatography*

The native form of TH is further purified by two consecutive DE52 column chromatographies in a manner similar to that described for the purification of TTH. When cultured cell lines are used as tissue source, the first DE52 column (with stepwise elution) can be omitted.

III.2.5 *Sucrose density gradient centrifugation*

The second DE52 eluate is next subjected to sucrose density gradient centrifugation. The linear density gradient between 0.3 and 20% sucrose is built in an SW 40.1 centrifuge tube. Approximately 0.3–0.5 ml of the TH preparation (protein concentration 10 mg/ml) is layered onto the gradient and centrifuged for 16 h. Fractions of 0.3 ml are then collected, starting from the top of the gradient, and 10–50 µl aliquots are assayed for TH activity.

Polyacrylamide gel electrophoresis of the most enzymatically active protein isolated from the sucrose gradient shows a single protein band which possesses TH activity. One or two minor contaminant proteins can be detected in some preparations.

III.2.6   *Heparin-sepharose CL-6B column chromatography*

Recently we have used heparin-linked Sepharose CL-6B column chromatography in order to replace sucrose density gradient centrifugation. This procedure also eliminates one DEAE-cellulose chromatography. The purification is effective and recovery is excellent. TH eluted from the first DEAE-cellulose column is dialysed against 10 mM Tris buffer, pH 7.4 and is subjected to a heparin Sepharose column which was previously equilibrated with 10 mM Tris buffer, pH 7.4. TH is then eluted with 20 mM Tris buffer, pH 8.6. With this purification, TH shows a single protein band on polyacrylamide gel electrophoresis.

IV   PURIFICATION OF DOPAMINE-β-HYDROXYLASE (DBH)

There are two basic procedures for the purification of DBH which are currently used in the authors' laboratory. One is designed for the isolation of soluble DBH from chromaffin granules of bovine adrenal medulla (Smith and Winkler, 1967) and the other is for the purification of total DBH (both soluble and membrane-bound DBH) from adrenal medulla (Goldstein *et al.*, 1965; Friedman and Kaufman, 1965). The former method requires fresh adrenal medullary tissue while the latter may also use frozen tissue. In general, the purification of DBH is the easiest of the catecholamine synthesizing enzymes.

IV.1.   Purification of Soluble DBH

Throughout the purification procedure the buffer referred to is potassium phosphate, pH 6.5, unless otherwise indicated. A schematic view of the procedure appears in Figure 3.

IV.1.1   *Homogenization of tissue*

Fresh bovine adrenal medulla (50 g) is gently homogenized in 150 ml of 5 mM buffer containing 0.3 M sucrose. As bovine adrenal medulla is difficult to homogenize in scintered glass, a Waring blender or Polytron tissue homogenizer can be used at the low-speed setting.

IV.1.2   *Isolation of chromaffin granules*

The pellet is gently suspended in 5 mM buffer containing 0.3 M sucrose using

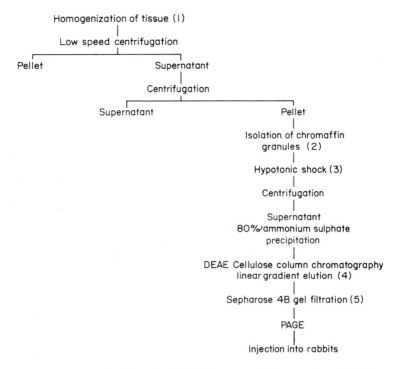

Figure 3   Purification of soluble dopamine-β-hydroxylase (DBH)

a smooth glass homogenizer with loose Teflon pestle. The final volume of the suspension is adjusted to 75 ml. Up to 6 ml of the suspension is carefully layered onto a 15 ml pad of 1.6 M ice-cold sucrose held in a tube for a Beckman 30 rotor. The layered tubes are then subjected to centrifugation at 55,000 g for 2 h. The total supernatant is aspirated and the walls of the centrifuge tubes are wiped clean with tissues. Approximately 1 ml of 1.6 M sucrose is added to each tube and the loosely adhering brownish layer on top of the pellet is resuspended by gentle shaking and is removed so that only the pink pellet remains. The pellet contains the isolated chromaffin granules which can be frozen for storage at this stage.

IV.1.3   *Hypotonic shock of chromaffin granules*

Soluble DBH is then released from the chromaffin granules by rupturing the granule membrane in a hypotonic solution. Each pink pellet is dissolved in 1 ml of water, suspensions are pooled (total volume 12 ml) and centrifuged in a Ti50 rotor at 110,000 g for 1 h. The supernatant is collected on ice. The pellets are resuspended in water to a total volume of 12 ml and they are centrifuged at 110,000 g for 1 h at 4 °C. All supernatants are pooled and protein is precipitated with powdered ammonium sulphate, added to 80% saturation. The 80% ammonium sulphate pellet is collected and can be frozen for storage. The pellet is suspended and dialysed against 5 mM buffer.

IV.1.4   *DEAE cellulose column chromatography*

A DE52 column is built (10 mg protein/20 ml bed volume) and equilibrated with 5 mM buffer. After the protein is loaded, the column is washed with 5 mM buffer. The enzyme is then eluted from the column with a linear concentration gradient between 5 mM and 300 mM buffer (total volume of gradient should be 10 times the column bed volume). Fractions containing the highest specific DBH activity are collected and proteins in these fractions are concentrated by 80% saturation with ammonium sulphate.

IV.1.5   *Sepharose 4B gel filtration*

The concentrated DE52 eluate is resuspended and dialysed against 10 mM buffer for subsequent molecular seiving on Sepharose 4B (30 mg protein/ 450 ml bed volume). Proteins are eluted with 10 mM buffer. With this gel filtration, a majority of proteins which ordinarily remain on the top of a PAGE gel are eliminated from the antigen preparation.

IV.2   Purification of Total Adrenal Medullary DBH

Total DBH from bovine or rat adrenal medulla is purified in a manner identical to that for the soluble form except that, instead of isolating chromaffin granules, DBH is released immediately from tissue by homogenizing in detergent and the enzyme is fractionated in ammonium sulphate before protein separation is performed on the first DE52 column.

IV.2.1   *Homogenization of tissue*

A 50 g portion of fresh or frozen bovine adrenal medulla is homogenized for 30 s in 0.25 M sucrose dissolved in 5 mM buffer, using a Waring blender at low speed. After the homogenate is passed through several layers of gauze, the filtrate is centrifuged at 40,000 g for 60 min. The sediment is collected and re-homogenized in 200 ml of 5 mM buffer containing 0.2% Triton X-100. The mixture is then allowed to stand at room temperature for 20 min with gentle shaking, after which it is centrifuged at 105,000 g for 90 min at 4 °C.

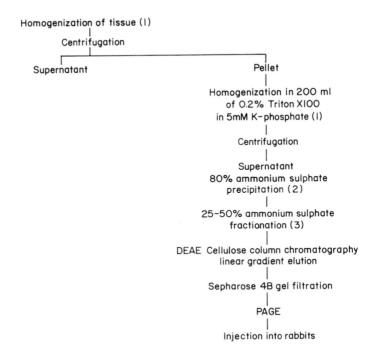

Homogenization of tissue (1)
    |
  Centrifugation
    |
┌───┐
Supernatant   Pellet
                                                 |
                                    Homogenization in 200 ml
                                     of 0.2% Triton X100
                                    in 5mM K-phosphate (1)
                                                 |
                                          Centrifugation
                                                 |
                                           Supernatant
                                      80% ammonium sulphate
                                         precipitation (2)
                                                 |
                                    25–50% ammonium sulphate
                                          fractionation (3)
                                                 |
                               DEAE Cellulose column chromatography
                                       linear gradient elution
                                                 |
                                   Sepharose 4B gel filtration
                                                 |
                                               PAGE
                                                 |
                                      Injection into rabbits

Figure 4   Purification of total medullary dopamine-β-hydroxylase (DBH)

IV.2.2 *Ammonium sulphate precipitation*

The collected supernatant is placed in the cold in a beaker with gentle stirring and powdered amonium sulphate is slowly added to a final saturation of 80%. The mixture is allowed to stand with continuous gentle stirring for 30 min followed by centrifugation at $15,000\,g$ for 15 min at 4 °C. Due to the addition of Triton X-100 in the homogenizing buffer, this ammonium sulphate pellet usually floats in the tube. To collect the protein, liquid is carefully aspirated from the bottom of the centrifuge tube. The pellet collected in this fashion is washed twice with an 80% saturated ammonium sulphate solution, suspended in, and dialyzed against, 5 mM buffer.

IV.2.3 *Ammonium sulphate fractionation*

Powdered ammonium sulphate is slowly added to the preparation with gentle stirring until 25% saturation in ammonium sulphate $(14.4\,g/100\,ml)$ is reached. After continuous stirring for 30 min the mixture is centrifuged at $15,000\,g$ for 15 min. The supernatant is collected and its volume measured.

Powdered ammonium sulphate is added to the supernatant, again with gentle stirring, to a final saturation of 50% (18.8 g/100 ml). After 30 min of continuous stirring in the cold, the precipitate is collected by centrifugation, suspended, and dialysed against 5 mM buffer.

Further purification of total adrenal medullary DBH involves DEAE cellulose column chromatography and Sepharose 4B gel filtration, as described for the isolation of soluble DBH.

V PHENYLETHANOLAMINE *N*-METHYLTRANSFERASE

V.1 Purification of Phenylethanolamine *N*-methyltransferase

Phenylethanolamine *N*-methyltransferase (PNMT) catalyses the production of epinephrine from norepinephrine and has been purified to homogeneity from adrenal medulla of bovine (Connet and Kirshner, 1970; Joh and Goldstein, 1973), rat (Park *et al.*, 1982; Pohorecky and Baliga, 1973), and several other species (Hyo-Sa *et al.*, 1978). However, species cross-reactivity of these antibodies is not complete, so that when immunohistochemical studies are pursued, the antibody raised, for example, against rat PNMT is used for staining rat tissues. The PAGE pattern of the bovine enzyme shows that PNMT exists as several charge isozymes which differ in electrophoretic mobility (Joh and Goldstein, 1973). Specific antibodies raised against bovine adrenal and rat adrenal PNMT have been produced in the authors' laboratory and others. These antibodies have been used for both immunocytochemical localization (Teitelman *et al.*, 1979; Hokfelt *et al.*, 1979) and immunotitration (Burke *et al.*, 1978).

Throughout the purification of PNMT, potassium phosphate buffer, pH 7.4, is used unless otherwise indicated. When bovine adrenal medulla is used, the sediment from the high-speed centrifugation of the tissue homogenate can be used for purification of the trypsin digested form of TH (see Section III.1.) or total DBH (see Sections IV.2). If one wishes to purify only PNMT, the 0.25 M sucrose should be omitted from the homogenizing buffer since isolation of protein from the supernatant after high-speed centrifugation is easier in the absence of sucrose. When purifying PNMT from rat adrenal glands, the supernatant from the high-speed centrifugation of the homogenate can be used for purification of both PNMT and native TH enzymes (see Section III.2). For dual isolation of enzymes, 10 mM buffer is recommended for homogenization.

V.1.1 *Homogenization of tissue*

Fresh or frozen bovine adrenal medulla (50 g) are homogenized in either 5 mM buffer containing 0.25 M sucrose (150 ml) or 10 mM buffer without

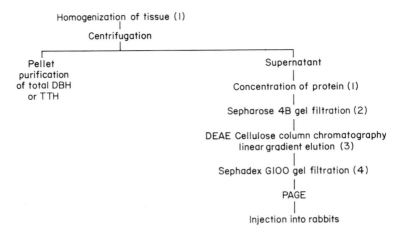

Homogenization of tissue (I)
|
Centrifugation
|
Pellet   Supernatant
purification |
of total DBH   Concentration of protein (I)
or TTH |
                                    Sepharose 4B gel filtration (2)
                                                     |
                                    DEAE Cellulose column chromatography
                                             linear gradient elution (3)
                                                     |
                                    Sephadex GIOO gel filtration (4)
                                                     |
                                                   PAGE
                                                     |
                                          Injection into rabbits

Figure 5   Purification of phenylethanolamine *N*-methyltransferase (PNMT)

sucrose using a Waring blender at low speed for 30 s. For purification of rat PNMT, approximately 500 pairs of rat adrenal glands (15 g) are homogenized in 10 mM buffer (300 ml). The homogenate is centrifuged at 105,000 g for 1 h and supernatant is collected, passed through several layers of gauze, and the filtrate is lyophilized to dryness. When 0.25 M sucrose is used, the protein is concentrated by addition of powdered ammonium sulphate to 80% saturation. The protein which has been either lyophilized or precipitated is dialysed against 10 mM buffer. When possible, lyophilization is preferred rather than ammonium sulphate precipitation as salting-out induces the appearance of more charge isozymes on PAGE gels and it becomes difficult to obtain a clearly defined protein band on PAGE once the enzyme is highly purified.

V.1.2   *Sepharose 4B gel filtration*

A Sepharose 4B column (5 × 85 cm) is equilibrated with 10 mM buffer and the dialysed protein is applied to the column. The protein is eluted with the same buffer. In order to ensure maximal purification on this column, the largest sample volume that can be used is 10 ml of a 20–25 mg protein/ml solution. Fractions containing highest specific activity of PNMT are collected and the protein is concentrated by lyophilization. The native form of TH (molecular weight 200,000 to 250,000) is completely separated from PNMT on this column. The concentrated protein is dialysed against 10 mM buffer.

V.1.3   *DEAE cellulose column chromatography*

A DE52 column (100 mg protein/50 ml bed volume) is equilibrated with

10 mM buffer and the Sepharose 4B eluate is applied to the column. Proteins not adhering to the column are washed out in 10 mM buffer. Protein is eluted by a linear concentration gradient ranging between 10 and 400 mM buffer. The total elution volume is 10 times the bed volume. Highest specific activity of PNMT is eluted in fractions around 180 mM buffer for rat PNMT and around 105 mM for the bovine enzyme. The most active protein is concentrated by lyophilization and the powder is suspended and dialysed against 10 mM buffer.

V.1.4   *Sephadex G100 gel filtration*

A 1 ml fraction (maximum concentration 20 mg protein/ml) of the DE52 eluate is then passed through a Sephadex G100 column (usually 1.6 × 86 cm) and proteins are eluted with the same buffer. PNMT activity is eluted in the fractions corresponding to a molecular weight around 40,000. Again, the most active fractions are concentrated by lyophilization and dialysed against 10 mM buffer.

VI   PRODUCTION OF ANTISERA

VI.1   Electrophoresis of Antigens

In the authors' laboratory, preparative tube gel electrophoresis is frequently used for the final isolation of enzyme antigens for immunization of rabbits. However slab gel electrophoresis can also be used.

Conditions for electrophoretic isolation of TH, TTH, DBH, and PNMT immunogens are as follows:

VI.1.1   *Acrylamide stock solution* (15% solution)

> acrylamide: 28.5 g
> bisacrylamide: 1.5 g
> distilled H$_2$O to a final volume of 200 ml.

After solids are completely dissolved the acrylamide solution is filtered through a sintered glass funnel. This solution can be stored in the cold (do not freeze) up to 6 months in a brown bottle.

VI.1.2   *Electrophoresis buffer and polyacrylamide gels*

For polymerizing gels, 1 litre of a 0.8 M glycine buffer, pH 8.2, is made by dissolving 60 g of glycine in approximately 800 ml of deionized water and pH is adjusted to 8.2 with concentrated Trizma base. Final volume is adjusted to 1 litre. Running buffer (0.4 M glycine, pH 8.2) for carrying out electrophoresis is produced by diluting the 0.8 M buffer 1:1. Ten centimeter tube gels of 7.5%

acrylamide with 5% cross-linking are made according to the method of Ornstein and Davis (1964) except that no stacking gel is used in this procedure.

VI.1.3 *Electrophoresis*

The upper and lower chambers of the electrophoretic apparatus are filled with 0.4 M glycine buffer, pH 8.2, tube gels (7.5%, 0.6 × 10 cm) are placed and 20 µl of a 0.01% solution of bromophenol blue is mixed with sucrose or 10 µl glycerol and layered onto each tube. Electrophoresis without protein (pre-run) is carried out for a minimum of 90 min at a current 3 mA/tube in a cooling water jacket (approximate temperature 10–15 °C). The dye should migrate through the gels as a single band. When the dye has moved out of the gels at the anode side, or at the end of 90 min, the buffer in each chamber is replaced with fresh buffer (0.4 M glycine buffer). Ten microlitres of either concentrated sucrose or glycerol are added to approximately 100 µg of protein (20–40 µl), 5 µl of bromphenol blue are added to each sample and the mixtures are applied to the top of each gel. Electrophoresis is run at 1.5 mA/tube for 5 min, at which time the current is increased to 3 mA/tube. The timing of electrophoresis for optimal separation and approximate position of the active band for each enzyme are shown in Table 1.

Table 1 Electrophoretic isolation of catecholamine synthesizing enzymes

Enzyme	Running time (min)	Approximate location of enzyme (cm)
TTH	90	5.5
Native TH	240	3.5–4.0
Bovine DBH	120	1.4
Bovine PNMT		
isozyme I	90	3.3
isozyme II	90	3.6
Rat PNMT	90	6.5

VI.1.4 *Isolation of enzyme from electrophoretic gels*

At least one gel is stained for protein in either Amido black or Coomassie blue, and one gel is cut into 2 mm slices. Gel slices are put into test tubes containing 50 µl of 0.1 M Na-acetate buffer, pH 5.6 for TTH, TH, or DBH or 0.1 M K phosphate buffer, pH 7.0, for PNMT. Gel slices are then cut into small pieces and are allowed to stand covered in a cold room overnight. Enzyme activities are assayed directly in the tubes with the gel slices.

The location of the stained protein band which contains peak enzymatic activity is identified. The region of the gel containing enzyme activity is cut out of each tube gel and slices are collected.

VI.2 Injection of Antigen into Rabbits

A minimum of 10 gel slices are homogenized in 0.9% NaCl (total volume approximately 1 ml) and an equal volume of complete Freund's adjuvant is added. These are vigorously mixed in a syringe and the emulsion is injected subcutaneously into the back of a rabbit. Approximately 0.2 ml is introduced per injection site for a total of 10 injection sites per animal.

Injection of antigen is repeated in the same manner, using incomplete Freund's adjuvant, every 2 weeks. Three or four immunizations are necessary to produce reasonably high titres of antibody. Presence of antibody in serum is determined immunochemically by immuno-double-diffusion, immunoelectrophoresis, and immunotitration. Antisera are harvested 5–7 days after the last injection.

REFERENCES

Baetge, E. E., Kaplan, B. B., Reis, D. J., and Joh, T. H. (1981). 'Translation of tyrosine hydroxylase from poly(A)mRNA in pheochromocytoma cells (PC12) is enhanced by dexamethasone.' *Proc. Natl. Acad. Sci.*, *USA*, **78**, 1269–1273.

Burke, W. J., Davis, J. W., Joh, T. H., Reis, D. J., Horenstein, S., and Bhagat, B. D. (1978). 'The effect of epinephrine on phenyl ethanolamine *N*-methyltransferase in cultured explants of adrenal medulla.' *Endocrinology*, **103**, 358–367.

Connet, R. J., and Kirshner, N. (1970). 'Purification of phenylethanolamine *N*-methyltransferase from bovine adrenal medulla.' *J. Biol. Chem.*, **245**, 329–334.

Coyle, J. T. (1972). 'Tyrosine hydoxylase in rat brain—cofactor requirements, regional and subcellular distribution.' *Biochem. Pharmacol.*, **21**, 1935–1944.

Friedman, S., and Kaufman, S. (1965). '3,4-Dihydroxyphenylethylamine-β-hydroxylase physical properties, copper content, and role of copper in catalytic activity.' *J. Biol. Chem.*, **240**, 4763–4773.

Goldstein, M., Lauber, E., and McKereghan, M. R. (1965). 'Studies on the purification and characterization of 3,4-dihydroxyphenylethylamine-β-hydroxylase.' *J. Biol. Chem.*, **240**, 2066–2072.

Hokfelt, T., Fuxe, K., Goldstein, M., and Joh, T. H. (1972). 'Immunohistochemical studies on the localization of three catecholamine synthesizing enzymes.' In Takeuchi, T., Ogawa, K., and Fujita, S. (eds), *Histochemistry and Cytochemistry*. Nakanishi Print Co., Kyoto, Japan.

Hokfelt, T., Fuxe, K., Goldstein, M., and Johansson, O. (1979) 'Immunohistochemical evidence for the existence of adrenaline neurons in the rat brain.' *Brain Res.*, **66**, 235–251.

Hyo-Sa, L., Schulz, A. R., and Fuller, R. W. (1978). 'Isolation and purification of rabbit adrenal norepinephrine *N*-methyltransferase isozymes.' *Arch. Biochem. Biophys.*, **185**, 222–227.

Joh, T. H., Kapit, R., and Goldstein, M. (1969). 'A kinetic study of particulate bovine adrenal tyrosine hydroxylase.' *Biochem. Biophys. Acta*, **17**, 378–380.

Joh, T. H., and Goldstein, M. (1973). 'Isolation and characterization of multiple forms of phenylethanolamine *N*-methyltransferase.' *Mol. Pharmacol.*, **9**, 117–129.

Joh, T. H., Park, D. H., and Reis, D. J. (1978). 'Direct phosphorylation of brain tyrosine hydroxylase by cyclic AMP-dependent protein kinases: a mechanism of enzyme activation.' *Proc. Natl. Acad. Sci.*, *USA*, **75**, 4744–4748.

Lowry, O. H., Rosebrough, N. J., Farr, A. L., and Randall, R. J. (1951). 'Protein measurement with the Folin phenol reagent.' *J. Biol. Chem.*, **193**, 265–276.

Ornstein, L., and Davis, B. J. (1964). Disc electrophoresis (parts I and II). *Ann. N.Y. Acad. Sci.*, **121**, 321–427.

Pohorecky, L. A., and Baliga, B. S. (1973). 'Purification and properties of rat adrenal phenylethanolamine *N*-methyltransferase.' *Arch. Biochem. Biophys.*, **156**, 701–711.

Park, D. H., and Goldstein, M. (1976). Purification of tyrosine hydroxylase from pheochromocytoma tumors.' *Life Sci.*, **18**, 55–60.

Park, D. H., Baetge, E. E., Kaplan, B. B., Albert, V. R., Reis, D. J. and Joh, T. H. (1982). 'Different forms of adrenal phenylethanolamine N-methyltransferase: species-specific posttranslational modification.' *J. Neurochem.*, **38**, 410–414.

Petrack, B., Sheppy, F., and Fetzer, V. (1968). 'Studies on tyrosine hydroxylase from bovine adrenal medulla.' *J. Biol. Chem.*, **243**, 743–748.

Pickel, V. M., Joh, T. H., Feild, P. M., Becker, C. G., and Reis, D. J. (1975a). 'Cellular localization of tyrosine hydroxylase by immunohistochemistry.' *J. Histochem. Cytochem.*, **23**, 1–12.

Pickel, V. M., Joh, T. H., and Reis, D. J. (1975b). 'Ultrastructural localization of tyrosine hydroxylase in noradrenergic neurons of brain.' *Proc. Natl. Acad. Sci., USA,* **72**, 659–663.

Pickel, V. M., Joh, T. H., and Reis, D. J. (1975c). 'Immunohistochemical localization of tyrosine hydroxylase in brain by light and electron microscopy.' *Brain Res.*, **85**, 295–300.

Pickel, V. M., Specht, L. A., Sumal, K. K., Joh, T. H., Reis, D. J., and Hervonen, A. (1981). 'Immunocytochemical localization of tyrosine hydroxylase in the human fetus.' *J. Comp. Neurol.*, **194**, 465–474.

Reis, D., and Molinoff, P. B. (1972). 'Brain dopamine-β-hydroxylase: regional distribution and effects of lesions and 6-hydroxydopamine on activity.' *J. Neurochem.*, **19**, 105–204.

Reis, D. J., Joh, T. H., and Ross, R. A. (1975). 'Effects of reserpine on activities and amounts of tyrosine hydroxylase and dopamine-β-hydroxylase in catecholamine neuronal systems in rat brain.' *J. Pharmacol. Exp. Ther.*, **193**, 775–784.

Rothman, T. P., Specht, L. A., Joh, T. H., Teitelman, G., Pickel, V. M., Gershon, M. D., and Reis, D. J. (1981a). 'Catecholamine biosynthetic enzymes are expressed in replicating cells of the peripheral but not central nervous systems.' *Proc. Natl. Acad. Sci., USA*, **77**, 6221–6225.

Shiman, R., Akino, M., and Kaufman, S. (1971). 'Solubilization and partial purification of tyrosine hydroxylase from bovine adrenal medulla.' *J. Biol. Chem.*, **246**, 1330–1340.

Smith, A. D., and Winkler, H. (1967). 'A simple method for the isolation of adrenal chromaffin granules on a large scale.' *Biochem. J.*, **103**, 480–482.

Teitelman, G., Baker, H., Joh, T. H., and Reis, D. J. (1979). 'Appearance of catecholamine synthesizing enzymes during development of rat sympathetic nervous system: possible role of tissue environment.' *Proc. Natl. Acad. Sci., USA*, **76**, 509–573.

Vulliet, P. R., Langar, T. A., and Weiner, N. (1980). 'Tyrosine hydroxylase: a substrate of cyclic AMP-dependent protein kinase.' *Proc. Natl. Acad. Sci., USA*, **77**, 192–196.

Wurtman, R. J., Axelrod, J., Vesell, E. S., and Ross, G. T. (1968). 'Species differences in inducibility of phenylethanolamine *N*-methyltransferase.' *Endocrinology*, **82**, 584–590.

Immunohistochemistry
Edited by A. C. Cuello
© 1983 IBRO

CHAPTER 6

Dopamine β-Hydroxylase (DBH) Immunohistochemistry and Immunocytochemistry

R. A. RUSH

Department of Human Physiology, School of Medicine, The Flinders University of South Australia, Bedford Park, South Australia, 5042

I INTRODUCTION

The first fluorescent micrographs identifying dopamine β-hydroxylase (DBH) within the cells of the adrenal medulla and sympathetic nervous system were published in 1969 (Geffen *et al.*, 1969). The initial success of the localization of this enzyme has helped to stimulate the now almost ubiquitous use of immunohistochemistry for the study of the nervous system. Consequently, it is not surprising that DBH localization continues to provide many research laboratories with a powerful technique even after becoming the ugly sister to the more recently discovered *Cinderella* peptides. I have attempted to provide in this chapter a complete laboratory manual that should allow most laboratories to perform the immunohistochemical and immunocytochemical localization of DBH independently and on a routine basis. Thus I have included sections on DBH purification, antibody production, antibody purification and modification, in addition to the procedures required for localization once the antiserum has been raised. References have been kept to an absolute minimum; complete bibliographies are available from several comprehensive reviews describing all aspects of the current state of knowledge of DBH that have appeared within the last 2 years (Skotland and Ljones, 1979; Weinshilboum, 1979; Winkler and Westhead, 1980; Rush and Geffen, 1980).

Dopamine β-hydroxylase is present within the catecholamine storage vesicles of the adrenal medulla and sympathetic nerves where it catalyses the conversion of dopamine to noradrenaline. This discrete subcellular localization makes DBH an ideal marker for the study of the dynamics of synaptic vesicles within sympathetic neurones.

Neuroanatomical mapping of catecholaminergic pathways was facilitated by the introduction of immunohistochemical localization of tyrosine hydroxylase, DBH, and phenolethanolamine *N*-methyl transferase, that allowed discrimination of dopaminergic, noradrenergic, and adrenergic pathways in a way not possible with the formaldehyde-induced catecholamine fluorescence procedures (see Hokfelt *et al.*, 1973; Hartman, 1973; Swanson and Hartman, 1975). More recently, the introduction of techniques utilizing *in vivo* antibody administration has added further impetus to several research areas including retrograde transport mechanisms, retrograde neuroanatomical tracing, synaptic vesicle utilization at the nerve terminal, and sympathetic neuropathy (Jacobowitz *et al.*, 1975; Costa *et al.*, 1976, 1979; Rush and Geffen, 1980).

An interesting and relatively new area of research where DBH immunohistochemistry should prove valuable is in developmental studies of the autonomic nervous system. Recent reports have suggested that some autonomic nerves have the capacity to produce both acetylcholine and noradrenaline synthetic enzymes *in vitro* (Patterson, 1978), whilst experiments *in vivo* have identified transient catecholamine-containing neuroblasts in young embryos (Kessler *et al.*, 1979). Furthermore, DBH immunohistochemistry has been used to visualize the enzyme in cholinergic parasympathetic nerves to the submandibular gland of the rat, although these cells apparently lack noradrenaline (Grzanna and Coyle, 1978). This is the only reported exception of the cellular localization of DBH outside noradrenaline synthesizing cells. It will be of interest to examine the development of this and other autonomic ganglia with DBH immunohistochemistry, as well as with antisera to tyrosine hydroxylase, choline acetylase, and various peptides.

It is clear that antibodies to DBH will continue to be useful in the future, as much is still to be learned in all of these important areas. The modern neuroscientist, having armed himself or herself with bottles of antisera, needs only to decide which problem to approach first!

II ASSAY OF DBH

II.1 Enzymatic Assay

Estimation of enzyme activity has been achieved with a variety of techniques including spectrophotometric, radioisotopic, and coupled enzymatic procedures (Weinshilboum and Axelrod, 1971; Nagatsu and Udenfriend, 1972; Nagatsu *et al.*, 1973; Joh *et al.*, 1974). At present, the most commonly used procedures are the coupled enzymatic assay of Weinshilboum and Axelrod (1971) that allows the most sensitive estimation of DBH but is also the most exacting procedure, and the spectrophotometric assay of Nagatsu and Udenfriend (1972) that is the simplest of all procedures. This simple spectrophotometric assay is ideal for enzyme purification analysis and for this reason the procedure is detailed below. Increased sensitivity can be obtained if required with modifications to the procedure as described by Kato *et al.* (1974, 1978).

Up to 400 μl of tissue homogenate or serum can be accommodated in the assay. The enzyme is added to 600 μl of reagent mix prepared as follows: 1 M sodium acetate buffer, pH 6.0 (200 μl), 0.2 M disodium fumarate (50 μl), 0.2 M ascorbate (50 μl), 1 mg/ml catalase (50 μl), 0.4 M tyramine hydrochloride (50 μl), 0.02 M pargyline hydrochloride (50 μl), and 0.2 M N-ethylmaleimide (50 μl). Incubation for 30 min at 37 °C is followed by 3 M trichloroacetic acid (200 μl), centrifugation, and column chromatography. Columns prepared from 0.2 ml of Dowex-50 (H^+ form, 200–400 mesh, Biorad) are washed successively with 2 ml each of water, 5 M HCl, water, 5 M HCl, water, water, before being loaded with the supernatant from the incubation mix. The octopamine formed in the reaction is eluted from the column with 1 ml of 4 M ammonium hydroxide and converted to *p*-hydroxybenzaldehyde with 2% sodium periodate (100 μl). After quenching of the excess periodate with 10% sodium metabisulphite (100 μl), the product is quantitated in a spectrophotometer at a wavelength of 330 nm.

II.2 Immunoassay

Measurement of DBH protein instead of, or in addition to, the estimation of DBH enzymatic activity has been performed in several laboratories with the aid of specific antisera. These studies were undertaken either to increase the sensitivity of detection or to assess whether the activity of the enzyme was a true indication of the amount of enzyme present. Results have generally confirmed that for serum and tissue extracts the level of enzyme activity correlates with the amount of enzyme protein present. However, for enzyme purification this has been shown not to be valid as many of the isolation procedures used inactivate some of the enzyme. For this reason the term homospecific activity was introduced (Rush *et al.*, 1975a) and defines the ratio of enzymatic activity to homologous enzyme protein.

In addition to its use in enzyme purification, the concept of homospecific activity has enabled differences in the activity of the membrane bound and soluble forms of DBH to be detected (Kirshner *et al.*, 1975; Rush *et al.*, 1975a), the demonstration of the stability of the enzyme activity following release into the circulation (Kirshner *et al.*, 1975), estimation of the number of DBH molecules present in synaptic vesicles (Klein *et al.*, 1977), and the detection of dissimilarities in enzyme above and below nerve ligations (Nagatsu and Kondo, 1975; Nagatsu *et al.*, 1976). However, the use of quantitative immunoassay is not essential for the development of DBH immunohisto-chemistry, and consequently the methodology is not described here.

III PURIFICATION OF SOLUBLE BOVINE ADRENAL DBH

Immunohistochemistry of DBH, like any other compound, has as absolute requirement for monospecific antisera. The simplest way of satisfying this requirement is to first produce pure antigen and fortunately this is not difficult for DBH. The ease of isolation is possible largely because of two factors. Firstly, a high concentration of the enzyme is packaged within chromaffin vesicles of the adrenal medulla (Smith and Winkler, 1967) and secondly, DBH is the only soluble protein of the vesicle that will interact with Concanavalin A (Rush *et al.*, 1974). The isolation procedure outlined below and in Figure 1 takes advantage of these facts, allowing the production of 3–10 mg of pure DBH from 50–60 bovine adrenal glands in a single day. Other procedures have been developed to increase the total production to 100 mg from a correspondingly longer time and greater numbers of adrenal medullae (Ljönes *et al.*, 1976). However, 10 mg of the enzyme will provide antigen for the production of large quantities of antiserum.

Protocol

Fresh (not frozen) adrenal glands must be used and all procedures are carried out on ice or at 2 °C.

(1) Fifty to sixty bovine adrenal glands are obtained fresh from the slaughterhouse and brought back to the laboratory on ice.
(2) The glands are defatted and the medullae removed from the cortex by gross dissection with scissors.

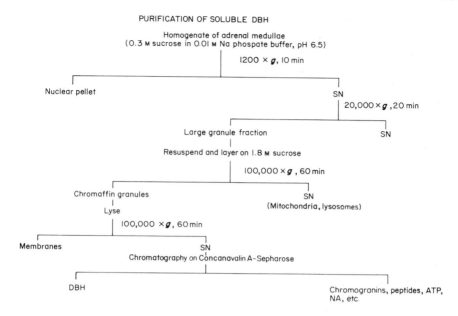

Figure 1　Purification of soluble DBH

(3) After finely chopping with scissors the medullae are homogenized in 5–10 volumes of 0.3 M sucrose in 0.01 M sodium phosphate buffer, pH 6.5. Homogenization can be either in a loosely fitting (clearance, 0.1 mm) Potter–Elvehjem glass-Teflon homogenizer, using four or five complete strokes. Alternatively, a Waring blender operated for 30 s at top speed or a stainless-steel shafted homogenizer (Ultra-turrax) also operated at top speed for 30 s may be used.

(4) Centrifuge at low speed 1200 *g* for 10 min, to remove unbroken cells, cell nuclei, and debris.

(5) Centrifuge the low-speed supernatant at 20,000 *g* for 20 min.

(6) The supernatant is decanted carefully and the sediment resuspended in ice-cold 0.3 M sucrose in 0.01 M sodium phosphate buffer, pH 6.5. Care must be taken to exclude the erythrocytes that are present in small numbers at the bottom of the sediment. The volume of buffer required is such that 1 ml of the resuspended sediment ('large granule fraction') corresponds to 1–2 g of original medulla. A homogeneous suspension can be achieved by gentle hand homogenization using a loosely fitting Teflon–glass homogenizer.

(7) Ten millilitres of the resuspended large granule fraction is layered onto 33 ml of 1.8 M sucrose buffered with 0.01 M sodium phosphate, pH 6.5

in high-speed centrifuge tubes. The addition of catalase to the 1.8 M sucrose (0.1 mg/ml) prevents loss of DBH enzymatic activity during the high-speed centrifugation. Centrifugation at 100,000 *g* for 60 min at 4 °C results in the sedimentation of intact chromaffin vesicles at the bottom of the tube with lysosomes and mitochondria in layers above.

(8) The total supernatant is discarded and the pink chromaffin granules left at the bottom of the tube lysed by suspension in ten volumes of ice-cold 0.005 M sodium phosphate buffer, pH 6.5.

(9) The vesicles are further disrupted by homogenization and recentrifuged at 100,000 *g* for 30 min at 4 °C.

(10) The supernatant is removed from the membranes and diluted with an equal volume of 100 mM phosphate buffer, pH 6.5 containing 0.4 M sodium chloride. This lysate is then applied to a 4.0 × 0.7 cm column of Concanavalin A–Sepharose 4B (Pharmacia, Australia) previously equilibrated with 50 mM phosphate buffer, pH 6.5 containing 0.2 M sodium chloride. The flow rate is kept at approximately 0.3 ml/min.

(11) After the lysate has been applied, the column is extensively washed with buffer until the absorbance of the effluent at 280 nm returns to the blank value.

(12) DBH is eluted with the same buffer but with the addition of 10% α-methyl D-mannoside. Elution at 0.1 ml/min allows the collection of the enzyme in approximately 20 ml.

(13) The purified DBH is concentrated and dialysed by negative pressure dialysis against 50 mM phosphate buffer, pH 6.5 containing 0.02% sodium azide. Storage is best in liquid nitrogen at a protein concentration of about 1 mg/ml.

DBH purified to homogeneity by this method has been shown to incur no loss of enzymatic activity and has a specific activity of about 20 μmoles of tyramine converted per minute per mg of protein (Rush *et al.*, 1974).

IV   PREPARATION OF DBH FROM OTHER SOURCES

Although the production of monospecific antisera to DBH has most commonly involved the use of the soluble form of the bovine adrenal enzyme several other enzyme preparations have also been used. Generally these alternate routes for antiserum production have been initiated to overcome the problem of cross-reactivity differences seen when the use of the antiserum is required in a species other than that from which the antigen was originally isolated (see Section X). Thus, some workers have found that antiserum produced to rat adrenal DBH has advantages over anti-bovine DBH for studies in the rat (Grzanna and Coyle, 1976; Grzanna *et al.*, 1977, 1978; Olschowka *et al.*, 1981). Disadvantages are generally greater for immunochemical studies such as radioimmunoassay, than for immunohistochemical studies where adequate staining can usually be achieved in selected species without the need for the difficult purification from rat adrenal glands. Isolation and purification of the enzyme has so far been achieved from the adrenal glands of sheep (Rush and Geffen, 1972), humans (Rush *et al.*, 1975c) and rats (Grzanna and Coyle, 1976, Helle *et al.*, 1979). Phaeochromocytoma, a tumour of the adrenal gland (Stone *et al.*, 1974; Markey *et al.*, 1980) and human serum (Miras-Portugal *et al.*, 1976; Lovenberg *et al.*, 1975; Ikeno *et al.*, 1977; Frigon and Stone, 1978) have also provided useful alternate sources for the isolation.

The soluble form of DBH from the bovine adrenal medulla represents only 50% of the total enzyme present. The remaining, membrane-bound enzyme can also be purified (Huber *et al.*, 1979) and used as antigen. Recently we have prepared antiserum to this form of the enzymes and found that the titre produced in a single rabbit is considerably higher than that seen as a result of immunization with the soluble enzyme. Most of the DBH in sympathetic nerves appears to be of the membrane form (see Winkler and Westhead, 1980).

A further source of DBH that may prove useful in the future is mouse or rat phaeochromocytoma tissues either grown as tumours in host animals or in tissue culture as clonal cell lines such as the PC 12 cells (Greene and Tischler, 1976). Sufficient material can be grown to enable a reasonable amount of the enzyme to be purified (Markey *et al.*, 1980).

V PRODUCTION OF ANTISERA

V.1 In Rabbits

The production of antiserum to DBH is a relatively simple task as the high molecular weight (approx. 290,000 daltons) and the presence of carbohydrate (approx. 4% by weight) make the enzyme an ideal antigen. Monospecific antisera to DBH have been produced in a number of laboratories around the world and each laboratory has generally utilized a different injection schedule. In our laboratory the following procedure has proved reliable for more than 20 animals used over the last 12 years. Every animal subjected to this regimen has produced an antiserum with sufficient titre for immunohisto-chemistry as well as for other immunochemical techniques. Several animals have provided a continual supply of antiserum for more than 3 years without loss of specificity of useful antibody titre.

Protocol
(1) DBH antigen, prepared as outlined in Section IV, is thawed, diluted to 100 μg/ml and mixed with an equal volume of Freund's complete

adjuvant (CSL, Australia). Mixing is achieved by continual transfer between two 5 ml glass syringes connected by a 40 mm long, 19-gauge needle. The needle is fitted with a luer lock at each end. Mixing is continued until a homogeneous emulsion is produced; a suitable test for complete emulsification is for a drop of the mixture to be added to the surface of a saline solution where it will not disperse if emulsification is complete.

(2) Two millilitres (i.e. 100 μg of DBH) of the emulsion is injected into several sites on the back of a young (3–6-month) rabbit of either sex. Topical application of antibiotic will control any abscess that may result. The injection of this antigen into footpads should be avoided as it is not required for the production of high-titre antisera and causes the animals unnecessary discomfort.

(3) Two further 100 μg doses are given in a similar manner 14 and 28 days after the initial injections. However, Freund's complete adjuvant is replaced by incomplete adjuvant.

(4) Bleeding is begun on the 10th day following the third injection, at which time 50 ml of blood can be taken, usually from the marginal ear vein. Routinely, a booster dose of 100 μg of antigen is given in Freund's incomplete adjuvant every 6 weeks and the animals bled (50 ml) after a further 10–14 days.

(5) The blood is allowed to clot for 1 h at room temperature and is then stored at 4 °C overnight to aid contraction of the clot. Serum can be decanted, or occasionally centrifuged away from the clot and is stored in aliquots at −70 °C. Lyophilization or liquid nitrogen storage has also proved to be satisfactory.

(6) The presence of antibodies to DBH in the sera samples can be most easily identified by gel diffusion analysis. Dilution of the antiserum around a 1 mg/ml antigen sample will result in precipitin lines forming after 24 h at room temperature. Reactions at a dilution of 1 in 8 of the serum indicate a titre sufficiently high to allow immunohistochemical staining.

V.2 In Other Species

Antisera useful for immunohistochemistry have also been produced in several other species. In goats, it has been found necessary to increase the antigen dose to between 1 and 3 mg. However, several hundred ml of antiserum can be obtained at each bleed; more than all the serum that has ever been applied to all sections ever stained for DBH!

Guinea-pigs and mice have been successfully immunized with 3 × 50 μg of DBH although even smaller quantities may be possible for the mouse. Mice have been used for the production of monoclonal antibodies in our laboratory but no comparative data are yet available (for immunization of small rodents see Chapter 9, Section III.1).

VI PURIFICATION OF ANTIBODY

Routine immunohistochemistry of DBH is normally performed with whole serum diluted to appropriate levels. However, specialized procedures requiring, for example F(ab)$'_2$ (bivalent antigen binding) fragments or horseradish peroxidase coupled antibodies may need or even demand a purified IgG fraction or purified DBH-specific antibody. Details of these purification procedures are described below.

VI.1 Preparation of IgG

Many techniques are available; however, in our laboratory it has been found that the use of Protein A–Sepharose (Pharmacia) affinity chromatography provides a simple and reliable method. Five millilitres of antiserum are dialysed overnight at 4 °C against 100 ml 0.05 M sodium phosphate buffer pH 7.4 and loaded at a rate of 0.5 ml/min onto a 6.5 × 1.2 cm column of Protein A–Sepharose pre-equilibrated with the same buffer. The column is then washed extensively with the buffer until the optical density at 280 nm of the eluant has dropped to the blank value. Bound IgG molecules are eluted with 1 M acetic acid and collected as 1.0 ml fractions into 0.5 ml of 2.0 M Tris-glycine buffer, pH 8.6 to prevent denaturing of the IgG molecules in the 1 M acetic acid. Protein containing fractions are pooled and dialysed against phosphate buffered saline, pH 7.4 (PBS).

VI.2 Preparation of DBH-specific Antibody

Although this method requires considerable amounts of purified DBH, the resulting antibody has proved extremely valuable for retrograde tracing studies (Lees *et al.*, 1981a) and for localization of DBH at the electron microscope level (see Section IX).

Five milligrams of pure DBH is coupled to 1 g of CH–Sepharose (Pharmacia) using the standard procedure suggested by the manufacturer. Briefly, 1 g of CH–Sepharose is swollen in 200 ml of 0.001 M ice-cold HCl. DBH previously dialysed against 0.005 M sodium phosphate buffer pH 7.4 is added to 0.1 M sodium bicarbonate, pH 8.0 at a concentration of at least 1 mg/ml and coupling is achieved by tumble-mixing the gel (with excess HCl solution removed) and the DBH solution together for 4 h at 4 °C. Excess DBH is removed by washing the gel successively with coupling buffer, 0.05 M Tris buffer pH 8.0 containing 0.5 M NaCl and 0.05 formate buffer, pH 4.0 containing 0.5 M NaCl.

Affinity chromatographic purification of the antibody is carried out on the DBH–Sepharose column at 4 °C. After equilibration of the column in PBS, pH 7.4, 2 ml of antiserum diluted equally with PBS is run slowly through the column (0.5 ml/min). Washing continues until the optical density 280 nm of the eluant has reached background level and the purified DBH-antibody molecules are eluted in 1 M acetic acid, collected as for normal IgG molecules described previously and immediately dialysed against PBS. The column may be stored for reuse if the acetic acid is rapidly replaced by PBS containing 0.1% sodium azide.

VII   PRODUCTION OF F(ab)$'_2$ FRAGMENTS

Fragments of antibody molecules have been used for localization studies by many workers as it was reasoned that a reduction in size of the molecules, without loss of antigen binding ability, would aid the penetration of the antibody across cell membranes. Although fragments have proved effective for other studies no clear advantage for DBH localization has been reported, with the single exception of the *in vivo* localization in the guinea-pig that is required to prevent degeneration of the noradrenergic nerve terminals (see Rush and Geffen, 1980). However, a simple method for the production of F(ab)$'_2$ fragments of the antibody molecules is outlined below for use in guinea-pig, and to pre-empt its possible use in immunocytochemical studies.

Protocol
Purified IgG or specific anti-DBH molecules prepared according to the method outlined in the previous section are dialysed at 4 °C overnight against 0.01 M sodium acetate buffer, pH 4.5 containing 0.05 M sodium chloride. The dialysed antibody molecules are then treated with pepsin (1% w/w) at 37 °C for 20 h followed by centrifugation (26,000 *g*, 30 min) and the supernatant transferred to a second tube containing sufficient 1 M sodium hydroxide to raise the pH to 8.0. Non-digested IgG molecules and Fc fragments are removed by chromatography on Protein A–Sepharose; the F(ab)$'_2$ fragments and other small peptides produced by the hydrolysis are eluted in the void volume and concentrated by ultrafiltration on a YM 10 filter (Amicon). After dialysis against 0.01 M sodium phosphate buffer pH 7.4, the preparation is stored frozen until required. The F(ab)$'_2$ fragments can be further purified on Sephadex G-100 to remove unwanted peptides and pepsin molecules, although in practice this has been found not to be necessary.

VIII   IMMUNOHISTOCHEMISTRY

VIII.1   *In vitro* Localization

Light microscopical analysis of DBH in all tissues can be performed after staining with either fluorescent-labelled second antibody (see Chapter 2) or the PAP (see Chapter 4) method of Sternberger (1974). In deciding which procedures to use, it should be noted that the sensitivities of both procedures are sufficiently similar to make other criteria more important. One possible exception has been noted by Jones and Hartman (1978) who have suggested that for examination of fine varicose terminals of the CNS, the fluorescent method allows better resolution, presumed to be due to diffusion barriers to the bulky PAP complex. However, with the use of homologous antisera (Grzanna *et al.*, 1978) this distinction between the two methods appears not to exist. If long-term storage of the stained tissue is required, then the PAP method is clearly indicated, whereas for rapid screening of many samples, use of the fluorescent antisera facilitates the programme. Both procedures are described below.

VIII.1.1 *Tissue preparation*

For tissues other than those suitable for stretch preparations (see below) the best method of fixation has been found to be formaldehyde perfusion (for details of procedure see Chapter 11, Section III). Cryostat sections of 5–10 μm are cut and allowed to air-dry on Chrom-alum coated glass microscope slides for a minimum of 30 min. Good results have also been achieved following fixation by immersion of tissue blocks in ice-cold 4% formaldehyde buffered in 0.1 M sodium phosphate, pH 7.4. The tissue is cut into small pieces no thicker than 2–3 mm and fixed overnight, after which the tissue is treated as for the perfused material.

Many tissues can be stretched unfixed onto glass slides and stained directly without further treatment. The advantages of stretch preparations include simplification (because the fixation procedures are not required) and better visualization of the terminal plexus in the thicker tissue. Details of the stretching process and a discussion of the advantages and disadvantages are outlined in Chapter 14. After drying of the stretched tissue, staining can proceed as outlined above.

Neurones grown in culture may also be stained for DBH after fixation in 4% formaldehyde buffered with 0.1 M sodium phosphate, pH 7.4. The concentration of Triton X-100 must be reduced, however, as high levels of the detergent lift the cells of the substratum. The antibody can be diluted in 0.1% Triton X-100 and the detergent in the washing buffer reduced to 0.3%.

VIII.1.2 *Fluorescent antibody staining* (see also Chapter 8)

After two 5-min washes in phosphate buffered saline the tissue sections are incubated in antiserum to DBH, diluted in PBS containing 0.3% Triton X-100. Routinely, the incubation is allowed to continue overnight as this allows the use of higher dilutions of the serum. The next morning the slides

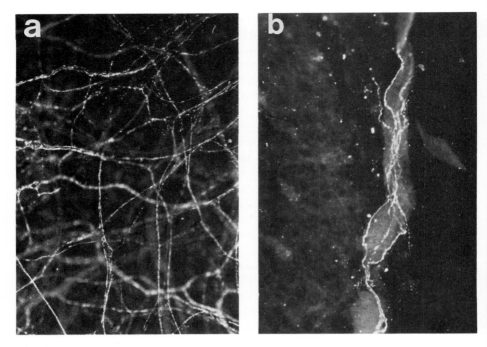

Figure 2 (a) Dopamine β-hydroxylase localization of antibodies bound by nerve terminals in the guinea-pig iris following systemic administration of antiserum 24 h earlier. *In vitro* localization of DBH in (b) cerebral blood vessel

are washed with three changes (3 × 5 min) of PBS containing 2% Triton X-100, followed by a 60-min incubation of appropriately diluted, fluorescently labelled anti-rabbit globulin (see Figure 2).

VIII.1.3 *Peroxidase–antiperoxidase staining*

Following overnight incubation in anti-DBH as described above, the sections are washed (3 × 5 min, PBS + 2% Triton X-100), and incubated with developing antibodies as for the PAP procedure (see Chapter 4, Section IV, and Chapter 11, Section III).

VIII.1.4 *Controls*

Specificity problems appear to be rare with DBH antisera, primarily because the extensive studies on DBH function over the past two decades have generated purification procedures that allow the isolation of DBH in a highly purified form with few contaminants. Thus, only the simplest controls seem necessary. Two control procedures are routinely used: firstly, substitution of the anti-DBH incubation with an equally diluted pre-immune serum; and secondly, incubation with anti-DBH that has been previously reacted with 10–50 μg of purified DBH (per ml of diluted anti-DBH). Although other interpretations are possible, absence of fluorescence in control sections is taken as specificity of the anti-DBH reaction (see Chapter 1).

VIII.2 *In vivo* Localization

Jacobowitz and his co-workers (1975) reported that following the systemic administration of DBH antiserum to rats, antibody molecules could be localized by immunohistochemistry within the terminals of sympathetic nerves. This specific uptake of the antibody has been confirmed in the guinea-pig and extended to demonstrate a complement-mediated lysis of nerve terminals (Costa *et al.*, 1976; Rush *et al.*, 1976). The administration of antibodies *in vivo* leads to a selective binding of only those membrane-bound DBH molecules present in the membrane of synaptic vesicles undergoing exocytosis, as exposure of DBH within the vesicle membrane to the outside of the cell is thought to occur only during the release process. Advantage has been taken of this phenomenon to study, at the electron microscope level, the involvement and subsequent fate of synaptic vesicles in the release of transmitter (see below).

A fortunate consequence of these *in vivo* studies has been the demonstration of a retrograde transport mechanism for the return of synaptic vesicle membranes from nerve terminals to the cell soma (Ziegler *et al.*, 1976). In addition to providing information concerning the ultimate fate of synaptic vesicles, the retrograde transport of DBH antibodies allows neuroanatomical mapping of catecholaminergic pathways by a method that combines the sensitivity of the popular HRP retrograde transport technique with an absolute specificity for DBH containing fibres (Fillenz *et al.*, 1976; Lees *et al.*, 1981a,b). Availability of antisera against other neuronal components will undoubtedly extend the technique to other chemically specified neurons. Several other molecules known to be transported retrogradely, such as tetanus toxin and certain lectins, are also available for this purpose. Localization of the transported molecules is usually achieved with immunohistochemical techniques, but can also be visualized by autoradiography of radioactively labelled material, enzymatic reaction if the molecule has first been coupled to HRP, or quantitated by determination of the accumulation of radioactively tagged molecules.

VIII.3 Protocol for Anti-DBH Administration *in vivo*

Subcutaneous, intraperitoneal, and intravenous administration of DBH antiserum have all proved equally effective for the localization of DBH within terminals of noradrenergic neurones. Usually 250 μl of whole antiserum given to an adult rat or guinea-pig achieves maximal labelling. Intra-ocular injection into the anterior chamber of the eye requires only 10–50 μl of serum. Uptake of antibody molecules into nerve terminals is slow, requiring approximately 24 h for maximum binding to occur. However, the antibody level remains high for at least 2 more days before slowly declining during the following weeks. In the guinea-pig, $F(ab)'_2$ fragments of the antiserum must be used to prevent degeneration of nerve terminals in most tissues (Lewis *et al.*, 1977; Furness *et al.*, 1977).

IX   IMMUNOCYTOCHEMISTRY

At the time this chapter was written only seven publications (for references see Rush and Geffen, 1980) have reported the successful identification of antigen at the electron microscope level since the first antibodies were produced in 1967 (Gibb *et al.*, 1967). This paucity of data is clearly due to technical difficulties encountered by all workers in gaining adequate penetration of the antibodies through two membranes (plasma and synaptic vesicle) to combine with DBH within the synaptic vesicle, whilst preserving the ultrastructural features of the nerve. Support for this suggestion comes from immunocytochemical studies of tyrosine hydroxylase that has proved to be more straightforward (Pickel *et al.*, 1976). This enzyme is found only in the cytoplasm of catecholaminergic neurons, and consequently disruption of the synaptic vesicle membrane is unnecessary.

Partial resolution of this (frustrating) difficulty has been achieved by *in vivo* administration of anti-DBH covalently linked with HRP. This technique allows good ultrastructural identification of a selected population of DBH molecules: those molecules located within the membrane of synaptic vesicles undergoing exocytosis and therefore exposed to antibody molecules in the extracellular fluid (Rush *et al.*, 1979). The localization of only a selected population of DBH molecules may be a disadvantage for some studies but is an obvious advantage for functional analysis. Thus it has been possible to identify synaptic vesicles that have previously participated in the release process and to trace their subsequent transport to the cell soma (see Rush and Geffen, 1980).

These studies have used anti-DBH coupled to HRP by the method of Nakane and Kawaoi (1974) without modification, so the procedure is not reproduced here (for coupling of HRP to antibodies see Chapter 3).

Procedure for localization with anti-DBH-HRP

Adult guinea-pigs are injected subcutaneously with 9 mg/kg of the anti-DBH-HRP complex in PBS. Twenty-four hours later the animals are anaesthetized, perfused briefly with heparinized saline (5 IU/ml), followed for 8 min with 4% formaldehyde plus 1% glutaraldehyde in 0.1 M cacodylate buffer, pH 7.4 containing 0.1 M sucrose and then flushed for a further 8 min with cacodylate buffer. Tissues to be examined are removed, cut into small blocks, rinsed in buffer, then incubated for 20 min at room temperature in a freshly prepared solution of 5 mg diaminobenzidine in 10 ml of cacodylate buffer, containing 0.02% hydrogen peroxide. After extensive washing in 0.1 M cacodylate buffer, tissue blocks are post-fixed in cacodylate-buffered 2% osmium tetroxide, rinsed in distilled water, dehydrated with ethanol and acetone, and embedded in TAAB embedding resin. Ultrathin sections are stained with lead citrate. Control animals are injected with non-immune IgG-HRP (9 mg/kg) and treated as for the anti-DBH-HRP injected animals (see Figure 3).

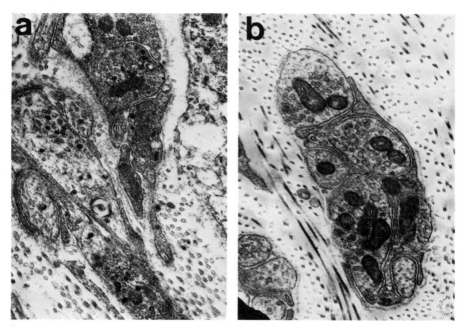

Figure 3 (a) Immunocytochemical localization of DBH–HRP complex within nerve terminals of the guinea-pig iris. The DBH–HRP complex was administered systemically 24 h earlier. (b) Control section taken from animal treated similarly but injected with HRP–IgG (normal serum). See text for more details

X CROSS-REACTIVITY

Most studies using DBH as an antigen have begun with the isolation of the enzyme from the bovine adrenal medulla. Unfortunately, antisera raised

Table 1 Summary of maximum antiserum dilution possible for positive staining of adrenal medulla and DBH enzyme activity levels using one particular anti-bovine DBH antiserum. See text for more details

	Maximum dilution for positive stain	DBH activity (μmole/h/g ww)
Sheep	1:4000	64
Pig	1:2000	28
Guinea-pig	1:64,000	19
Rat	1:8000	11
Mouse	1:32,000	46
Cow	1:256,000	21
Dog	1:2000	17

against the bovine enzyme show ability to react with DBH from other species. This is illustrated in Table 1, which summarizes findings from our laboratory. Using a single batch of antiserum it was possible to stain the adrenal medullary cells of all species tested. However, the level to which serum could be diluted and still produce a positive reaction was vastly different. Since no clear correlation could be discerned between the dilution level and evolutionary distance, estimation of the DBH enzymatic activity was also performed. Although some trends were discerned (for example the correlation between rat and mouse activity and dilution levels) no obvious pattern could be identified. This might have been predicted because several other variables are certainly important, such as the concentration of DBH within each cell (high levels of DBH activity may be due to more DBH per cell, or more cells containing DBH). In the rat adrenal, for example, we have consistently observed groups of cells that are less intensely stained than the majority of medullary cells.

To overcome the lack of reactivity of anti-bovine DBH with DBH of other species, we have repeatedly immunized a few rabbits hoping to increase the number of antigenic determinants recognized, thereby increasing the reactivity with DBH from other species. This has apparently been achieved, as sera taken from animals receiving many doses of the antigen have generally proved more useful for immunohistochemical staining of rat and mouse tissue than the sera of newly immunized animals having similar antibody titre.

Despite these shortcomings, the results provide a guide for the use of anti-bovine DBH serum in other species. We have consistently found that the guinea-pig is a better animal for immunohistochemical studies than either rat or mouse. Kato *et al.* (1978) have reported that this species has higher levels of enzyme activity than the rat in all tissues, and the better immunohistochemistry may therefore be the result of better cross-reactivity or greater antigen levels, or both. One final point to make is that, fortunately, the loss of sensitivity in cross-species analysis does not appear to be associated with a loss of specificity as the staining is always restricted to known sites of noradrenaline synthesis (see also Chapter 7, Section VII.1 for species-specificity of anti-GAD antibodies).

XI SUMMARY

Twelve years of immunohistochemical visualization of DBH has produced much valuable information concerning all aspects of the role of this important molecule in neuronal function. Knowledge of neuronal differentiation, innervation of target tissues, maturation, response to available central drive and to hormonal and trophic stimuli, intracellular transport, and transmitter release has been gained, supplementing and confirming details obtained by other techniques. However, much is still to be learned from the technique not only of fundamental neuronal mechanisms but also clinically by analysis of complex neurological disorders such as autonomic dysautonomia (Black and Petito, 1976) and Alzheimer's disease (Cross *et al.*, 1981) or the autonomic neuropathy found in diabetic patients.

The stated aim of this review was to provide a manual that would enable neuroscience laboratories to pursue the localization of DBH independently. If this has been achieved I shall enjoy learning of the new findings that will certainly be made.

ACKNOWLEDGEMENTS

Much of this work has been supported by the National Heart Foundation of Australia and the National Health and Medical Research Foundation. I also wish to acknowledge the contribution of Professor Laurie Geffen, with whom I have collaborated over many years.

REFERENCES

Black, I. B. and Petito, C. K. (1976). 'Catecholamine enzymes in the degenerative neurological disease idiopathic orthostatic hypotension.' *Science*, **192**, 910–912.

Costa, M., Geffen, L. B., Rush, R. A., Bridges, D., Blessing, W. W., and Heath, J. W. (1979). 'Immune lesions of central noradrenergic neurons produced by antibodies to DBH.' *Brain Res.*, **173**, 65–78.

Costa, M., Rush, R. A., Furness, J. B., and Geffen, L. B. (1976). 'Histochemical evidence for degeneration of peripheral noradrenergic axons following intravenous injection of antibodies to dopamine β-hydroxylase.' *Neurosci. Lett.*, **3**, 201–207.

Cross, A. J., Crow, T. J., Perry, E. K., Perry, R. H., Blessed, G., and Tomlinson, B. E. (1981). 'Reduced dopamine β-hydroxylase activity in Alzheimer's disease. *Br. Med. J.*, **282**, 93–94.

Fillenz, M., Gagnon, C., Stoeckel, K., and Thoenen, H. (1976). 'Selective uptake and retrograde axonal transport of dopamine β-hydroxylase antibodies in peripheral adrenergic neurons.' *Brain Res.*, **114**, 293–303.

Frigon, R. P. and Stone, R. A. (1978). 'Human plasma dopamine β-hydroxylase: purification and properties.' *J. Biol. Chem.*, **253**, 6780–6786.

Furness, J. B., Lewis, S. Y., Rush, R., Costa, M., and Geffen, L. B. (1977). 'Involvement of complement in degeneration of sympathetic nerves after administration of DBH antibodies.' *Brain Res.*, **136**, 67–75.

Geffen, L. B., Livett, B. G., and Rush, R. A. (1969). 'Immunological localization of chromogranins in sheep sympathetic neurons and their release by nerve impulses'. *J. Physiol.*, **204**, 598–605.

Gibb, J. W., Spector, S., and Udenfriend, S. (1967). 'Production of antibodies to dopamine β-hydroxylase of bovine adrenal medulla.' *Mol. Pharmacol.*, **3**, 473–478.

Greene, L. A. and Tischler, A. S. (1976). 'Establishment of a noradrenergic clonal line of rat adrenal phaeochiomocyloma cells which respond to nerve growth factor.' *Proc. Natl. Acad. Sci.*, **73**, 2424–2428.

Grzanna, R. and Coyle, J. T. (1976). 'Rat adrenal dopamine β-hydroxylase; purification and immunologic characteristics.' *J. Neurochem.*, **27**, 1091–1096.

Grzanna, R. and Coyle, J. T. (1978). 'Dopamine β-hydroxylase in rat submandibular ganglion cells which lack norepinephrine.' *Brain Res.*, **151**, 206–214.

Grzanna, R., Molliver, M. E., and Coyle, J. T. (1978). 'Visualization of central noradrenergic neurons in thick sections by the unlabelled antibody method; a transmitter specific Golgi image.' *Proc. Natl. Acad. Sci.*, **75**, 2502–2506.

Grzanna, R., Morrison, J. H., Coyle, J. T., and Molliver, M. E. (1977). 'The immunohistochemical demonstration of noradrenergic neurons in the rat brain: the use of homologous antiserum to DBH.' *Neurosci. Lett.*, **4**, 127–134.

Hartman, B. K. (1973). 'Immunofluorescence of dopamine β-hydroxylase.' *J. Histochem. Cytochem.*, **21**, 312–332.

Helle, K. B., Fillenz, M., Stanford, C., Pihl, K. E., and Srebro, B. (1979). 'A simplified method for raising antibodies to rat dopamine β-hydroxylase. *J. Neurochem.*, **32**, 1351–1355.

Hokfelt, T., Fuxe, K., Goldstein, M., and Joh, T. H. (1973). 'Immunohistochemical localization of three catecholamine synthesizing enzymes: aspects on methodology.' *Histochemie*, **23**, 231–254.

Huber, E., Konig, P., Schuler, G., Aherer, W., Plattner, H., and Winkler, H. (1979). 'Characterization and topography of the glycoproteins of adrenal chromaffin-granules.' *J. Neurochem.*, **32**, 35–47.

Ikeno, T., Hashimoto, S., Kuzuya, H., and Nagatsu, T. (1977). 'Purifications and properties of human serum dopamine β-hydroxylase.' *Mol. Cell. Biochem.*, **18**, 117–123.

Jacobowitz, D. M., Ziegler, M. G., and Thomas, J. A. (1975). '*In vivo* uptake of antibody to dopamine β-hydroxylase into sympathetic elements.' *Brain Res.*, **91**, 165–170.

Joh, T. H., Ross, R. A., and Reis, D. J. (1974). 'A simple and sensitive assay for dopamine β-hydroxylase. *Anal. Biochem.*, **62**, 248–254.

Jones, E. G. and Hartman, B. K. (1978). 'Recent advances in neuroanatomical methodology.' *Ann. Rev. Neurosci.*, **1**, 215–296.

Kato, T., Kuzuya, H., and Nagatsu, T. (1974). 'A simple and sensitive assay for dopamine β-hydroxylase: activity by dual-wavelength spectrophotometry.' *Biochem. Med.*, **10**, 320–328.

Kato, T., Wakui, Y., Nagatsu, T., and Ohnishi, T. (1978). 'An improved dualwave-length spectrophotometric assay for DBH.' *Biochem. Pharmacol.*, **27**, 829–831.

Kessler, J. A., Colchard, P., and Black, I. B. (1979). 'Nerve growth factor alters the fate of embryonic neuroblasts.' *Nature (Lond.)*, **280**, 141–142.

Kirshner, N., Schanberg, S. M., and Sage, H. J. (1975). 'Homospecific activity of serum and tissue DBH.' *Life Sci.*, **17**, 423–430.

Klein, R. L., Kirksey, D. F., Rush, R. A., and Goldstein, M. (1977). 'Preliminary estimates of the DBH content and activity in purified noradrenergic vesicles.' *J. Neurochem.*, **28**, 81–86.

Lees, G. J., Geffen, L. B., and Rush, R. A. (1981a). 'Phentolamine increases neuronal binding and retrograde transport of dopamine β-hydroxylase antibodies.' *Neurosci. Lett.*, **22**, 115–118.

Lees, G. J., Chubb, I. W., Freeman, C., Geffen, L. B., and Rush, R. A. (1981b). 'Effect of nerve activity on transport of nerve growth factor and dopamine β-hydroxylase antibodies in sympathetic nerves.' *Brain Res.*, **214**, 186–189.

Lewis, S. Y., Rush, R. A., and Geffen, L. B. (1977). 'Biochemical effects on guinea-pig iris of local injections of DBH antibodies and Fab$_2'$ fragments.' *Brain Res.*, **134**, 173–179.

Ljönes, F., Skotland, T., and Flatmark, T. (1976). 'Purification and characterisation of dopamine β-hydroxylase from bovine adrenal medulla.' *Europ. J. Biochem.*, **61**, 525–533.

Lovenberg, W., Goodwin, J. R., and Wallace, E. F. (1975). 'Molecular properties and regulation of dopamine β-hydroxylase. In Mandell, A. J. (ed.), *Neurobiological Mechanisms of Adaptation and Behaviour*, pp. 77–93.

Markey, K. A., Fong, J. C., Shenkman, L., Burroughs, V. J., Ebstein, R., and Goldstein, M. (1980). 'Purification, characterization and quantitation of rat phaeochromocytoma, tyrosine hydroxylase and of dopamine β-hydroxylase'. In Usdin, E., Sourkes, T. L., and Youdim, M. B. H. (eds), *Enzymes and Neurotransmitters in Mental Disease*, chap. V.10. John Wiley, Chichester.

Miras-Portugal, M. T., Mandel, P., and Aunis, D. (1976). 'Amino acid and carbohydrate compositions of human serum dopamine β-hydroxylase.' *Neurochem. Res.*, **1**, 403–408.

Nagatsu, I. and Kondo, Y. (1975). 'Studies on axonal flow of DBH and TOH in sciatic nerves by immunofluorescent and biochemical methods.' *Acta Histochem. Cytochem.*, **8**, 279–287.

Nagatsu, I., Kondo, Y., Kato, T., and Nagatsu, T. (1976). 'Retrograde axoplasmic transport of inactive dopamine β-hydroxylase in sciatic nerves.' *Brain Res.*, **116**, 277–285.

Nagatsu, T., Thomas, P., Rush, R. A., and Udenfriend, S. (1973). 'A radioassay for dopamine β-hydroxylase activity in rat serum.' *Anal. Biochem.*, **55**, 615–619.

Nagatsu, T. and Udenfriend, S. (1972). 'Photometric assay of dopamine β-hydroxylase activity in human blood.' *Clin. Chem.*, **18**, 980–983.

Nakane, P. K. and Kawaoi, A. (1974). 'Peroxidase labelled antibody; a new method of conjugation.' *J. Histochem. Cytochem.*, **22**, 1084–1091.

Olschowka, J. A., Molliver, M. E., Grzanna, R., Rice, F. L., and Coyle, J. T. (1981). 'Ultrastructural demonstration of noradrenergic synapses in the rat central nervous system by dopamine β-hydroxylase immunocytochemistry.' *J. Histochem. Cytochem.*, **29**, 271–280.

Patterson, P. (1978). 'Environmental determination of autonomic neurotransmitter functions.' *Ann. Rev. Neurosci.*, **1**, 1–17.

Pickel, B. M., Joh, T. H., and Reis, D. J. (1976). 'Monoamine-synthesizing enzymes in central dopaminergic, noradrenergic and serotonergic neurons. Immunocytochemical localization by light and electron microscopy.' *J. Histochem. Cytochem.*, **24**, 792–806.

Rush, R. A., Costa, M., Furness, J. B., and Geffen, L. B. (1976). 'Changes in tyrosine hydroxylase and dopamine β-hydroxylase activities during degeneration of noradrenergic axons produced by antibodies to dopamine β-hydroxylase.' *Neurosci. Lett.*, **3**, 209–213.

Rush, R. A. and Geffen, L. B. (1972). 'Radioimmunoassay and clearance of circulating dopamine β-hydroxylase.' *Circ. Res.*, **31**, 444–452.

Rush, R. A. and Geffen, L. B. (1980). 'Dopamine β-hydroxylase in health and disease.' *CRC Crit. Rev. Clin. Lab. Sci.*, **12**, 241–247.

Rush, R. A., Kindler, S. H., and Udenfriend, S. (1975a). 'Homospecific activity, an immunologic index of enzyme homogeneity; changes during the purification of dopamine β-hydroxylase.' *Biochem. Biophys. Res. Commun.*, **61**, 38–44.

Rush, R. A., Kindler, S. H., and Udenfriend, S. (1975b). 'Solid-phase radioimmunoassay on polystyrene beads and its application to dopamine β-hydroxylase.' *Clin. Chem. (NY)*, **21**, 148–151.

Rush, R. A., Millar, T. J., Chubb, I. W., and Geffen, L. B. (1979). 'Use of DBH antibodies in study of vesicle dynamics.' In Usdin, E., Kopin, I. J., and Barchas, J. (eds), *Catecholamines: Basic and Clinical Frontiers*, p. 331. Pergamon Press, New York.

Rush, R. A., Thomas, P. E., Kindler, S. H., and Udenfriend, S. (1974). 'The interaction of dopamine β-hydroxylase with Concanavalin A and its use in enzyme purification.' *Biochem. Biophys. Res. Commun.*, **57**, 1301–1305.

Rush, R. A., Thomas, P. E., and Udenfriend, S. (1975c). 'Measurement of human dopamine β-hydroxylase in serum by homologous radioimmunoassay.' *Proc. Natl. Acad. Sci.*, **72**, 750–752.

Skotland, T. and Ljones, T. (1979). 'Dopamine β-mono-oxygenase; structure, mechanism, and properties of the enzyme-bound copper. *Inorg. Perspect. Biol. Med.*, **2**, 151–180.

Smith, A. D. and Winkler, H. (1967). 'A simple method for the isolation of adrenal chromaffin granules on a large scale.' *Biochem. J.*, **103**, 480–482.

Sternberger, L. A. (1974). *Immunocytochemistry, Immunohistochemistry*. In *Foundations of Immunology* series. Prentice-Hall, New Jersey.

Stone, R. A., Kirshner, N., Reynolds, J., and Vanaman, T. C. (1974). 'Purification and properties of dopamine β-hydroxylase from human phaeochromocytoma.' *Mol. Pharmacol.*, **10**, 1009–1015.

Swanson, L. W. and Hartman, B. K. (1975). 'The central adrenergic system: an immunofluorescence study of the localization of cell bodies and their efferent connections in the rat, utilizing dopamine β-hydroxylase as a marker.' *J. Comp. Neurol.*, **163**, 467–505.

Weinshilboum, R. M. (1979). 'Serum dopamine β-hydroxylase.' *Pharmacol. Rev.*, **30**, 133–166.

Weinshilboum, R. and Axelrod, J. (1971). 'Serum dopamine-beta-hydroxylase activity.' *Circ. Res.*, **28**, 307–315.

Winkler, H. and Westhead, E. (1980). 'The molecular organization of adrenal chromaffin granules.' *Neuroscience*, **5**, 1803–1823.

Ziegler, M. G., Thomas, J. A., and Jacobowitz, D. M. (1976). 'Retrograde axonal transport of antibody to dopamine β-hydroxylase.' *Brain Res.*, **104**, 390–395.

Immunohistochemistry
Edited by A. C. Cuello
© 1983 IBRO

CHAPTER 7

Preparation of Glutamic Acid Decarboxylase as Immunogen for Immunocytochemistry

JANG-YEN WU

Department of Cell Biology, Baylor College of Medicine, Texas Medical Center, Houston, Texas 77030

I INTRODUCTION

There are many lines of evidence to suggest that GABA is an inhibitory neurotransmitter at the crustacean neuromuscular junction and that it probably also is the major inhibitory neurotransmitter in the vertebrate central nervous system (Bazemore *et al.*, 1957; Florey, 1957; Krnjevic, 1974; Roberts *et al.*, 1976; Wu *et al.*, 1981a,b).

L-Glutamate decarboxylase (EC 4.1.1.15) (GAD), which catalyses α-decarboxylation of L-glutamate to form GABA and CO_2, is believed to be the rate-limiting enzyme that normally determines the steady-state levels of GABA in vertebrate and invertebrate nervous systems (Kravitz, 1967; Roberts and Kuriyama, 1968). Furthermore, it has been shown that there is a good correlation between GABA levels and GAD activity in vertebrate nervous system (Kuriyama *et al.*, 1966, 1968; Baxter, 1970). Hence GAD is a better marker for GABAergic neurons than GABA *per se*, which may redistribute or be metabolized during the preparation of the tissues (Baxter, 1970; Fonnum, 1975).

Perhaps the most direct and sensitive means of identifying GABAergic neurons is to visualize GAD-containing neurons by immunocytochemical methods. One of the prerequisites of using immunocytochemical methods for localizing GAD is to obtain a monospecific GAD antiserum which in turn requires an homogeneous GAD preparation.

This review discusses mainly the progress to date dealing with various purification procedures, and assay methods for GAD and criteria of purity of GAD preparations. In addition, immunochemical characterization of anti-GAD serum and the application of anti-GAD serum to species- and tissue-specificities and immunocytochemical studies of GAD are included.

II ASSAY METHOD

For the study of any enzyme it is essential to use an assay method for monitoring the enzyme activity. A good assay should be simple, rapid, sensitive, and specific. Numerous methods for assaying GAD have been reported in the literature (Roberts and Frankel, 1950, Roberts *et al.*, 1964; Kravitz *et al.*, 1965; Chude and Wu, 1976; Wu, 1976a, 1978). They are based on measurement of either CO_2 formation or GABA formation.

II.1 CO_2 Method

The CO_2 method, which is based on the formation of $^{14}CO_2$ from either L-[1-^{14}C]- or L-[U-^{14}C]glutamate, has been widely used (Roberts *et al.*, 1964; Wu *et al.*, 1973; Wu, 1976a). In a typical assay, the incubation vessel contained 0.1 ml of 0.208 M L-glutamic acid (0.74 μCi L-[1-^{14}C]glutamate) in

0.1 M potassium phosphate buffer containing 0.2 mM pyridoxal phosphate, pH 7.2. The reaction is started by injecting 1 ml enzyme solution in 50 mM potassium phosphate buffer, pH 7.2, containing 0.2 mM pyridoxal phosphate and 1 mM 2-aminoethylisothiouronium bromide (AET) (standard buffer) into the incubation vessel. The incubation is performed in a Dubnoff metabolic incubator for 30 min at 37 °C at approximately 150 rpm and terminated by injecting 0.1 ml of 8 N H_2SO_4 into the reaction mixture. The vessels are incubated for another 60 min to ensure a complete release of CO_2 and absorption in the Hyamine base.

Recently, we have simplified the above procedure by substituting the special two-arm incubation vessels with the ordinary disposable culture tubes (15 × 85 mm) (Fisher Scientific Co., Pittsburgh, Pa.) sealed with a serum tube rubber stopper. A plastic centre well (Kontes, Vineland, N.J.) that contained hyamine solution, is inserted through the centre of the rubber stopper to absorb the CO_2 formed in the reaction mixture.

The volume of the reaction mixture was also reduced by five-fold. The rest of the procedure was the same as described above.

II.2 GABA Method

For the GABA method, we (Chude and Wu, 1976) have modified the method of Molinoff and Kravitz (1968) by combining the speed of vacuum filtration and the selectivity of ion exchange resins for assaying any enzyme whose substrate and product differ by charge. For instance, in GAD assay the substrate, glutamate, which is negatively charged at neutral pH, is therefore retained by anion exchanger, while the product, GABA, is not charged at neutral pH and hence passes through the resin without retention. The apparatus of this vacuum filtration-ion exchange assay is shown in Figure 1.

Briefly, the filter manifold (Hoefer Scientific Instruments, San Francisco, Calif.) is set up with test tubes or counting vials to collect the filtrate and Millipore filters, pore size 8 μm, or Whatman No. 1 filter paper over the steel screens to act as a support for the resin. Five millilitres of the aqueous resin suspension (0.4 g of BioRad AG 1 × 8 per ml; BioRad Laboratory, Richmond, Calif.) is pipetted into each filter receptacle. The water is allowed to drain into the test tubes without the use of the vacuum pump and discarded. The GAD reaction mixture is then carefully applied on top of the resin. The solution is allowed to drain and 1 ml of water is then added to wash the resin. After the water has drained, the vacuum is turned on to remove the last traces of solution in the resin. The resin cake is dislodged into a 1 mM HCl solution in order to recover the glutamate and resin later. Fifteen millilitres of Aquasol is added to each filtrate in a scintillation vial and mixed thoroughly before counting.

The identity of the reaction product in the filtrate is identified as GABA by

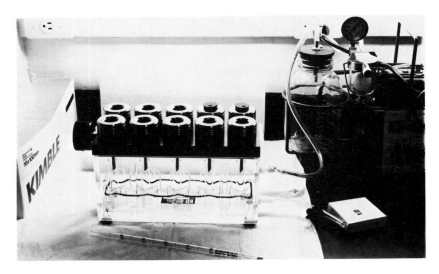

Figure 1   Principle of a simple and sensitive assay method for any enzyme system whose substrate and product differ by charge. The device consists of a pump and a ten-lace steel filter manifold capable of collecting the filtrate

comparing with the authentic GABA in high-voltage electrophoresis and amino acid analysis.

The vacuum filtration–ion exchange technique possesses the following advantages: First of all, it is a simple and rapid method that allows one to do up to 100 assays a day easily and, when it becomes desirable, reaction mixtures can be frozen and assayed later. Second, it is a more direct method as it measures the GABA formation instead of CO_2 formation. Third, the availability of tritiated glutamate with a very high specific activity may further increase methods sensitivity. Furthermore, the tritiated compound is much more economical than the ^{14}C-labelled substrate. Fourth, the resin and substrate used in this method can be regenerated and reused. Because in the GAD reaction only a small percentage of the labelled substrate is converted to GABA, it is highly desirable to be able to recover the unused labelled substrate.

Another important point is that the principle of this method can be applied to the assay of any enzyme whose substrate and product differ by charge, such as decarboxylases, transaminases, kinases, phosphorylases, and many other enzyme systems. In fact, this method has been routinely used in the author's laboratory for assaying various transmitter enzymes, e.g. GAD (Chude and Wu, 1976), GABA–T (Wu *et al.*, 1978b), choline acetyltransferase (CAT) (Brandon and Wu, 1978), and cysteic acid decarboxylase (Wu *et al.*, 1979a).

III PURIFICATION PROCEDURES

III.1 Preparation of Crude Extract

Crude mitochondrial fraction is used as the starting material because the transmitter synthesizing enzymes are believed to be concentrated at the nerve terminals. In a typical preparation, 300 mice are killed by cervical dislocation, the whole brain minus the brainstem is removed rapidly, and a 15% homogenate is made in ice-cold, N_2-saturated, 0.32 M sucrose in a motor-driven glass homogenizer with a Teflon pestle. The homogenate is centrifuged at 900 g for 15 min. All operations and centrifugations are carried out at 0–4 °C and all buffer solutions contain 0.2 mM pyridoxal phosphate and 1 mM AET, unless otherwise mentioned. The supernatant liquid is centrifuged at 23,000 g for 15 min. The pellet thus obtained is again centrifuged at 73,000 g for 20 min, and the supernatant liquid is poured off. The pellet was suspended in 144 ml of glass-distilled H_2O and stirred slowly at 4 °C for 20 min; the suspension is centrifuged at 105,600 g for 75 min. The supernatant fluid thus obtained is called the 'crude extract'. Additional enzyme activity could be obtained with a second water extraction on the residue. Concentrated potassium phosphate buffer, AET, and pyridoxal phosphate is added to the extract to give the following concentrations: potassium phosphate, 50 mM; AET, 1 mM; and pyridoxal phosphate, 0.2 mM. The final pH is 7.2. About 25% of GAD activities is recovered in the crude extract with a more than 7-fold increase in specific activity. The crude extract was stable for many months at −20 °C and served as the starting material for further purification of GAD.

III.2 Ammonium Sulphate Fractionation

Five batches of the crude GAD extract prepared as above are combined, and ultra-pure solid ammonium sulphate (157 g/l) is added gradually to the well-stirred solution to give approximately 27% saturation. The pH of the solution is monitored continuously with a pH meter and maintained at 7.2 by gradual addition of 0.1 N NH_4OH during the addition of ammonium sulphate (approximately 0.5 ml of 0.1 N NH_4OH per gram of ammonium sulphate is needed to maintain the pH at 7.2). After the addition of ammonium sulphate, the solution is stirred for another 15–20 min. The solution is then centrifuged at 13,200 g for 30 min. The pellet is discarded, and more ammonium sulphate (234 g/l) is added to the supernatant fluid to give approximately 62% saturation. The precipitate is dissolved in a minimal volume (40–50 ml) of the standard buffer. The solution is centrifuged at 105,600 g for 30 min and the supernatant is applied to Sephadex G200 column directly. When storage is desirable, it is dialysed against a large volume of the standard buffer to remove ammonium sulphate and stored at −20 °C. About 70% of GAD activity is recovered in 27–62% ammonium sulphate fraction with a twofold increase in specific activity.

III.3   Chromatography on Sephadex G200

Sephadex G200 gel is equilibrated with the standard buffer and packed into a column of 5.0 × 60 cm. Approximately 40–50 ml (800–1000 mg of protein) of GAD solution from step 2 above is applied to the column. The column is eluted with the standard buffer at a flow rate of 25 ml/h (Figure 2). Fractions

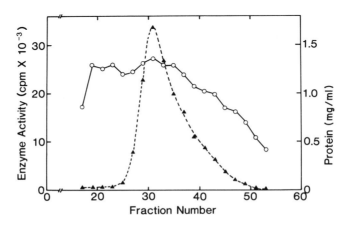

Figure 2   First Sephadex G200 gel filtration of GAD from the first ammonium sulphate fractionation. The details of chromatography are described in the text. Protein concentration (○) was in mg/ml. GAD activity (▲) was in terms of counts/min/ml. Samples of 18 ml per fraction were collected

of approximately 18 ml are collected and stored at −20 °C. All the GAD activities are recovered with a three- to four-fold purification obtained at the peak fraction. Three batches of G200 fractions with specific activity of between 0.05 and 0.17 unit/mg of protein are pooled and ammonium sulphate fractionation is carried out as before. The precipitate between 30 and 68% saturation (176–455 g of ammonium sulphate per litre) is collected and dissolved in a minimal volume of 1 mM potassium phosphate buffer, pH 7.2, and dialysed against the same buffer overnight with two changes.

III.4   Chromatography on Calcium Phosphate Gel

The amount of calcium phosphate gel needed to adsorb all of the GAD activity, and the ionic strength needed to elute the enzyme, are determined in small-scale batchwise experiments. A slight excess of calcium phosphate gel was packed in a column (2.5 × 50 cm) with adapters to give a bed volume of 2.5 × 20 cm. The enzyme solution from the preceding steps is applied to a column which had been equilibrated with 1 mM potassium phosphate buffer, pH 7.2. After the application of the solution, an equal volume of the same buffer solution is introduced and the column is washed further with 100–150 ml of 25 mM potassium phosphate buffer, pH 7.2. A linear gradient made from 300 ml of 25 mM and 300 ml of 0.15 M potassium phosphate buffer, pH 7.2, is then employed. The enzyme activity starts to appear after the beginning of the gradient, and the peak fraction appears at 75 mM (Figure 3).

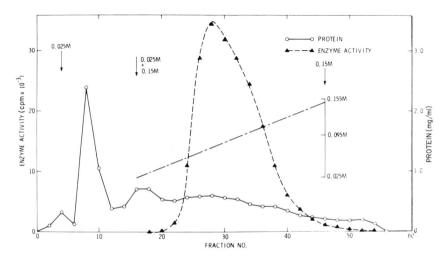

Figure 3 Calcium phosphate gel chromatography of GAD from the second ammonium sulphate fractionation. See text for details of chromatograph. First arrow, application of 0.025 M standard buffer; second arrow, application of a linear gradient from 0.025 to 0.15 M standard buffer; third arrow, application of 0.15 M standard buffer. Protein concentration (○) was in mg/ml. GAD activity (▲) was in terms of counts/min/ml. Gradient (—·—) was in molarity

The position of the peak fraction shifts toward higher ionic strength when the washing step is incomplete or when a larger amount of calcium phosphate gel is used. After the gradient, elution is continued with 0.15 M phosphate buffer. Another four- to five-fold purification is obtained with calcium phosphate gel column. Three batches of calcium phosphate gel fractions containing enzyme with a specific activity of 0.25 unit/mg of protein or higher are pooled and fractionated with ammonium sulphate. The precipitate coming out between 33 and 70% saturation (196–472 g of ammonium sulphate per litre) is collected, dissolved in a minimal volume of the standard buffer, and dialysed against the buffer. Fractions with a specific activity lower than 0.25 unit/mg protein are concentrated and reapplied to calcium phosphate column.

III.5 Chromatography on DEAE–Sephadex

DEAE–Sephadex A–50 is equilibrated with the standard buffer and packed into a column of 2.5×50 cm. The GAD solution from the preceding step is applied. An equal volume of the standard buffer is introduced after the sample and the column is washed with 100 ml of 0.1 M potassium phosphate buffer, pH 7.2. A linear gradient of potassium phosphate made from 160 ml of 0.1 M, pH 7.2, and 160 ml of 0.3 M, pH 6.4, is used for elution. The enzyme activity starts to appear shortly after the gradient and peaks at 0.19 M phosphate buffer (Figure 4).

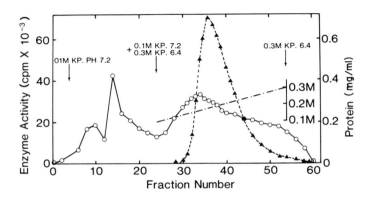

Figure 4 DEAE–Sephadex chromatography of GAD from the third ammonium sulphate fractionation. See text for details of chromatography. First arrow, application of 0.1 M standard buffer; second arrow, application of a linear gradient from 0.1 M, pH 7.2 to 0.3 M, pH 6.4 standard buffer; third arrow, application of 0.3 M standard buffer, pH 6.4. Protein concentration (○) was in mg/ml. GAD activity (▲) was in terms of counts/min. Gradient (—·—) was in molarity

Additional fourfold purification is obtained at the peak fraction. Fractions with specific activities above 1.2, between 0.5 and 1.19, and below 0.5 unit/mg of ptotein are pooled separately into three fractions, and concentrated by precipitation with $(NH_4)_2SO_4$ at 75% saturation (516 g/l). The precipitates are dissolved in 3.5 ml of the standard buffer. Fractions containing the highest specific activities are used for the last step of purification. Fractions containing the specific activities between 0.5 and 1.19, and below 0.5 unit/mg of protein, are reapplied to DEAE–Sephadex and calcium phosphate gel columns, respectively.

III.6 Second Chromatography of GAD on Sephadex G200

Sephadex G200 is prepared and packed as before except for the column size, which is reduced to 2.5 × 50 cm. Samples of 3.5 ml of the highest specific activity from the DEAE–Sephadex column at a concentration of 4.8 mg/ml are applied to the column. The column is eluted with the standard buffer at a flow rate of 22 ml/h, and fractions are collected at 22 min intervals (Figure 5).

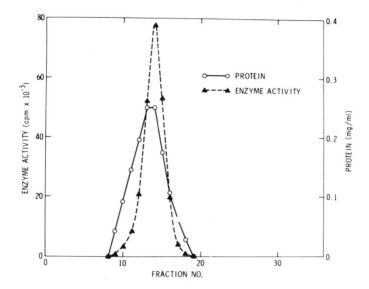

Figure 5 Second Sephadex G200 gel filtration of GAD from the fourth ammonium sulphate fractionation. The details of chromatography are described in the text. Protein concentration (○) was in mg/ml. GAD activity (▲) was in terms of counts/min/ml

About twofold purification is additionally obtained at the peak fraction. Two peak fractions which have the same specific activity, 3.3 units/mg protein, are concentrated with $(NH_4)_2SO_4$ as described above. The precipitates are dissolved and dialysed against a large volume of the standard buffer.

The successive steps in the purification of GAD from 9000 mouse brains are summarized in Table 1. In that purification, eleven steps were employed and approximately 1.2% of the total activity was recovered as a purified enzyme preparation representing 940-fold purification over the original homogenate (Wu, 1976a).

In addition to the conventional procedures, we have also employed affinity column chromatographies for GAD purification. The following compounds: L-glutamic acid, D-glutamic acid, β-aminoglutaric acid, α-, γ-diaminoglutaric

Table 1   Purification of GAD from mouse brain[a]

Sample	Volume (ml)	Total activity (units)[b]	Total protein (mg)	Specific activity (units/mg $\times 10^3$)	Yield (%)
Sucrose homogenate	30,000	1,680	480,000	3.5	100
Crude extract	4,800	429	16,500	26	26
First $(NH_4)_2SO_4$ (27–62%)	300	300	6,000	50	18
First Sephadex G200	1,080	180	1,500	120[c]	11
Second $(NH_4)_2SO_4$ (30–68%)	126	147	980	150	8.8
Calcium phosphate gel (pool)	290	88	195	450[d]	5.2
Third $(NH_4)_2SO_4$ (33–70%)	23	66	120	550	3.9
DEAE–Sephadex (pool)	60	31	18	1,720	1.8
Fourth $(NH_4)_2SO_4$ (0–75%)	3.5	29	17	1,700[e]	1.7
Second Sephadex G200	16.0	20	6	3,300	1.2
Fifth $(NH_4)_2SO_4$ (0–75%)	2.0	20	6	3,300	1.2

[a] Purification of GAD was made from 9000 brains.
[b] One unit = 1 μmol of product formed per minute at 37 °C under standard conditions.
[c] Peak fraction specific activity of 170.
[d] Peak fraction specific activity of 650.
[e] Peak fraction specific activity of 2100.

acid and L-aspartic acid which are either substrates, substrate analogues, or competitive inhibitors (Wu, 1976a), have been covalently linked through the amino group to the 'arm' or the matrix of the Sepharose gel. All of the above affinity resins showed only weak affinity towards GAD and hence gave poor purification. The best result we have obtained so far for GAD purification was with the affinity columns using either anti-GAD IgG or *p*-chloromercuribenzoate (PCMB)/*p*-hydroxymercuribenzoate (PHMB) as ligands, as detailed below.

III.7   Anti-GAD IgG Sepharose 4B Affinity Column

100 ml Sepharose 4B (Pharmacia Fine Chemicals, Piscataway, N.J.) is washed extensively with 0.1 M NaCl and then glass-distilled water. This gel is activated with 100 ml cyanogen bromide (50 mg CNBr per ml water) for 10 min. The pH of the reaction mixture is maintained at pH 11 by the gradual addition of 5 M NaOH. The gel is then washed with 2 litres of cold 0.1 M NaHO₃ solution on a sintered-glass funnel. 4 ml Anti-GAD IgG (5 mg/ml) is dialysed against 100 ml 0.05 M potassium phosphate–0.1 M sodium bicarbonate buffer, pH 9.5, at 4 °C for 4 h. After dialysis, anti-GAD IgG solution is mixed with the cyanogen bromide-activated gel. The reaction is carried out at 4 °C for 20 h with gentle shaking. The reaction is terminated by filtration through a glass filter (C-grade). The anti-GAD IgG–Sepharose 4B complex is then washed with 2 litres of 0.05 M potassium phosphate–0.14 M sodium chloride,

pH 7.2, followed by 4 litres of 0.05 M potassium phosphate buffer, pH 7.2, containing 1 mM AET and 0.2 mM pyridoxal phosphate. The anti-GAD IgG–Sepharose 4B affinity gel is stable for several months at 4 °C in the presence of 0.02% sodium azide. Anti-GAD IgG-Sepharose 4B affinity gel is packed into a 1.5 × 25 cm column and the column is equilibrated with the standard buffer as described before; 5 ml crude GAD extract is applied to the column and 8.0 ml per fraction is collected. The column is first washed with 100 ml standard buffer, followed by 70 ml 0.1 M potassium phosphate standard buffer and finally eluted with 0.1 M acetic acid, pH 2.8, containing 1 mM AET and 0.2 mM pyridoxal phosphate. One mole of potassium phosphate, pH 8.0, is introduced through a separate tubing to the fractions simultaneously to neutralize acetic acid to maintain the pH in the fractions around 6.7. The elution profile is shown in Figure 6. In that preparation, a 36-fold purification was obtained with about 25% of GAD activity retained. The inactivation of GAD appeared to occur at the time of the brief exposure of GAD to a low pH environment during elution with acetic acid. The use of other conditions such as high salt concentrations to dissociate GAD–anti-GAD complex may give a

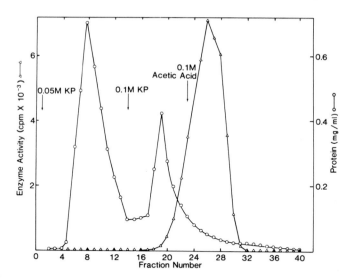

Figure 6 Affinity chromatography of GAD on anti-GAD IgG-Sepharose 4B column. About 5 ml of the crude enzyme solution (64 mg of protein) was applied to a column (1.5 × 10 cm) which had been equilibrated with 0.05 M potassium phosphate standard buffer. The column was first eluted with standard buffer, followed by 0.1 M potassium phosphate standard buffer and finally with 0.1 M acetic acid containing 1 mM of AET and 0.2 mM pyridoxal phosphate, pH 2.81. A concentrated potassium phosphate buffer (1 M), pH 8.0 was introduced directly to the fraction in a separate tubing to neutralize acetic acid. (O——O), protein (mg/ml); (△——△). GAD activity (counts per min)

better result than the use of acid. Another approach is to use anti-GAD IgG with low affinity towards GAD as ligand, so that the GAD–anti-GAD complex can be easily dissociated by gentle treatments such as slightly alkali or acidic solutions, low concentration of urea, or other denatured reagents.

III.8   PCMB (or PHMB)–Sepharose 4B Affinity Column

Sepharose 4B was activated with cyanogen bromide as described above. The activated gel is aminated by incubating with diaminodipropyl amine (8.0 g in 100 ml H_2O, pH 10) for 16 h at 4 °C with gentle shaking. 6 mmoles of sodium *p*-hydroxymercuribenzoate and the aminated gel are suspended in a total volume of 150 ml of 40% (v/v) dimethylformamide. Three grams of 1-ethyl-3-(3-dimethylaminopropyl) carbodi-imide are added, and the pH of the reaction mixture is maintained at 5.0 for 3 h. The reaction mixture is shaken overnight at 4 °C. About 15 litres of 0.1 M $NaHCO_3$, pH 8.8, solution is used to wash the PHMB-substituted gel over an 8 h period. The PHMB–Sepharose 4B affinity resin is stored in 0.1 M $NaHCO_3$, pH 8.8, containing 0.02% sodium azide. Three millilitres of PHMB–Sepharose 4B is packed in a small column $(0.9 \times 10\,cm)$ and the column is equilibrated with 0.05 M potassium phosphate, pH 7.2, containing 0.2 mM pyridoxal phosphate. Three millilitres of crude GAD extract is dialysed in 0.05 M potassium phosphate, pH 7.2, containing 0.2 mM pyridoxal phosphate and 0.01 mM AET. The column is first washed extensively with 0.1 M potassium phosphate, Ph 7.2, containing 0.2 mM pyridoxal phosphate, followed by 30 ml each of 0.1 M potassium phosphate, 0.2 mM pyridoxal phosphate, pH 7.2, and of the same solution containing 50 mM dithiothreitol (DTT). The elution profile is shown in Figure 7. About ten-fold purification was obtained, with a recovery of about 60%. Although the affinity columns that we have employed in the purification of GAD have not produced the results which were as dramatic as those reported in the literature for some other proteins (Cuatrecasas and Anfinsen, 1971; Cuatrecasas, 1972), the anti-GAD IgG–Sepharose 4B affinity column did give a much better result than any other single step of conventional methods that we have employed. By selecting the proper ligands, the length of the 'arm', and the elution conditions, we may improve further the affinity chromatography and obtain an optimal separation. The combination of conventional procedures and affinity chromatography also may prove to be effective and practical in the large-scale purification of the enzymes. Recently, we have also purified GAD from catfish brain (Su *et al.*, 1979) and GAD and taurine-synthesizing enzyme, cysteic/cysteine sulphinic acids decarboxylase (CAD/CSAD) from bovine brain (Wu *et al.*, 1980; also Figure 8a,b) using preparative polyacrylamide gel electrophoresis in addition to the procedures that we have used for the purification of GAD from mouse brain.

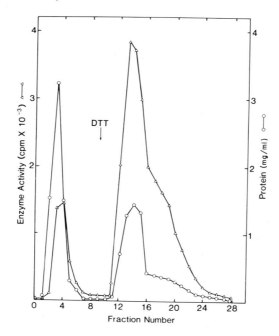

Figure 7 Affinity chromatography of GAD in PHMB-Sepharose 4B column. Three millilitres of the crude enzyme solution (38 mg of protein) was applied to a column, 0.5 × 5 cm, which had been equilibrated with 0.05 M potassium phosphate buffer, pH 7.2 containing 0.2 mM of pyridoxal phosphate. All the elution buffers contained 0.2 mM pyridoxal phosphate unless otherwise mentioned. The column was first eluted with 0.05 M potassium phosphate buffer, followed by 0.1 M of the same buffer and finally eluted with a linear gradient of dithiothreitol which was made of 30 ml of 0.1 M potassium phosphate buffer, pH 7.2 and 30 ml of the same buffer containing 50 mM of dithiothreitol. (O——O), ptotein (mg/ml); (△——△), GAD activity (counts/min)

IV CRITERIA OF PURITY

Since an homogeneous enzyme preparation is a prerequisite for obtaining a monospecific antibody, this in turn is essential for meaningful results in immunocytochemical techniques. We have employed several physical and chemical methods to vigorously test the purity of GAD preparations (Wu *et al.*, 1973; Wu, 1976a; Wu *et al.*, 1980).

The homogeneity of GAD preparations which were used as antigen for antibody production were established based on the following criteria:

IV.1 Polyacrylamide Gel Electrophoresis

Twenty-five to seventy micrograms of the purified enzyme revealed a single

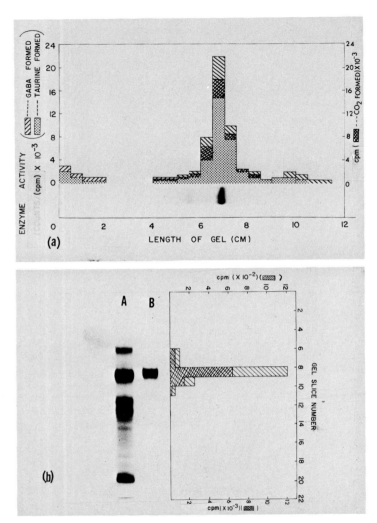

Figure 8 (a) Polyacrylamide gel electrophoresis of bovine GAD: a 25 μg aliquot of the most purified GAD solution was applied to a 5% polyacrylamide slab gel. The protein pattern is at the bottom. Migration was from left (cathode) to right (anode). Enzyme activity was measured in slices of a parallel gel. GAD activity (▨), CAD activity (▦) and CSAD activity (▩) were expressed as counts per minute. (b) Preparative gel electrophoresis: 500 μl of the concentrated partially purified CAD solution was applied to a 7% polyacrylamide slab gel. The enzyme solution was in 10% glycerol containing bromphenol blue as marker. Before application of the sample, a current of 20 mA was passed through the gel for 30 min with buffer containing 0.025 M tris, 0.192 M glycine, 0.065 mM reduced glutathione, 0.2 mM pyridoxal phosphate, and 0.1% β-mercaptoethanol, pH 8.4. Electrophoresis was carried out at 4 °C at 15 mA for

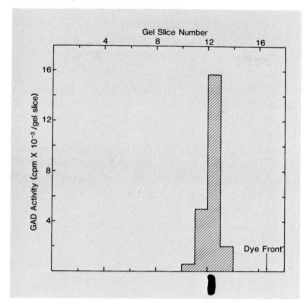

Figure 9 Polyacrylamide gel electrophoresis of GAD purified from mouse brain. The protein pattern is at the bottom. A 40 μg aliquot of the most purified GAD solution was applied to a 5% polyacrylamide separating gel slab. Migration was from left (cathode) to right (anode). Enzyme activity obtained from a parallel gel slab was in terms of counts/min per gel slice (5 mm)

protein band with the location of the enzyme activity corresponding to the location of the protein band on polyacrylamide gel electrophoresis (Figures 8a,b and 9), suggesting that GAD preparations were homogeneous in terms of size and charge. The purified GAD preparation from bovine brain also displayed CAD and CSAD activities (Figure 8a). However, the purified CAD/CSAD did not possess any GAD activity (Figure 8b).

Gradient polyacrylamide gel electrophoresis, which differs from the regular (uniform pore size) polyacrylamide gel electrophoresis in that the latter separates proteins according to their charge and size and the former is based

the first hour and 20 mA for an additional hour using the same buffer system as described except that no β-mercaptoethanol was present. After electrophoresis, one gel strip (1 cm wide) was stained for protein with Coomassie (A) and another gel strip was sliced into 1 cm squares and assayed for CAD activity (▨) and CSAD activity (▩). The bands which contained CAD activity were pooled together. CAD was extracted from the gel by homogenizing the gel (about 200 μl/cm^2 of gel) in 0.1 M potassium phosphate buffer containing 1 mM AET, 0.2 mM pyridoxal phosphate, pH 6.0. Gel was removed by a brief centrifugation. CAD solutions thus obtained were concentrated and analysed for protein pattern (B) and enzyme activities on polyacrylamide gel as described above

on size only, has also been used to check the purity of GAD from catfish. On 3.7–15% gradient polyacrylamide gel electrophoresis, the purified catfish enzyme preparation also migrated as a sharp, single protein band which contained all the enzyme activity suggesting that GAD preparation is homogeneous in terms of size (Su *et al.*, 1979).

IV.2   Sedimentation Equilibrium Analysis

The purified mouse brain GAD preparation appeared to be homogeneous in size under various conditions as judged from the linear plot of the logarithm of concentrations (c) against the squares of the distances (r) from the centre of rotation to points of interest in high-speed sedimentation equilibrium runs in both H_2O and D_2O solutions (Figure 10). Furthermore, GAD preparations treated with dissociating reagents—e.g., guanidine HCl and 2-mercaptoethanol—also appeared to be monodisperse in the high-speed

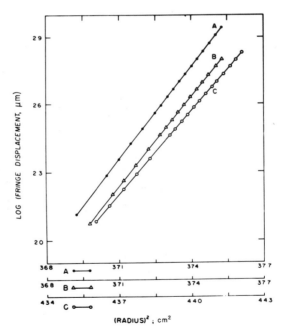

Figure 10   Sedimentation equilibrium plot of GAD. Rayleigh fringe displacement (log) plotted against the square of the distance from the centre of rotation. **A**: 40 h after the rotor had reached 24,630 rpm at 4 °C with a protein concentration of 0.25 mg/ml in aqueous buffer solution. **B**: 40 h after the rotor had reached 27,690 rpm at 4 °C with a protein concentration of 0.25 mg/ml in D_2O buffer solution. **C**: 45 h after the rotor had reached 42,040 rpm at 20 °C with a protein concentration of 0.20 mg/ml in 6 M guanidine HCl containing 0.1 M β-mercaptoethanol

sedimentation equilibrium runs (Figure 10). A molecular weight of $84,000 \pm 2000$ was obtained for mouse brain GAD with a partial specific volume of 0.732. The molecular weight of GAD in the presence of 6 M guanidine HCl and 0.1 M 2-mercaptoethanol was reduced to $44,000 \pm 2000$, which was about half of the size of the native enzyme, suggesting that GAD may consist of two identical or closely related subunits.

IV.3 Ouchterlony Double Immunodiffusion Tests

Antibodies against the purified GAD preparations appeared to be specific only to GAD, as demonstrated in immunodiffusion experiments in which a sharp, single precipitin band was obtained with GAD antisera and crude enzyme preparations (Figure 11). Furthermore, the precipitin band also

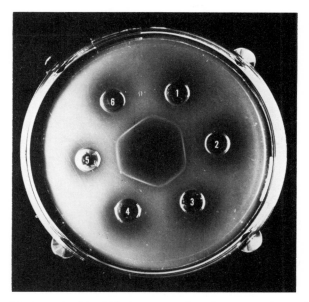

Figure 11 Ouchterlony double diffusion tests of crude preparations of GAD from brain of different mouse strains. In all cases, 30 µl of antisera against the purified enzymes from brains of Swiss mice was placed in the centre well and 30 µl of a concentrated solution of the enzymes from the different strains in the outer wells. GAD from (1) C57BL, (2) Swiss, (3) CBA, (4) Swiss, (5) CE, (6) Swiss

contained GAD activities, while a comparable piece of gel did not show any enzyme activity, suggesting that the precipitin band was indeed a GAD–anti-GAD complex. Immunoelectrophoresis of the crude enzyme preparations also showed a single precipitation band with anti-GAD (Wong *et al.*, 1974). Furthermore, antibodies against partially purified GAD also formed a sharp,

single band with the purified GAD preparations, whereas the crude preparations showed multiple bands in immunodiffusion tests (Matsuda *et al.*, 1973)
suggesting that the purified GAD preparation is immunochemically
homogeneous.

V   PRODUCTION OF ANTIBODIES

Once we had established the purity of GAD preparations from physical and
chemical criteria as described above, we would inject various amounts of the
purified protein solutions into rabbits and follow the titre of the antibodies
periodically. In the past, we were able to obtain high-titre antibodies with
microgram quantities of antigens. In general, rabbits were injected biweekly
with 3–180 µg of antigen in complete Freund's adjuvant into subscapular
muscles. Animals were bled after the fifth injection. The use of microgram
instead of milligram quantities of protein as antigen, as has been used in the
conventional method of immunizing animals for the production of antibody,
is essential because of the scarcity of the purified protein from the nervous
tissues. Furthermore, the chance of producing antibodies against trace
impurities which might still be associated with the purified preparations and
escape detection by sensitive physical and chemical techniques, is much less
because of the small amount (microgram quantities) of antigen used in the
immunization of animals. This technique has been successfully used in our
laboratory for the production of antibodies against various proteins purified
from the nervous system. For instance, a total of 15, 50, 50, 7, and 75 µg of
purified GABA-transaminase (GABA–T) (Saito *et al.*, 1974b) and GAD
from mouse brain (Figure 11; also Saito *et al.*, 1974c), choline acetyl
transferase from the electric organ of *Torpedo* (Brandon and Wu, 1977),
neurofilament protein from *Myxicola* (Lasek and Wu, 1976) and GAD and
CAD from bovine brains (Wu *et al.*, 1979b) respectively, were able to evoke
production of specific antibodies in rabbits.

An alternative method is to inject the gel slice which contains the protein of
choice into the rabbit. This is particularly useful in those cases where trace
impurities are co-purified with the protein of choice, but they can be clearly
separated by the gel electrophoresis system. We have used this technique to
prepare antibody against sodium dodecyl sulphate–polyacrylamide gel electrophoresis (SDS–PAGE) purified clathrin, and have shown that the antibody is specific to clathrin (Garbern and Wu, 1981).

Since we obtained specific antibody against GAD, one way to produce
more antibody is to isolate precipitating antigen–antibody complexes from
immunodiffusion or immunoelectrophoresis gels and use these precipitates
for immunization. Because of the enhanced antigenicity of such antigen–
antibody precipitates, nanogram quantities of antigen are sufficient to
provoke antibody production (Krøll and Andersen, 1976). One drawback of
this otherwise sensitive method is the possibility of contamination, and hence

it is necessary to wash the precipitates extensively to remove all the non-specific proteins before they can be used as immunogens. The anti-GAD sera used in all the subsequent immunochemical and immunocytochemical studies were obtained from rabbits which had been immunized with a total of 50–150 μg of purified GAD over a period of 2 months.

VI CHARACTERIZATION OF ANTIBODIES

VI.1 Immunodiffusion and Immunoelectrophoresis Tests

When antiserum against the purified GAD was tested with a crude GAD preparation, a single precipitin band was obtained (Figure 11). Furthermore, this precipitation band contained GAD activity suggesting that the precipitation band is GAD–anti-GAD complex and the antiserum is specific to GAD. Similar results were obtained with immunoelectrophoresis in which a single precipitation band was formed, when crude GAD preparations which had been electrophoresed in agarose gel were incubated with anti-GAD serum (Wong *et al.*, 1974).

For immunodiffusion and immunoelectrophoresis tests, we employed either the serum or γ-globulin fraction which was obtained from serum at 50% saturation of ammonium sulphate. In order to increase the sensitivity of immunodiffusion and immunoelectrophoresis, the immunodiffusion plate or immunoelectrophoresis gel after an extensive wash can be stained for protein with Coomassie blue or by autoradiographic technique using ^{125}I-labelled protein A because of the affinity of protein A with the Fc (constant fragment) portion of the mammalian IgG. We have used this technique to visualize the precipitin band which may be too faint to be photographed as in the case of clathrin and anti-clathrin (Garbern and Wu, 1981). We have also used the peroxidase-labelled antibody method which was introduced by Nakane and Pierce (1966, 1967) for localizing tissue antigens to stain the precipitin bands formed in agar immunodiffusion tests (Matsuda *et al.*, 1973). Briefly, crude GAD preparations were incubated with anti-GAD serum, followed by extensive wash, incubation with peroxidase-labelled goat anti-rabbit IgG, and finally, the agar plate was stained with 0.01% (v/v) H_2O_2 and 2.5 mM 3,3′-diaminobenzidine in 0.05 M Tris-HCl, pH 7.6.

VI.2 Enzyme Inhibition Test

GAD activity was inhibited to a maximum of bout 50% by incubating with excess of anti-GAD serum for 24 h at 4 °C (Saito *et al.*, 1974c). Almost all of the enzyme activity was precipitated, presumably in the form of GAD–anti-GAD complex, when GAD (17 μg protein) was incubated with an approximately equal amount of anti-GAD serum (Matsuda *et al.*, 1973). The activity of the enzyme in the precipitates was a linear function of incubation time for at least 30 min at 37 °C, an indication that the enzymatic activity in the precipitates was stable and that it was possible to employ the usual assay procedure for GAD on these precipitates. The K_m value for glutamic acid of the control enzyme which was incubated with unimmunized rabbit serum was 0.6 mM and that of the precipitates was 1.8 mM. In similar experiments we found that the K_m values for pyridoxal phosphate of the control enzyme and of precipitates were 2×10^{-8} M and 10×10^{-8} M, respectively. Thus, the affinities of the precipitates for both substrate and co-enzyme were significantly less than those of the control enzyme.

Substrate, co-enzyme, and competitive inhibitors, e.g. D-glutamate and Cl⁻ could only slightly protect the enzyme from inhibition by anti-GAD, suggesting either that the antigenic site and the catalytic site are different or the affinity between GAD and anti-GAD is much higher than affinities between GAD and L-glutamate, pyridoxal phosphate, or competitive inhibitors.

VI.3   Microcomplement Fixation Test

Since serum from unimmunized rabbits also interfered with the fixation of complement, it was necessary to employ IgG for microcomplement fixation tests. IgG was obtained either from serum or from the γ-globulin fraction by DEAE chromatography as described by Fahey (1967). A typical fixation curve is shown in Figure 12A. Fifty per cent fixation of complement was obtained with about 6 μg of anti-GAD IgG and 40 ng of GAD. Previously, we have shown that the fixation curves obtained with the partially purified GAD and the purified GAD preparations became superimposable when the amount of GAD protein was estimated from the specific activities of GAD preparations, suggesting that the antiserum is specific to GAD only (Saito *et al.*, 1974c). Micro-complement fixation can be employed to determine the actual quantity of antigen protein in a crude preparation. For instance, in case of GAD, the extent of complement fixed was roughly proportional to the amount of GAD in the range of 15–50 ng of GAD (Figure 12A). In addition, microcomplement fixation test can be used to distinguish antigens with subtle differences in their structure. For instance, microcomplement fixation has been reported to be capable of distinguishing lactate dehydrogenases with a single amino acid difference (Wilson *et al.*, 1964).

VI.4   Enzyme Immunoassay

Although microcomplement fixation is a sensitive method for quantitation of antigens, this method cannot be applied to those antigens which do not fix complements in microcomplement fixation reactions or do that only to a small extent, although they cross-react with the specific antibody. For instance, GAD from brain of frog and bird does not show any complement fixation,

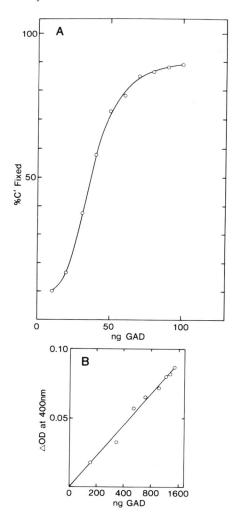

Figure 12 (**A**) Microcomplement fixation curve of GAD. The amounts of complement fixed (in percentages) are plotted against the amounts of GAD (ng). The amount
of GAD was calculated from the protein concentrations and the specific activities of
the samples by expressing the latter as a percentage of the specific activity of the
purified enzyme. Six micrograms of anti-GAD IgG was used in each tube. (**B**) Enzyme
immunoassay of GAD. Anti-GAD IgG was coupled to Sepharose 4B to form an
immobilized complex. The Sepharose–anti-GAD IgG complex was incubated with
peroxidase-labelled GAD and various amounts of free GAD at 4 °C for 18 h. After
the incubation the peroxidase activity in the precipitate was measured. The inhibition
of the binding of peroxidase–GAD to Sepharose–anti-GAD IgG by free GAD was
expressed as the difference of OD in the precipitate at 400 nm. The plot shows the OD
at 400 nm versus the amount of free GAD in logarithms

although they cross-reacted with antibody against the purified mouse brain GAD as shown in immunodiffusion tests (Saito *et al.*, 1974c; also see Section VII.1). Recently, we have developed an enzyme immunoassay for GAD, which it is hoped will enable us to determine the actual quantity of GAD proteins from various sources in addition to the enzyme activity. The basic principles of the enzyme immunoassay are the same as those for radioimmunoassay. Thus, the method involves incubation of a determined quantity of enzyme-labelled antigen with increasing concentration of unlabelled one, in the presence of a given amount of antibody directed against this antigen. The extent of binding of the enzyme-labelled antigen in the presence of known varying amounts of unlabelled antigen allows the establishment of a reference curve from which unknown concentrations of the antigen in samples can be determined. Several enzymes have been used to label antigens for the quantitation of the corresponding antigens, e.g., glucoamylase-labelled insulin (Ishikawa, 1973), peroxidase-labelled human IgG (Avrazmeas and Guilbert, 1972). Such a method will be particularly useful for detecting GAD which cross-react with anti-mouse GAD, but which do not show any complement fixation or do so only to a small extent, as in the case for GAD from several other species. With peroxidase-labelled GAD and immobilized anti-GAD IgG (see Section III.7 for details of the coupling procedures), we could detect GAD in nanogram quantities, a sensitivity that is comparable to that of the microcomplement fixation procedure (Figure 12B). We believe that the sensitivity of enzyme immunoassay still can be greatly increased by selecting an enzyme with a high turnover number and a substrate that forms a product with a high extinction coefficient, e.g. alkaline or acid phosphatase, and by optimizing the assay conditions.

VII APPLICATION OF ANTIBODIES

VII.1 Species-Specificity

The species-specificity of GAD was examined by the double diffusion, enzyme inhibition, and microcomplement fixation tests employing the concentrated crude GAD preparations (150–300 μg of protein) from various species. In immunodiffusion tests, single precipitation bands were observed with anti-mouse brain GAD serum and crude GAD preparations from rat, rabbit, quinea-pig, quail, pigeon, human, calf, and frog (Figure 13). The precipitation bands with the preparations from quail, pigeon, and frog brain showed spurs; no precipitation band was obtained with the preparation from trout brain. Recently, we have purified GAD from catfish brain and obtained antibodies against the fish enzyme (Su *et al.*, 1979). Antibodies against catfish GAD were found to cross-react with GAD from goldfish, chick, frog, turtle, *Drosophila*, and crayfish (Su *et al.*, 1980). Thus, the combination of anti-

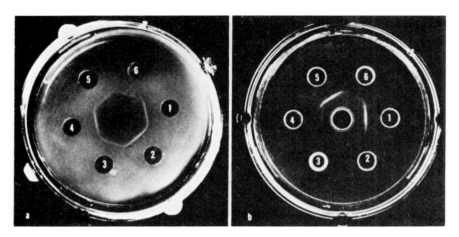

Figure 13 Ouchterlony double diffusion test with GAD from various species. Centre well contained 30 μl of anti-GAD serum in both (a) and (b). Outer wells contained 30 μl of crude GAD preparations from brain of the following species: (**a**) Mouse (well 1), rat (2), rabbit (3), guinea-pig (4), quail (5), and pigeon (6). (**b**) Mouse (wells 1 and 5), bovine (2), trout (3), frog (4), and human (6)

mouse GAD and anti-catfish GAD would enable us to use immunological methods to examine the GABAergic system in almost all the vertebrate species and also some invertebrate species (see also Chapter 6, section X for species-specifity of anti-DBH antibodies).

In enzyme inhibition tests a crude GAD preparation from mouse and rat brain was inhibited maximally to the extent of 50% and 35% by anti-GAD IgG, respectively. GAD preparations from other species were only slightly inhibited (5–10%) with the exception of that prepared from pigeon, which was inhibited to an extent of 20% (Table 2). These results are quantitatively comparable, for the GAD had similar specific activities in all of the preparations except for those from human and calf brain. A two-fold increase of antibody did not affect the extent of inhibition, indicating that antibody was in excess. IgG from a non-immunized rabit did not inhibit GAD activities from any of the species tested.

In microcomplement fixation tests, the fixation curves obtained with the crude GAD preparation and purified GAD solution became superimposable when the plots were made on the basis of the amount of antigen (the crude extract had a specific activity of 0.03 units/mg protein, which is 1% of the content of the purified enzyme). The complement fixation curves obtained with crude GAD preparations from mouse, rat, and human were very similar. The maximal degree of fixation with GAD from calf, rabbit, and guinea-pig was about 40–65% (Figure 14). GAD from quail, pigeon, frog, and trout did not react at all under these conditions.

Table 2 Inhibition of GAD from different species by antibody against mouse brain enzyme[a]

Species	Specific activity (units/mg × 10^2)[b]	Inhibition by antibody (%)
Mouse	2.5–3.0	50
Rat	2.9	35
Rabbit	2.0	13
Guinea-pig	2.0	0
Calf	0.45	8
Human	0.16	8
Quail	29	0
Pigeon	2.0	22
Frog	3.1	0
Trout	3.3	7

[a] The enzyme was incubated with an excess of antibody (IgG) at 4 °C for 18 h before the enzyme activity was measured.
[b] 1 unit = 1 μmol of GABA formed per minute at 37 °C under standard conditions.

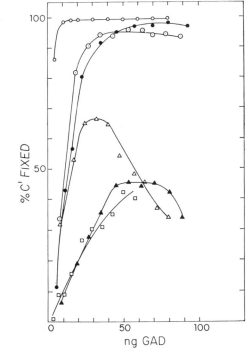

Figure 14 Microcomplement fixation curves with crude GAD preparations from brain of various species: Mouse (○), human (⊙), rat (●), rabbit (△), calf (▲) and guinea-pig (□) crude enzymes. Results are plotted in terms of complement fixed (percentage) as a function of the amount of antigen. Fixation was 40 h at 4 °C with 5 μg of anti-GAD IgG

VII.2 Tissue-Specificity

Although GABA and GAD were originally believed to exist exclusively in the central nervous system in vertebrate (Roberts and Frankel, 1950), with more sensitive methods, GABA has been detected in kidney and GAD activity has also been detected in glia and non-neural tissues such as kidney, heart, liver, and blood vessels (Zachmann *et al.*, 1966; Haber *et al.*, 1969; Whelan *et al.*, 1969; Kuriyama *et al.*, 1970; Wu *et al.*, 1974; Wu, 1976b, 1977; Wu *et al.*, 1978a). We have used five methods, namely radiometric CO_2 method (Roberts *et al.*, 1963), the rapid filtration–ion exchange method (Chude and Wu, 1976), the ion exchange column method (Kravitz *et al.*, 1965), the electrophoretic separation, and amino acid analysis (Chude and Wu, 1976), to measure GAD activity in brain, heart, kidney, and liver. Results from the latter four methods agreed well, showing that brain had the highest activity, 4.27 nmol/min/mg protein (100%), followed by heart (7.4%), kidney (6.3%), and liver (1.5%) (Wu *et al.*, 1978a). Measurement of brain GAD using the radio-metric CO_2 assay method agreed with the other techniques. However, in heart, kidney, and liver the GAD activities measured by the CO_2 method were about 3–4 times higher than those obtained by the GABA method, suggesting that the CO_2 method does not give a valid measurement of GAD activity in a crude non-neural tissue preparation (Table 3).

The identity or non-identity of GAD from various tissues has also been examined immunochemically using antibodies against the purified GAD from mouse brain. In immunodiffusion tests, anti-GAD serum was shown to cross-react with the crude GAD preparations from whole mouse brain and spinal cord, while no precipitin band could be seen with GAD preparations from mouse heart, kidney, and liver. All the precipitin bands were fused together and no spur was observed.

In enzyme inhibition tests, the GAD activities of brain and spinal cord preparations were inhibited by anti-GAD IgG to an extent of about 70%. GAD preparations from heart, kidney, and liver were not inhibited by anti-GAD IgG under the same conditions as those employed for brain and spinal cord. The amount of anit-GAD IgG used in each experiment was in excess as a three-fold increase of anti-GAD IgG did not change the degree of inhibition.

In microcomplement fixation tests, GAD preparations from spinal cord and brain showed similar complement fixation curves in both the extent of fixation and the shape of the curve, and no fixation was observed with GAD preparations from heart, kidney, and liver. Fifty per cent fixation of complement was obtained with about 20 ng of GAD and 5 µg of anti-GAD IgG.

From the above discussion, it is clear that at least in the mammalian system, GAD in the non-neural tissues is different from the neuronal GAD. The

Table 3 Distribution of L-glutamate decarboxylase activity in various tissues of mouse

Activity (units = 10^3/mg protein)

| Tissue | CO_2 Method | GABA Method | | | | Activity assigned (units × 10^3) mg protein | Percentage[e] |
		Column separation[a]	Electrophoresis separation[b]	Filtration method[c]	amino acid analysis[d]		
Brain	4.63	4.55	4.68	4.25	3.60	4.27	100
Heart	0.82	0.35	0.30	0.29	0.32	0.315	7.4
Kidney	1.00	0.17	0.35	0.22	0.33	0.268	6.3
Liver	0.22	—	—	0.06	0.07	0.065	1.5

[a] GABA was measured as total counts in the eluate after subtracting the counts in the control sample.
[b] GABA was calculated based on the ratio of the area of GABA peak to total area in electrophoresis.
[c] GABA was calculated from counts in the filtrate after subtracting counts in the control sample.
[d] GABA was calculated from counts in fractions corresponding to GABA peak in the standard.
[e] GAD activity in brain homogenate was used as reference, 100%.

functional aspect of GABA and GAD in non-neural tissues is totally unknown.

VII.3 Immunocytochemical Studies

Another important aspect of immunochemical studies is to apply the antibodies specific to GAD for immunocytochemical localization of GAD at precise cellular and subcellular levels. In the past, we chose to use peroxidase-labelled antibody method (Nakane and Pierce, 1966, 1967; see also Chapter 3) to localize GAD on tissue sections. In principle, rabbit antibody reacts with the tissue antigen and after the removal of the unreacted globulin by washing, the antibody antigen complex is localized by reacting the tissue with peroxidase-labelled sheep anti-rabbit γ-globulin. With the peroxidase-labelled antibody method, it was possible to visualize GAD at light and electron microscopic levels in various regions of rat central nervous system (Saito *et al.*, 1974a; McLaughlin *et al.*, 1974, 1975a,b).

More recently, we have modified the peroxidase–antiperoxidase procedure of Sternberger *et al.* (1970) by substituting the second antibody, goat anti-rabbit IgG, with protein A, and we have localized GAD in habenula (Gottesfeld *et al.*, 1980) and retina (Lam *et al.*, 1979; Brandon *et al.*, 1979, 1980; Wu *et al.*, 1981a). Briefly, rats were anaesthetized and perfused via intracardiac perfusion with the periodate–lysine–paraformaldehyde fixative (0.01 M periodate, 0.075 M lysine, 2% formaldehyde, and 0.037 M sodium phosphate, pH 6.2) of McLean and Nakane (1974). The perfusion procedure was taken from Palay and Chan-Palay (1974). After perfusion, tissues were removed and fixed overnight at 4 °C in 2% formaldehyde in PBS. Tissues were sectioned with a vibratome to give 40–50 μm sections.

For staining, sections were incubated in 20×60 mm plastic Petri dishes on an orbital rotator at room temperature, in the following sequence: (for conventional PAP protocol see Chapter 4, section IV, for light microscopy, and Chapter 11, section III for electron microscopy)

—20% dimethylsulphoxide in 25 mM sodium phosphate/130 mM NaCl, pH 7.2 (PBS), 1 h, *OR*
 0.025% digitonin in PBS, 2 h (aids antibody penetration), *OR*
 0.2% Triton X-100 in PBS (solubilizes membrane lipids extensively).
—10% normal goat serum in PBS, 2 h (blocks 'non-specific' IgG binding).
—PBS, 30 min (wash)
—anti-GAD or control (preimmune serum or antiserum pre-absorbed with the purified antigen) serum dilutions of 1:250 to 1:500, in PBS containing 0.1% normal goat serum. 16 h, 4 °C with orbital agitation.
—PBS, 2×60 min (wash).
—protein A solution (50 μg/ml), 1.5 h.
—PBS, 2×60 min (wash).

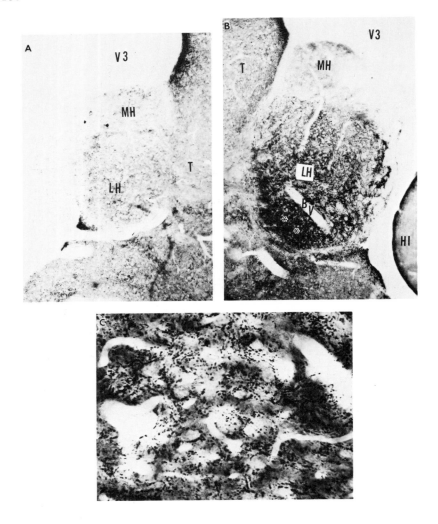

Figure 15 Immunocytochemical localization of GAD in the habenula. (**A**) Contra-lateral habenula, 5 months after stria medullaris lesion. GAD reaction product is markedly diminished in the lateral habenula (LH), while staining in the medial habenula (MH) is unaffected. The size of the nucleus is dramatically reduced as a result of the lesion. (**B**) Control side. Dense punctate reaction product fills the LH, especially its ventrolateral aspect. The MH is lightly stained. (**C**) High-magnification view of the punctate staining observed in a portion of the intact LH. (**A,B**: Magnification ×137; **C**, ×550; BV, blood vessel; HI, hippocampus; T, thalamic region; V3, third ventricle)

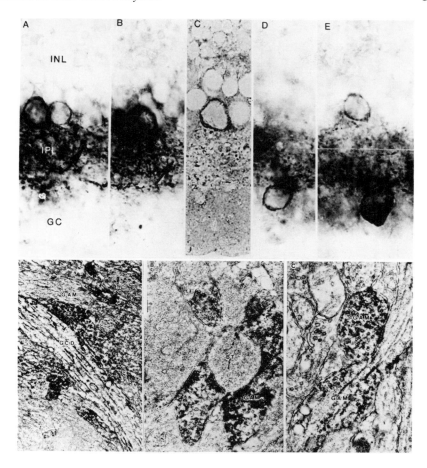

Figure 16 Localization of GAD in rabbit retina.
Upper pictures (**A** and **B**): 50 μm sections showing amacrine processes descending into the IPL (arrowheads). (**C**) One-micron section through a similarly stained cell. (**D**) A probable misplaced GAD-containing amacrine cell, (**E**) An unidentified stained cell body lying in the ganglion cell layer beneath a labelled amacrine cell (×550).
Lower pictures: a GAD-positive process presynaptic to a large ganglion cell dendrite (**A**, ×15,500), to a bipolar cell terminal (**B**, ×21,590), and to an amacrine process (**C**, ×28,765).

—peroxidase–antiperoxidase complex (1:100 dilution or 45 μg/ml), 1.5 h
—PBS, 2 × 60 min (wash).
—30 mg diaminobenzidine tetrahydrochloride in 50 ml PBS + 0.015% H_2O_2, 5–8 min, to develop reaction product.
Figures 15 and 16 illustrate typical results obtained following this protocol.

VIII   CONCLUDING REMARKS

This brief review described the approaches that have been taken in the author's laboratory in the elucidation of GABAergic pathways in various parts of the vertebrate central nervous system, starting with the purification of the GABA-synthesizing enzyme, GAD, to homogeneity, followed by production and characterization of anti-GAD serum and finally the visualization of GAD-containing neurons at light and electron microscopic levels by immunocytochemical techniques. This approach has proved to be very fruitful, at least in our hands.

ACKNOWLEDGEMENTS

This work was supported in part by grant NS 13224 from the National Institutes of Health, US. Contributions from Drs T. Matsuda, K. Saito, C. Brandon, and T. Y. Y. Su are gratefully acknowledged.

REFERENCES

Avrameas, S. and Guilbert, B. (1972). 'Enzyme-immunoassay for the measurement of antigens using peroxidase conjugates.' *Biochimie*, **54**, 837–842.

Baxter, C. F. (1970). 'The nature of γ-aminobutyric acid.' In Lajtha, A. (ed.),: *Handbook of Neurochemistry*, vol. 3, pp. 289–353. Plenum Press, New York.

Bazemore, A. W., Elliott, K. A., and Florey, E. (1957). 'Isolation of factor I.' *J. Neurochem.*, **1**, 334–339.

Brandon, C., Lam, D. M. K., and Wu, J.-Y. (1979). 'The γ-aminobutyric acid system in rabbit retina: localization by immunochemistry and autoradiography.' *Proc. Natl. Acad. Sci. USA*, **76**, 3557–3561.

Brandon, C., Lam, D. M. K., Su, Y. Y. T., and Wu, J.-Y. (1980). 'Immunocytochemical localization of GABA neurons in the rabbit and frog retina.' *Brain Res. Bull.*, **5**, (Suppl. 2), 21–29.

Brandon, C. and Wu, J.-Y. (1977). 'Electrophoretic and immunochemical characterization of choline acetyltransferase from *Torpedo*.' *Society of Neuroscience, Abstract*, vol. **3**, 404.

Brandon, C. and Wu, J.-Y. (1978). 'Purification and properties of choline acetyltransferase from *Torpedo*.' *J. Neurochem.*, **30**, 791–797.

Chude, O. and Wu, J.-Y. (1976). 'A rapid method for assaying enzymes whose substrates and products differ by charge: Application to brain L-glutamate decarboxylase.' *J. Neurochem.*, **27**, 83–86.

Cuatrecasas, P. (1972). 'Affinity chromatography of macromolecules.' *Adv. in Enzymol.*, **36**, 29–90.

Cuatrecasas, P. and Anfinsen, C. (1971). 'Affinity chromatography.' *Ann. Rev. Biochem.*, **40**, 259–280.

Fahey, J. L. (1967). 'Chromatographic separation of immunoglobulins.' In Williams, C. A. and Chase, M. W. (eds), *Methods in Immunology and Immunochemistry*, vol. 1, p. 321. Academic Press, New York.

Florey, E. (1957). 'Further evidence for the transmitter-function of factor I.' *Naturwissenschaften*, **44**, 424–425.

Fonnum, F. (1975). 'The localization of glutamate decarboxylase, choline acetyltransferase, and aromatic amino acid decarboxylase in mammalian and invertebrate nervous tissue.' In Berl, S., Clarke, D. D., and Schneider, D. (eds), *Metabolic Compartmentation and Neurotransmission*, pp. 99–122. Plenum Press, New York.

Garbern, J.-Y. and Wu, J.-Y. (1981). 'Purification and characterization of clathrin from bovine brain.' *J. Neurochem.* **36**, 602–612.

Gottesfeld, Z., Brandon, C., Jacobowitz, D. M., and Wu, J.-Y. (1980). 'The GABA system in the mammalian habenula.' *Brain Res. Bull.*, **5**, (Suppl. 2), 1–6.

Haber, B., Kuriyama, K., and Roberts, E. (1969). 'Decarboxylation of glutamate by tissues other than brain, non-identity with CNS GAD.' *Fedn. Proc. Fedn. Am. Socs. Exp. Biol.*, **28**, 577.

Ishikawa, E. (1973). 'Enzyme immunoassay of insulin by fluorimetry of the insulin-glucoamylase complex.' *J. Biochem.*, **73**, 1319–1321.

Kravitz, E. A. (1967). 'Acetylcholine, γ-aminobutyric acid and glutamic acid: physiological and chemical studies related to their roles as neurotransmitter agents.' In Quarton, G. C., Melnechuk, T., and Schmitt, F. O. (eds), *The Neurosciences*, pp. 433–444. Rockefeller University Press, New York.

Kravitz, E. A., Molinoff, P. B., and Hall, Z. W. (1965). 'A comparison of the enzymes and substrates of gamma-aminobutyric acid metabolism in lobster excitory and inhibitory axons.' *Proc. Natl. Acad. Sci. USA*, **54**, 778–782.

Krnjevic, K. (1974). 'Chemical nature of synaptic transmission in vertebrates.' *Physiol. Rev.*, **54**, 418–540.

Krøll, J. and Andersen, M. M. (1976). 'Specific antisera produced by immunization with precipitin lines.' *J. Immunol. Methods*, **13**, 125–130.

Kuriyama, K., Haber, B., and Roberts, E. (1970). 'Occurrence of a new L-glutamic acid decarboxylase in several blood vessels of the rabbit.' *Brain Res.*, **23**, 121–133.

Kuriyama, K., Haber, B., Sisken, T., and Roberts, E. (1966). 'The γ-aminobutyric acid system in rabbit cerebellum.' *Proc. Natl. Acad. Sci. USA*, **55**, 846–849.

Kuriyama, K., Sisken, T., Haber, B., and Roberts, E. (1968). 'The γ-aminobutyric acid system in rabbit retina.' *Brain Res.*, **9**, 165–168.

Lam, D. M. K., Su, Y. Y. T., Swain, L., Marc, R. E., Brandon, C., and Wu, J.-Y. (1979). 'Immunocytochemical localization of glutamic acid decarboxylase in goldfish retina.' *Nature*, **278**, 565–567.

Lasek, R. J. and Wu, J.-Y. (1976). 'Immunochemical analysis of the proteins comprising myxicola (10 nm) neurofilaments.' *Abstract of the Sixth Annual Meeting of Society for Neuroscience*, p. 40.

Matsuda, T., Wu, J.-Y., and Roberts, E. (1973). 'Immunochemical studies on glutamic acid decarboxylase from mouse brain.' *J. Neurochem.*, **21**, 159–166.

McLaughlin, B. J., Barber, R., Saito, K., Roberts, E., and Wu, J.-Y. (1975a). 'Immunocytochemical localization of glutamate decarboxylase in rat spinal cord.' *J. Comp. Neural.*, **164**, 305–322.

McLaughlin, B. J., Wood, J. G., Saito, K., Barber, R., Vaughn, J. E., Roberts, E., and Wu, J.-Y. (1974). 'The fine structural localization of glutamate decarboxlase in synaptic terminals of rodent cerebellum.' *Brain Res.*, **76**, 377–391.

McLaughlin, B. J., Wood, J. G., Saito, K., Roberts, E., and Wu, J.-Y. (1975b). 'The fine ultrastructural localization of glutamate decarboxylase in developing axonal processes and presynaptic terminals of rodent cerebellum.' *Brain Res.*, **85**, 355–371.

McLean, I. W. and Nakane, P. K. (1974). 'Periodate-lysine-paraformaldehyde fixative: a new fixative for immunoelectron microscopy.' *J. Histochem. Cytochem.*, **22**, 1077–1083.

Molinoff, P. B. and Kravitz, E. A. (1968). 'The metabolism of γ-aminobutyric acid (GABA) in the lobster nervous system—glutamic decarboxylase.' *J. Neurochem.*, **15**, 391–409.

Nakane, P. K. and Pierce, G. B., Jr. (1966). Enzyme-labeled antibodies: preparation and application for the localization of antigens.' *J. Histochem. Cytochem.*, **14**, 929–931.

Nakane, P. K. and Pierce, G. B., Jr. (1967). 'Enzyme-labeled antibodies for the light and electron microscopic localization of tissue antigens.' *J. Cell Biol.*, **33**, 307–318.

Palay, S. and Chan-Palay, V. (1974). In: *Cerebellar Cortex*, pp. 322–331. Springer-Verlag, New York.

Roberts, E., Chase, T. N., and Tower, D. B. (eds) (1976). *GABA in Nervous System Function*. Raven Press, New York.

Roberts, E. and Frankel, S. (1950). 'γ-Aminobutyric acid in brain.' *Fed. Proc.*, **9**, 219.

Roberts, E. and Kuriyama, K. (1968). 'Biochemical–physiological correlations in studies of the γ-aminobutyric acid system.' *Brain Res.*, **8**, 1–35.

Roberts, E., Wein, J., and Simonsen, D. G. (1964). 'γ-Aminobutyric acid (GABA), vitamin B_6, and neuronal function: a speculative synthesis.' *Vitamin. Horm.*, **22**, 503–559.

Saito, K., Barber, R., Wu, J.-Y, Matsuda, T., Roberts, E., and Vaughn, J. E. (1974a). 'Immunohistochemical localization of glutamic acid decarboxylase in rat cerebellum.' *Proc. Natl. Acad. Sci. USA*, **71**, 269–273.

Saito, K., Schousboe, A., Wu, J.-Y., and Roberts, E. (1974b). 'Some immunochemical properties and species specificity of GABA-α-ketoglutarate transaminase from mouse brain.' *Brain Res.*, **65**, 287–296.

Saito, K., Wu, J.-Y., and Roberts, E. (1974c). 'Immunochemical comparisons of vertebrate glutamate decarboxylase.' *Brain Res.*, **65**, 277–285.

Sternberger, L. A., Hardy, P. H., Jr., Cuculis, J. J., and Meyer, H. G. (1970). 'The unlabeled antibody enzyme method of immunohistochemistry. Preparation and properties of soluble antigen antibody complex (horseradish peroxidase–antihorseradish peroxidase) and its use in identification of spirochetes.' *J. Histochem. Cytochem.*, **18**, 315–333.

Su, Y. Y. T., Wu, J.-Y., and Lam, D. M. K. (1979). 'Purification of L-glutamic acid decarboxylase from catfish brain.' *J. Neurochem.*, **33**, 169–179.

Su, Y. Y. T., Wu, J.-Y., and Lam, D. M. K. (1980). 'Immunochemical comparisons of L-glutamic acid decarboxylase from different species.' *Soc. Neurosci., Abstract*, **6**, 542.

Whelan, D. T., Scriver, C. R., and Mohyuddin, F. (1969). 'Glutamic acid decarboxylase and gamma-aminobutyric acid in mammalian kidney.' *Nature*, **224**, 916–917.

Wilson, A. C., Kaplan, N. O., Levine, L., Pesce, A., Reichlin, M., and Allison, W. S. (1964). 'Evolution of lactic dehydrogenases.' *Fed. Proc.*, **23**, 1258–1266.

Wong, E., Schousboe, A., Saito, K., Wu, J.-Y., and Roberts, E. (1974). 'Glutamate decarboxylase and GABA-transaminase from six mouse strains.' *Brain Res.*, **68**, 133–139.

Wu, J.-Y. (1976a). 'Purification and properties of L-glutamate decarboxylase (GAD) and GABA-aminotransferase (GABA–T).' In Roberts, E., Chase, T., and Tower, D. (eds), *GABA in Nervous System Function*, pp. 7–55. Raven Press, New York.

Wu, J.-Y. (1976b). 'Comments on evidence for GAD II.' In Roberts, E., Chase, T., and Tower, D. (eds), *GABA in Nervous System Function*, pp. 59–60. Raven Press, New York.

Wu, J.-Y. (1977). 'Comparative study of L-glutamate decarboxylase from brain and heart with purified preparations.' *J. Neurochem.*, **28**, 1359–1367.

Wu, J.-Y. (1978). 'Microanalytical methods for neuronal analysis.' *Physiol. Rev.*, **58**(4), 863–904.

Wu, J.-Y., Brandon, C., Su, Y. Y. T., and Lam, D. M. K. (1981a). 'Immunocyto-chemical and autoradiographic localization of GABA system in the vertebrate retina.' *Molec. Cell. Biochem.* **39**, 229–238.

Wu, J.-Y., Chude, O., Wein, J., and Roberts, E. (1978a). 'Glutamate decarboxylase from neural and non-neural tissues.' *J. Neurochem.*, **30**, 849–857.

Wu, J.-Y., Matsuda, T., and Roberts, E. (1973). 'Purification and characterization of glutamate decarboxylase from mouse brain.' *J. Biol. Chem.*, **248**, 3029–3034.

Wu, J.-Y., Moss, L. G., and Chen, M. S. (1979a). 'Tissue and regional distribution of cysteic acid decarboxylase in bovine brain: a new assay method.' *Neurochem. Res.*, **4**, 201–212.

Wu, J.-Y., Moss, L. G., and Chude, O. (1978b). 'Distribution and tissue specificity of GABA-2-ketoglutarate transaminase: a new assay method.' *Neurochem. Res.*, **3**, 207–219.

Wu, J.-Y., Saito, K., Wong, E., and Roberts, E. (1974). 'Studies of L-glutamate decarboxylase and γ-aminobutyric transaminase from various tissues and species.' *Trans. Am. Soc. Neurochem.*, **5**, 112.

Wu, J.-Y., Su, Y. Y. T., Brandon, C., Lam, D. M. K., Chen, M. S., and Huang, W. M. (1979b). 'Purification and immunochemical studies of GABA-, acetylcholine-, and taurine-synthesizing enzymes from bovine and fish brains.' *Seventh International Meeting of the ISN*, p. 662.

Wu, J.-Y., Su, Y. Y. T., Lam, D. M. K., Brandon, C., and Denner, L. (1980). 'Purification and regulation of L-glutamate decarboxylase.' *Brain Res. Bull.*, **5** (Suppl. 2). 63–70.

Wu, J.-Y., Su, Y. Y. T., Lam, D. M. K., Schousboe, A., and Chude, O. (1981b). 'Assay methods, purification and characterization of L-glutamate decarboxylase and GABA-transaminase.' *Res. Methods Neurochem.*, **5**, 129–177.

Zachman, M., Tocci, P., and Nyhan, W. L. (1966). 'The occurrence of γ-aminobutyric acid in human tissues other than brain.' *J. Biol. Chem.*, **241**, 1355–1358.

Immunohistochemistry
Edited by A. C. Cuello
© 1983 IBRO

CHAPTER 8

Antibodies to Serotonin for Neuroimmunocytochemical Studies: Methodological Aspects and Applications

H. W. M. STEINBUSCH, A. A. J. VERHOFSTAD*, and H. W. J. JOOSTEN*

Department of Pharmacology, Free University, Van der Boechorststr 7, 1081 BT Amsterdam, The Netherlands
*Department of Anatomy and Embryology, University of Nijmegen, PO Box 9101, 6500 HB Nijmegen, The Netherlands

I INTRODUCTION

The presence of serotonin (5-hydroxytryptamine, 5-HT) in the central nervous system of many species has been demonstrated by a variety of bio-chemical and histochemical methods. Serotonin and its biosynthetic enzymes have been demonstrated first biochemically (Twarog and Page, 1953; Amin *et al.*, 1954; Bogdansky *et al.*, 1956). The formaldehyde-induced fluorescence method introduced in the early 1960s (Falck, 1962; Falck *et al.*, 1962; Falck and Owman, 1965) brought up the possibility of visualization of serotonin and catecholamines in histological sections of brain and spinal cord. Recently, many modifications of the original technique have been introduced, such as the use of glyoxylic acid instead of formaldehyde (Björklund *et al.*, 1972; Furness and Costa, 1975; Bloom and Battenberg, 1976; de la Torre and Surgeon, 1976), the combined use of glyoxylic acid and formaldehyde (Nygren, 1976), the combination of formaldehyde and glutaraldehyde (Furness *et al.*, 1977) and more recently, the aluminium–formaldehyde (ALFA) method (Ajelis *et al.*, 1979; Lorén *et al.*, 1980). However, in spite of all these improvements the induced fluorescence methods are rather insensitive with regard to serotonin. Moreover, its demonstration by, e.g., photomicrography is complicated by the rapid fading of the fluorescence light. In addition, since serotonin and other monoamines like DA, NA, and A are demonstrated at the same time, the induced fluorescence techniques are not quite specific. In fact, microspectrofluorimetry and pharmacological manipulations, e.g., by enzyme inhibitors or by selective destruction of serotoninergic or catecholaminergic neurons with 5,7-dihydroxytryptamine (Jonsson *et al.*, 1978) or 6-hydroxydopamine (Thoenen and Tranzer, 1973) respectively, are needed to improve sensitivity and specificity.

The introduction of immunocytochemistry using specific antibodies to enzymes involved in the synthesis of serotonin opened new possibilities to overcome this lack in specificity. Antibodies both to tryptophan hydroxylase and DDC have been used (Hökfelt *et al.*, 1973; Pickel *et al.*, 1976; Hökfelt *et al.*, 1978). However, this approach suffers from several limitations. First, isolation of these enzymes is time-consuming and needs expensive technical equipment. Second, antibodies to these enzymes are rather species-specific, which means that a certain antibody can only be used for immunocytochemical purposes in a limited number of species. Third, another, although minor disadvantage, is that localizing an enzyme by immunocytochemistry does not provide information on the question whether the enzyme studied is in its active or inactive state.

In this chapter we want to discuss the immunocytochemical approach using antibodies to serotonin. Since the serotonin molecule is too·small to be antigenic itself it needs to be coupled to a carrier protein like bovine serum albumin (BSA). In the past, several studies have been published regarding the production of antibodies to serotonin (Fillip and Schneider, 1964; Ranadive and Sehon, 1967; Peskar and Spector, 1973; Spector *et al.*, 1973; Grota and Brown, 1974; Kellum and Jaffe, 1976). However, the antibodies raised were only used in immunodiffusion tests or in radioimmunoassay. In this chapter different procedures for coupling of serotonin to BSA will be described. It will be demonstrated that antibodies to such conjugates can be used in immunocytochemical studies on the central nervous system of various species.

II PREPARATION OF THE IMMUNOGENS

Three different types of serotonin–immunogens were synthesized. In all cases BSA was used as the carrier protein.

II.1 Serotonin–Immunogen A

This was prepared according to the Mannich reaction using formaldehyde as a coupling reagent. The procedure was modified after the descriptions of Ranadive and Sehon (1967) and Grota and Brown (1974). In brief, 9.2 mg serotonin–creatinine sulphate (Sigma) in 1 ml aquadest was mixed with 28.1 mg BSA (Sigma) also dissolved in 1 ml aquadest, 1 ml 3 M sodium acetate buffer, and 1 ml 7.5% formaldehyde (Merck). In order to study the influence of the pH on the coupling reaction sodium acetate buffers with different pH were used. The reaction mixture was incubated at room temperature in a shake water-bath. The pH was readjusted after 30 min. Incubation was continued for an additional 18 h. The reaction was then stopped by dialysis for 3 days against running tap water at 4 °C. The precipitate was removed by centrifugation at 20,000 *g*. The protein concentration was measured according to Lowry *et al.* (1951). Ultraviolet absorption spectra were determined in order to estimate the molar ratio of BSA and serotonin. The immunogen-containing solution was stored at −20 °C.

II.2 Serotonin–Immunogen B

This was synthesized via a mixed anhydride reaction, as has been described by Wurzburger *et al.* (1976) for the preparation of a melatonin immunogen. The coupling procedure consists of three steps. First, diazotization of para-aminobenzoic acid (PABA): 1 mmol PABA (Sigma) was dissolved in 5 ml 1.0 N HCl at room temperature; 1 mmol sodium nitrite was dissolved in 1 ml aquadest and added dropwise to the PABA solution. After an incubation for 20 min at 4 °C the reaction was stopped by adding 0.5 M ammonium sulphamate. Second, coupling of the diazotized PABA to serotonin: 1 mmol serotonin creatinine sulphate was dissolved in 1 ml 0.1 N NaOH at room temperature. The solution was adjusted to pH 1.0. The diazotized PABA (±6 ml) was added dropwise and the reaction was continued for 2 h at 4 °C. The precipitate was removed by centrifugation at 12,000 *g* and washed several times with aquadest. The precipitate was lyophilized until further use. Third, conjugation to BSA: 0.26 mmol PABA–serotonin was dissolved in 2 ml dry dioxane, obtained by purifying this solution over a basic aluminium oxide column. Then 0.26 mmol triethylamine (Merck) at 8–10 °C was added to the PABA–5-HT solution followed by 0.26 mmol isobutylchloroformate (Sigma). The reaction was continued for 20 min at 8–10 °C; 300 mg BSA was dissolved in 1.0 ml aquadest at room temperature, after which 8 ml dry dioxane was added dropwise. The pH was readjusted to 9.0 with 0.1 N NaOH and the mixed anhydride solution was added. The reaction mixture was kept for 30 min at 8–10 °C, under constant stirring and then further stored overnight at 4 °C. The solution was dialysed for 3 days against dioxane–water (1:1) and finally for 1 day against aquadest. The immunogen was lyophilized until further use. The molar ratios of BSA to serotonin were estimated from ultraviolet absorption spectra.

II.3   Serotonin–Immunogen C

This was prepared by means of a carbodiimide reaction previously described by Holloway *et al.* (1980) for the conjugation melatonin to BSA. The first steps in the preparation of immunogen C are similar to the first and second part of the procedure followed for immunogen B. However, the final step, i.e. conjugation to BSA, is different: 200 mg PABA–serotonin in 10 ml 10 mM PBS buffer, pH 6.5, was mixed with 400 mg BSA in 10 ml 10 mM PBS buffer and 200 mg 1-ethyl-3-(3-dimethylaminopropyl)-carbodiimide HCl (ECDI; Sigma) in 10 ml 10 mM PBS buffer. The reaction was heavily stirred for 4 h at room temperature. Then the reaction mixture was dialysed for 3 days against running tap water. The immunogen was lyophilized until further use. The molar ratio of BSA to serotonin was also estimated from ultraviolet absorption spectra.

III   PREPARATION OF THE ANTISERA

Antibodies were raised in rabbits. Each animal received 0.5 ml of an immunogen-containing solution (2 mg protein/ml) emulsified in 0.5 ml complete Freund's adjuvant (Difco) intracutaneously at eight different sides. Booster injections with incomplete Freund's adjuvant were given 3-weekly intramuscularly in the hind limb at four sides.

Serum samples were taken just before immunization (pre-immune serum) and 8 days after the booster injections. These samples were tested by immunodiffusion according to Ouchterlony (1967), immunoelectrophoresis, and immunofluorescence microscopy. Since antibodies with a high affinity to BSA caused unwanted staining of collagen-rich tissues, as i.e. blood vessel walls, all sera to be used for immunofluorescence or immunoperoxidase staining were previously purified by liquid-phase absorption with BSA (3–5 mg/ml) or by solid-phase absorption using a Sepharose 4B–CNBr-activated BSA column (for a more detailed description of the purification, see Steinbusch *et al.*, 1978).

IV   IMMUNOCYTOCHEMICAL STAINING PROCEDURES

Two different immunocytochemical staining techniques have been applied. Firstly, the indirect immunofluorescence staining according to Coons (1958; see Chapter 2) on cryostat sections and secondly, the peroxidase–antiperoxidase (PAP) method described by Sternberger and co-workers (1970; see Chapter 4) on Vibratome sections. Mostly, brains and spinal cords of untreated animals were used; however, where cell bodies or dendrites were studied, animals were pretreated with the monoamine oxidase inhibitor Nialamide (Sigma; 100 mg/kg body weight: intraperitoneally, 2 h before sacrificing). We have used male albino rats (Wistar strain) anaesthetized with sodium pentobarbital (60 mg/kg body weight, injected intraperitoneally). Trouts (*Salmo gairdneri*) and lampreys (*Lampetra fluviatilis*) were anaesthetized by adding MS-222 (Sandoz) to the water in which they were kept. All animals were perfused through the heart with 50 ml ice-cold oxygen-enriched, Ca^{2+}-free Tyrode's buffer, followed by 250 ml ice-cold 4% paraformaldehyde dissolved in 0.1 M sodium phosphate buffer, pH 7.3, in 30 min at a pressure of 50 mmHg. The brains and the spinal cords were rapidly removed and postfixed in the same fixative for 2 h at 4 °C. Tissue pieces were rinsed in 5% sucrose dissolved in 0.1 M sodium phosphate buffer, pH 7.3, for 24 h at 4 °C if they were studied by immunofluorescence. This step need not to be included in cases where Vibratome sections are processed with the PAP-technique.

IV.1 Immunofluorescence Staining of Cryostat Sections

Tissue pieces were frozen on cryostat chucks with carbon dioxide gas. Sections were cut at 10 μm thickness on a cryostat (Dittes, Heidelberg, GFR) at −25 °C and were mounted on glass slides coated with chrome–alum gelatine. The staining procedure was as follows:

—rinsing with 0.1 M phosphate buffered saline (PBS), pH 7.3, at room temperature (10–30 min);
—overnight incubation at 4 °C with antisera or pre-immune sera diluted 1:500 with PBS containing 0.1% Triton X-100;
—rinsing in PBS at room temperature (30 min);
—incubation at room temperature with fluorescein isothiocyanate (FITC) conjugated sheep antirabbit immunoglobulins (Statens Bakteriologiska Laboratorium, Stockholm, Sweden) diluted 1:16 with PBS also containing 0.1% Triton X-100 (30 min);
—rinsing in PBS at room temperature (30 min);
—mounting in a mixture of glycerine and PBS (3:1, vol/vol).

The sections were examined in a Zeiss Universal microscope equipped for fluorescence with incident illumination. Kodak Tri-X film was used for photomicrography. The slides were stored at −20 °C.

IV.2 Immunoperoxidase Staining of Vibratome Sections (see also PAP protocol in Chapter 9, Section IV.2)

Tissue pieces (8 mm in thickness) were mounted on chucks of a Vibratome

(Oxford Instruments) with a cyanoacrylate adhesive (Loctite, I.S. 495). After drying for 5 min the tissue slices were kept in ice-cold 0.1 M sodium phosphate buffer, pH 7.3, until sectioning. Serial sections of 50 or 100 μm thickness were cut at a vibration rate of 8–9 and a feeding speed of 2–4 scale units. The sections were collected in counting tubes up to a maximum of 10 sections in 2 ml 0.1 M PBS, pH 7.3, and kept at 4 °C. The staining procedure was as follows:

—incubation at 4 °C with an antiserum or a pre-immune serum diluted 1:1500 with PBS containing 0.2% (vol/vol) Triton X-100 (overnight);
—rinsing in PBS containing 0.2% Triton X-100, then in PBS containing 0.1% Triton X-100 and finally in PBS without Triton X-100 at room temperature (5 min each);
—incubation with goat anti-rabbit immunoglobulins (Fc specific; Nordic, Tilburg, The Netherlands) diluted 1:30 with PBS at room temperature (2 h);
—rinsing twice in PBS at room temperature (10 min each);
—incubation with rabbit-PAP (Dakopatts, Copenhagen, Denmark) diluted 1:90 with PBS at room temperature (1 h);
—rinsing twice in PBS at room temperature (10 min each);
—pre-staining at room temperature in a solution containing 3,3-diamino-benzidine HCl (0.75 mg/ml, Sigma) and $CaCl_2$ (120 μm) in 50 mM Tris–HCl, pH 7.7;
—staining at room temperature in the same solution after adding H_2O_2 to a final concentration of 0.03% (15 min); mounting on glass slides coated with chrome alum gelatine; air-drying overnight and a postfixation for 10 min with 2% glutaraldehyde in 0.05 M Tris–HCl, pH 7.7;
—for permanent storage, sections were dehydrated and coverslipped with DepeX (Gurr). Agfapan-25 was used for photomicrography. The slides were stored at room temperature.

IV.3 Experiments

Three types of experiments were performed.

(a) Using the indirect immunofluorescence technique antisera raised with the immunogens A, B, and C were tested on cryostat sections of rat brains.
(b) The specificity of the antisera obtained after immunization with immunogen A was investigated by indirect immunofluorescence on cryostat sections of rat brain tissue. Several tests were performed. First, consecutive sections were incubated with either immune or pre-immune sera. Second, serum samples, previously absorbed with BSA, were incubated with increasing concentrations of serotonin, 5-methoxytryptamine (5-MT), DA, NA, A, octopamine (OCT), synephrine (SYN), or hista-

mine (HIST). These samples were first incubated for 1 h at 37 °C and then kept at 4 °C overnight. Third, with a similar procedure serum samples were absorbed with different immunogens, viz. BSA–5-HT (immunogen A), BSA–5-MT, BSA–DA, BSA–NA, and BSA–A.

(c) Finally, to test whether antibodies to serotonin can be used for neuro-immunocytochemical purposes irrespective of the species, brains of the lamprey (*Lampetra fluviatilis*), the trout (*Salmo giardneri*) and the rat were investigated by the indirect immunofluorescence or PAP technique on cryostat or Vibratome sections respectively. In these experiments only antibodies to immunogen A were used.

V PREPARATION, SPECIFICITY, AND APPLICATION OF SEROTONIN ANTIBODIES IN IMMUNOCYTOCHEMISTRY

Serotonin itself is not immunogenic. However, from the work of Land-steiner (1945) we know that such molecules might become immunogenic after linkage to proteins. In fact, this principle was adopted by those who reported on the preparation of antibodies against serotonin previously (Fillip and Schneider, 1964; Ranadive and Sehon, 1967; Peskar and Spector, 1973; Spector *et al.*, 1973; Grota and Brown, 1974; Kellum and Jaffe, 1976). These authors characterized their antisera by immunoprecipitation tests or radio-immunoassays only. However, we were able to show that these antibodies can be used for immunohistochemical localization of serotonin on the central nervous system (Steinbusch *et al.*, 1978).

In the following sections special attention will be given to: (1) the preparation of three types of serotonin–immunogens and some immunohisto-chemical characteristics of the antibodies raised by them; (2) specificity tests; and (3) some applications of serotonin antibodies in neuroimmunocyto-chemistry.

V.1 Preparation of Three Types of Serotonin–Immunogens and Antibodies Raised by Them

Serotonin was linked to BSA either directly or indirectly via PABA as a spacer molecule. Direct linkage (serotonin–immunogen A) was achieved by the Mannich reaction with formaldehyde as a coupling reagent. The coupling procedure was pH-dependent, as is shown in Figure 5. The highest molar ratio of about 54 was obtained at pH 6.8. It is most likely that with the procedure followed serotonin is coupled through the nitrogen atom of its indole nucleus to lysine or tyrosine residues of BSA (Figure 1). Sero-tonin–immunogens B and C were prepared differently, using PABA as a spacer molecule (indirect linkage). For serotonin–immunogen B the mixed

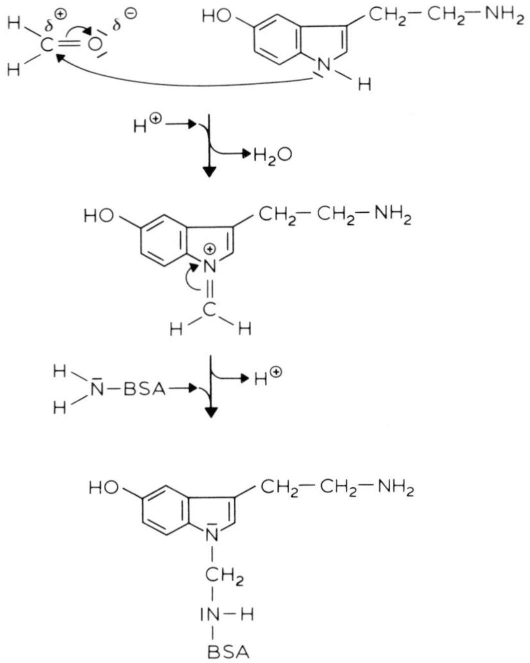

Figure 1 Preparation of the serotonin–immunogen A according to the Mannich reaction

anhydride method was adopted, isobutylchloroformate serving as a coupling reagent. Maximal molar ratios were of about 24. Probably, in this case serotonin is conjugated to BSA through its aromatic ring (Figure 2 a and b; Figure 3 A). In preparing serotonin–immunogen C coupling was achieved with a carbodiimide reagent. The highest molar ratio obtained was about 60. Most probably, serotonin–immunogens B and C have similar structures (Figure 3 A and B).

Antibodies raised by the immunogens A, B and C were tested by immunofluorescence on cryostat sections of rat brain. Antibodies to the immunogens A and B showed a similar distribution of immunoreactive cell bodies, nerve fibres, and nerve terminals after fixation by 4% para-formaldehyde dissolved in 0.1 M sodium phsophate buffer, pH 7.3. Anti-bodies to immunogen A were also tested under other fixation conditions. Thus, it was established that addition of a small amount of glutaraldehyde (0.5%) caused a decrease in the immunofluorescence intensity. Moreover, no fluorescence was obtained either in fresh-frozen tissue without fixation or after perfusion with 2% glutaraldehyde in 0.1 M cacodylate buffer, pH 7.3.

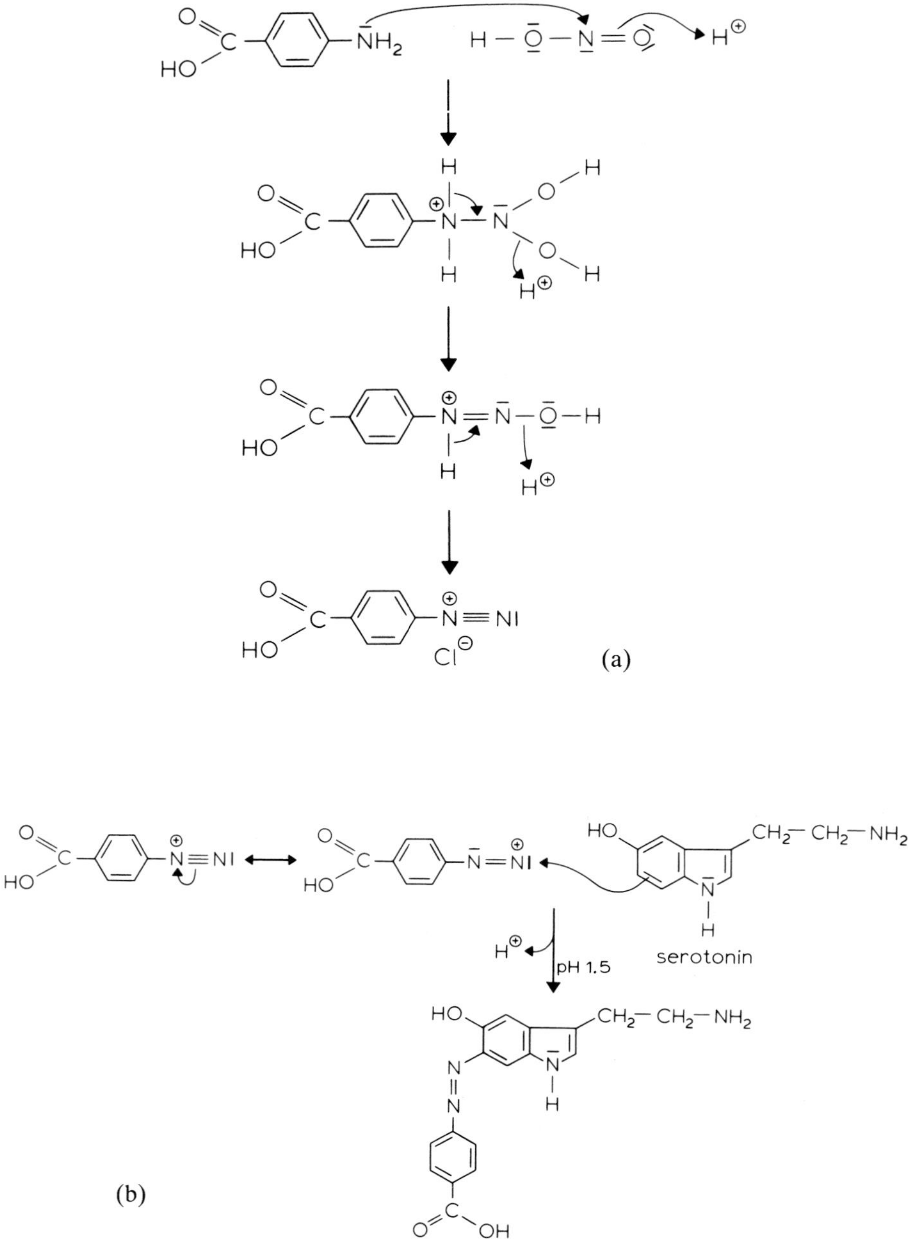

Figure 2 The first two steps in the preparation of the serotonin–immunogens B and C. (a): diazotization, (b): conjugation of PABA to serotonin

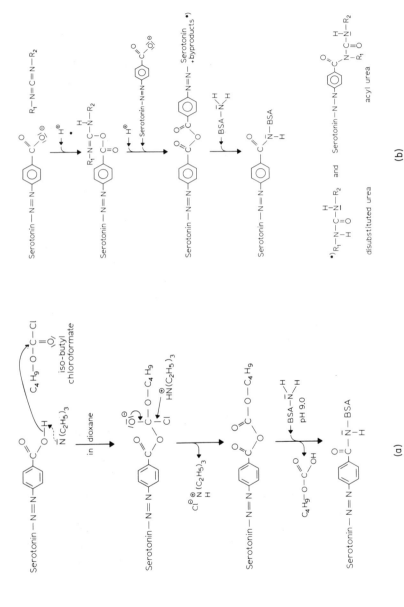

Figure 3 The last step in the preparation of the serotonin–immunogens B and C. C1: coupling to BSA by the mixed anhydride reaction (serotonin–immunogen B). C2: coupling to BSA via a carbodiimide reaction (serotonin–immunogen C)

Apparently, fixation is of utmost importance. The fixation efficiency of 4% paraformaldehyde was further demonstrated by Schipper *et al.* (1981). Using rat brain tissue and a non-biological model system, both incubated with radioactive serotonin, they showed that about 50% of the radioactivity was retained after fixation and several rinsing steps. These data, together with our findings with regard to the antibodies raised by the immunogens A and B, seem to support our supposition that antibodies to serotonin–immunogen A, first described in 1978 (Steinbusch *et al.*, 1978), are demonstrating serotonin rather than its β-carboline derivative.

No immunofluorescence was obtained with antibodies to immunogen C employing 4% paraformaldehyde fixation.

Recently, the application of antibodies to serotonin in immunohisto-chemistry was reported by two other groups. In both cases antibodies were raised by an immunogen prepared according to Peskar and Spector (1973). This immunogen, very much resembling our serotonin–immunogen C, was prepared by coupling of serotonin to a diazotized conjugate of BSA and aminophenylalanine. One group (Buffa *et al.*, 1980) reported on studies in the rat brain and spinal cord. Immunoreactive nerve axons and terminals, as well as immunoreactive cell bodies, were observed after fixation with 2% glut-araldehyde, or 2% glutaraldehyde plus 0.2% picric acid, both buffered at pH 7. However, the distribution of immunoreactive material differs from those obtained with antibodies to the presently described serotonin–immuno-gens A and B. A second group (Facer *et al.*, 1979) found immunostained cells in the gastrointestinal epithelium of several species employing *p*-benzo-quinone vapour fixation of freeze-dried material. In both cases no staining was seen after fixation by formaldehyde, which is in agreement with our findings.

If one assumes that the serotonin–immunogens B and C have similar structures the absence of immunostaining by antibodies to immunogen C in formaldehyde-fixed tissues is difficult to explain. One explanation might be a different steric configuration of the immunogens B and C due to the different coupling reactions used. Apparently, antibodies to serotonin–immunogen C do not recognize serotonergic structures as do antibodies to the immunogens A and B. Further, if serotonin–immunogen C does indeed resemble the serotonin–immunogen used by Buffa and co-workers (1980) one might suggest that the immunoreactivity they demonstrated in sections of rat brain and spinal cord is due to a different compound. Obviously, such antibodies are able to bind serotonin in a radioimmunoassay performance.

V.2 Specificity Tests

Antibodies to the immunogens B and C were obtained recently, whereas antibodies against serotonin–immunogen A have been used widely since 1978

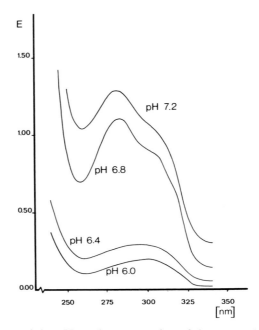

Figure 4   Influence of the pH on the preparation of the serotonin–immunogen A

(Steinbusch *et al.*, 1978). Hence, this paragraph will be devoted to the specificity of antibodies to immunogen A only. Using indirect immuno-fluorescence several tests were performed on cryostat sections of rat brain fixed by 4% paraformaldehyde. The results of these tests can be summarized as follows:

(1) Immunofluorescence could only be achieved with immune sera. No staining was seen using pre-immune sera.
(2) Serum samples incubated with increasing concentrations of different substances revealed that antibodies can be blocked by 5-MT and to a lesser extent also by DA (Table 1). From these data it may be concluded that there is a cross-reactivity of 2–3% to 5-3% to 5-MT and of less than 0.25% to DA in rat brain tissue under the conditions used for immuno-fluorescence microscopy. Cross-reactivity to the other compounds tested seems to be negligible.
(3) Immunofluorescence staining disappeared completely after absorption of the antiserum with serotonin–immunogen A. On the contrary, no reduc-tion of fluorescence intensity was observed after absorption with im-munogens to NA (BSA–NA) and A (BSA–A). These findings indicate once more that there is a negligible degree of cross-reactivity to NA and A, if any.

Table 1 Results of blocking experiments

µm	1	2	4	8	16	32	64	128	256	512	1024	2048	4096	8192
5-HT	+++	++	+	+	+	−	−	−	−	−	−	−	−	−
5-MT	+++	+++	+++	+++	+++	++	++	+	+	+	−	−	−	−
DA	+++	+++	+++	+++	+++	+++	+++	+++	+++	++	+	+	+	+
NA	+++	+++	+++	+++	+++	+++	+++	+++	+++	+++	+++	+++	+++	+++
OCT	+++	+++	+++	+++	+++	+++	+++	+++	+++	+++	+++	+++	+++	+++
A	+++	+++	+++	+++	+++	+++	+++	+++	+++	+++	+++	+++	+++	+++
SYN	+++	+++	+++	+++	+++	+++	+++	+++	+++	+++	+++	+++	+++	+++
HIST	+++	+++	+++	+++	+++	+++	+++	+++	+++	+++	++	++	++	++

Fluorescence intensity in comparable cryostat sections of the rat medulla oblongata stained with samples of an antiserum to serotonin–immunogen A purified from BSA-antibodies. These samples were incubated with different concentrations of substances as indicated. +++: normal fluorescence; ++: some inhibition; +: strong inhibition, and −: no fluorescence. 5-HT: serotonin; 5-MT: 5-methoxy-tryptamine; DA: dopamine; NA: noradrenaline; OCT: octopamine; A: adrenaline; SYN: synephrine, and HIST: histamine.

There are additional observations relevant to the matter of specificity. Thus, immunofluorescence staining in rat brain sections could be abolished or strongly reduced by treatment with the serotonin neurotoxins 5,7-dihydroxy-tryptamine (Hökfelt *et al.*, 1978; Köhler *et al.*, 1981) and parachloro-amphetamine (Köhler *et al.*, 1981) or by treatment with reserpine. Further, in the rat there is a close correlation between the distribution of serotonin immunoreactivity as revealed by antibodies to immunogen A and observations obtained by other histochemical methods, e.g., immunofluorescence microscopy using antibodies to DDC (Goldstein *et al.*, 1971; Hökfelt *et al.*, 1978) and the induced fluorescence techniques (Dahlström and Fuxe, 1964).

Although the value of each single parameter might be questioned, the combined use of the presented data strongly supports the conclusion that antibodies to serotonin–immunogen A are highly specific tools for demonstrating serotonergic neuronal structures of the rat brain and spinal cord. It seems reasonable to assume that a similar degree of specificity applies also to other species, especially if there is a good correspondence between immunohistochemical findings and previous observations made, e.g., by the induced fluorescence techniques.

V.3   Applications of Serotonin Antibodies in Neuroimmunocytochemistry

Immunoreactivity of antibodies to biosynthetic enzymes is mostly species-specific. Apparently, proteins with similar enzymatic functions may have different immunogenic properties. Therefore, application of these antibodies in immunohistochemistry is often limited to certain species. However, it may be expected that antibodies to small molecular substances like serotonin can be used irrespective of the species studied. In order to test this assumption the central nervous system of three species, viz. lamprey, trout, and rat were examined employing antibodies to the serotonin–immunogen A. Immunoreactive neuronal structures could be demonstrated clearly in all species, either by immunofluorescence on cryostat sections or by immunoperoxidase staining of Vibratome sections (Figures 5–7). In general, the distribution of the immunoreactivity corresponds well with earlier observations made by, for example, induced fluorescence techniques in the lamprey (Baumgarten, 1972), the trout (Terlou *et al.*, 1978) and the rat (Dahlström and Fuxe, 1964). In addition, cell bodies, nerve fibres and nerve terminals were also observed in other, hitherto undescribed areas, indicating the high sensitivity of the presented method. The matter of sensitivity was investigated recently by Schipper and co-workers (1981). Using model preparations it was estimated that the presently described immunofluorescence method for serotonin is approximately 1000 times as sensitive as the formaldehyde-induced fluorescence technique. Detailed descriptions of the serotonin–immunoreactivity in different species have been reported (Steinbusch *et al.*, 1978; Hökfelt *et al.*,

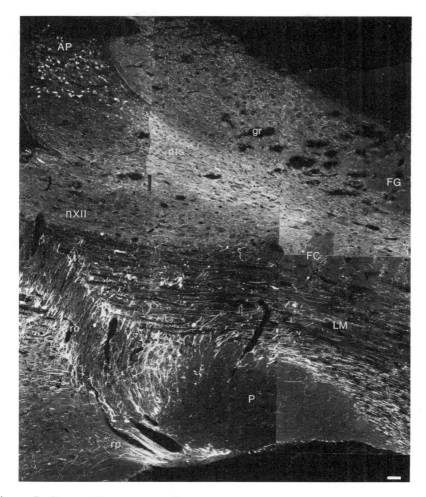

Figure 5 Immunofluorescence photomicrograph of a cryostat section midsagittal through the caudal brain stem of the rat incubated with an antiserum to serotonin–immunogen A. Numerous immunoreactive cell bodies are found in the nucleus raphe pallidus (rp), in the nucleus raphe obscurus (ro) and in the area postrema (AP). Note differences in the serotoninergic innervation of the nucleus gracilis (gr), the nucleus tractus solitarius (nts), the nucleus nervi hypoglossi (nXII), the fasciculus gracilis (FG), the fasciculus cuneatus (FC), the lemniscus medialis (LM), and the tractus corticospinalis (P). (Bar = 50 μm)

1978; Steinbusch and Verhofstad, 1979; Steinbusch and Nieuwenhuys, 1979; Köhler *et al.*, 1980; Yamamoto *et al.*, 1980; Steinbusch, 1981; Steinbusch and Nieuwenhuys, 1981; Köhler *et al.*, 1981; Frankenhuys, unpublished observations in the trout).

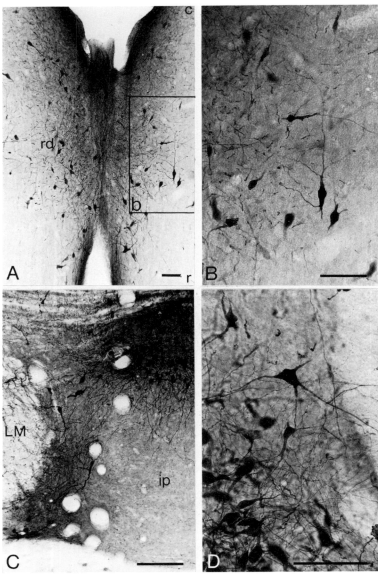

Figure 6 Photomicrographs of horizontal (A, B) transverse (C) and sagittal (D) immunoperoxidase-stained Vibratome sections through the midbrain of the rat incubated with an antibody to serotonin–immunogen A. Note in A and B the presence of immunoreactive neurons with long processes in the dorsal part of the nucleus raphe dorsalis (rd). Note in C the presence of serotonin-positive dendrites in the dorsal part of the nucleus interpeduncularis (ip) and in the region between the latter nucleus and the lemniscus medialis (LM). Note in D large, multipolar cells in the bilateral wings of the nucleus raphe dorsalis. (Bars = 50 μm)

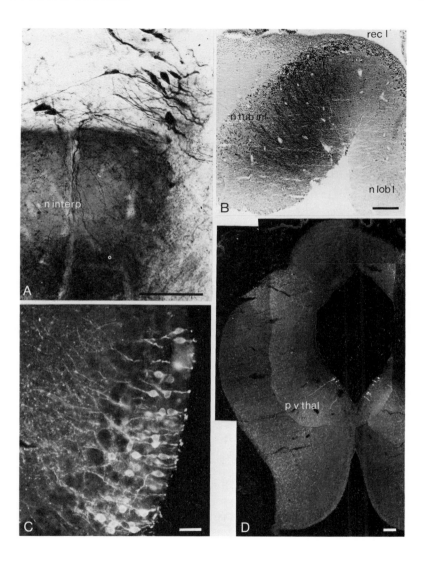

Figure 7 Photomicrographs of transverse, immunoperoxidase-stained Vibratome sections through the brain of the trout (*Salmo gairdneri*) (A, B) and transverse cryostat sections stained by immunofluorescence through the brain of the lamprey (*Lampetra fluviatilis*) (C, D), incubated with antibodies to serotonin–immunogen A. Note in A serotoninergic cell bodies in the raphe region and serotonin-positive terminals in the nucleus interpeduncularis (n interp). Note in B small cell bodies in the nucleus tuberis inferior, (n tub inf), which give rise to ventrolaterally oriented fibres (rec l: recessus lateralis; n lob l: nucleus lobis lateralis). Note in C and D liquor-contacting neurons situated in the pars ventralis thalami. (Bars = 50 μm)

Immunofluorescence results in a convenient and reliable method for the demonstration of serotoninergic neurons in general and serotoninergic fibres and terminals in particular. It can be easily combined with the fluorescent retrograde axonal labelling technique (Steinbusch *et al.*, 1980, 1981). On the other hand, immunoperoxidase-stained Vibratome sections are especially suited for morphological studies on nerve processes, such as examining the spatial orientation and the branching pattern of dendrites.

Virtually, due to the high sensitivity of the immunohistochemical method for serotonin no pharmacological treatment of the animals examined is needed. However, the demonstration of cell bodies and dendrites is facilitated by raising the endogenous serotonin concentration, e.g., by monoamine oxidase inhibitors.

VI CONCLUSIONS

Antibodies raised by the serotonin–immunogen A appeared to be well-suited for neuroimmunocytochemical studies on the central nervous system after fixation with 4% paraformaldehyde in 0.1 M sodium phosphate buffer, pH 7.3. The applicability of these antibodies seems *not to be limited to certain species*, as is the case with antibodies to biosynthetic enzymes.

Antibodies to the serotonin–immunogen A appeared to be rather *specific*. Blocking experiments showed that there might be a cross-reactivity of about 2–3% to 5-methoxytryptamine and less than 0.25% to dopamine. Cross-reactivity to the other substances tested, *viz.* noradrenaline, adrenaline, octopamine, synephrine, and histamine, seemed to be negligible. Moreover, there was good correspondence with previously reported histochemical data concerning the distribution of serotonin. Therefore, it is concluded that the immunoreactivity demonstrated is indeed due to serotonin.

In the three species studied immunoreactivity was also observed in areas where earlier histochemical techniques failed to do so, indicating the high *sensitivity* of the present method. This assumption seems to be supported by recent experiments using model preparations. These experiments showed that the immunohistochemical procedure is about 1000 times more sensitive than the classical formaldehyde-induced fluorescence technique.

Both immunofluorescence on cryostat sections and immunoperoxidase staining of Vibratome sections can be used. *Immunofluorescence on cryostat sections* appears to be a convenient and reliable method for the visualization of serotoninergic neurons, in particular serotoninergic fibres and terminals. *Immunoperoxidase-stained Vibratome sections* are especially suited for examining the dendrites of serotoninergic neurons.

Besides serotonin–immunogen A, two other immunogens (B and C) were synthesized, both containing PABA as a spacer molecule. Serotonin–immunogen B was prepared via a mixed anhydride reaction. For serotonin–immunogen C a carbodiimide reaction was used for coupling the PABA–serotonin complex to BSA. Probably both immunogens have a similar structure. In spite of this, immunoreactivity could only be revealed with antibodies to the serotonin–immunogen B. This unexpected observation might indicate differences in the steric configuration of the immunogens B and C, probably due to the different coupling reactions used. A similar distribution of immunoreactivity was observed employing antibodies to the serotonin–immunogens A and B. From this one might infer that antibodies to the immunogen A, currently used since our first report (Steinbusch *et al.*, 1978), are demonstrating serotonin rather than its β-carboline derivate.

ACKNOWLEDGEMENTS

We are most grateful to Miss Betsy Verburg, Mr Joan Berkeljon, and Mr Evert de Vries for their interest and help in the production of immunogens. The authors wish to thank Miss M. Sjak Shie for typing the manuscript.

REFERENCES

Ajelis, V., Björklund, A., Falck, B., Lindvall, O., Lorén, I., and Walles, B. (1979). 'Application of the aluminium–formaldehyde (ALFA) histofluorescence method for demonstration of peripheral stores of catecholamines and indolamines in freeze-dried paraffin-embedded tissue, cryostat sections and whole-mounts.' *Histochemistry*, **65**, 1–15.

Amin, A. H., Crawford, T. B. B., and Gaddum, J. H. (1954). 'The distribution of substance P and 5-hydroxytryptamine in the central nervous system of the dog.' *J. Physiol., Lond.*, **126**, 596–618.

Baumgarten, H. G. (1972). 'Biogenic amines in the cyclostome and lower vertebrates brain.' *Progr. Histochem. Cytochem.*, **4**, 1–90.

Björklund, A., Lindvall, O., and Svensson, L.-A. (1972). 'Mechanisms of fluorophore formation in the histochemical glyoxylic acid method for monoamines.' *Histochemie*, **32**, 113–131.

Bloom, F. E. and Battenberg, E. L. F. (1976). 'A rapid, simple and sensitive method for the demonstration of central catecholamine-containing neurons and axons by glyoxylic acid-induced fluorescence. II. A detailed description of methodology.' *J. Histochem. Cytochem.*, **24**, 561–571.

Bogdansky, D. F., Pletscher, A., Brodie, B. B., and Udenfriend, S. (1956). 'Identification and assay of serotonin in brain.' *J. Pharmacol. Exp. Ther.*, **117**, 82–88.

Buffa, R., Crivelli, O., Lavarini, C., Sessa, F., Verme, G., and Solcia, E. (1980). 'Immunohistochemistry of brain 5-hydroxytryptamine.' *Histochemistry*, **68**, 9–15.

Coons, A. H. (1958). 'Fluorescent antibody methods.' In Danielli, J. F. (ed.), *General Cytochemical Methods*, pp. 399–422. Academic Press, New York.

Dahlström, A. and Fuxe, K. (1964). 'Evidence for the existence of monoamine-containing neurons in the central nervous system. I. Demonstration of monoamines in cell bodies of brain neurons.' *Acta Physiol. Scand.*, **62** (Suppl. 232), 1–55.

Facer, P., Polak, J. M., Jaffe, B. M., and Pearse, A. G. E. (1979). 'Immunocyto-chemical demonstration of 5-hydroxytryptamine in gastrointestinal endocrine cells.' *Histochem. J.*, **11**, 117–121.

Falck, B. (1962). 'Observations on the possibilities of the cellular localization of monoamines by a fluorescence method.' *Acta Physiol. Scand.*, **56**, Suppl. 197.

Falck, B., Hillarp, N. Å., Thieme, G., and Torp, A. (1962). 'Fluorescence of catecholamines and related compounds with formaldehyde.' *J. Histochem. Cytochem.*, **10**, 348–354.

Falck, B. and Owman, C. (1965). 'A detailed methodological description of the method for the cellular demonstration of biogenic monoamines.' *Acta Univ. Lund*, Sect. II, **7**, 1–23.

Fillip, G. and Schneider, H. (1964). 'Die Synthese der Serotoninazoproteins. Experimente zur Frage der Serotoninimmunität.' *Acta Allergol.*, **19**, 216.

Furness, J. B. and Costa, M. (1975). 'The use of glyoxylic acid for the fluorescence histochemical demonstration of peripheral stores of noradrenaline and 5-hydroxytryptamine in whole mounts.' *Histochemistry*, **41**, 335–352.

Furness, J. B., Costa, M., and Blessing, W. W. (1977). 'Simultaneous fixation and production of catecholamine fluorescence in central nervous tissue by perfusion with aldehydes.' *Histochem. J.*, **9**, 745–750.

Goldstein, M., Fuxe, K., Hökfelt, T., and Joh, T. H. (1971). 'Immunohistochemical studies on phenylethanolamine-N-methyltransferase, DOPA-decarboxylase, and dopamine-β-hydroxylase.' *Experientia*, **27**, 951–952.

Grota, L. J., and Brown, G. M. (1974). 'Antibodies to indolealkylamines: serotonin and melatonin.' *Can. J. Biochem.*, **52**, 196–202.

Hökfelt, T., Fuxe, K., and Goldstein, M. (1973). 'Immunohistochemical localization of aromatic-L-aminoacid decarboxylase (DOPA-decarboxylase) in central dopamine and 5-hydroxytryptamine nerve cell bodies of the rat brain.' *Brain Res.*, **53**, 175–180.

Hökfelt, T., Ljungdahl, Å., Steinbusch, H., Verhofstad, A., Nilsson, G., Brodin, A., Pernow, B., and Goldstein, M. (1978). 'Immunohistochemical evidence of substance-P like immunoreactivity in some 5-hydroxytryptamine containing neurons in the rat central nervous system.' *Neuroscience*, **3**, 517–538.

Holloway, W. R., Grota, L. J., and Brown, G. M. (1980). 'Determination of immunoreactive melatonin in the colon of the rat by immunocytochemistry.' *J. Histochem. Cytochem.*, **28**, 255–262.

Jonsson, G., Pollare, T., Hallman, H., and Sachs, Ch. (1978). 'Development plasticity of central serotonin neurons after 5,7-dihydroxytryptamine treatment.' In Jacoby, J. and Lytle, L. (eds), *Serotonin Neurotoxins*, pp. 150–167. *Proc. N.Y. Acad. Sci. Symp.*

Kellum, J. M. and Jaffe, B. M. (1976). 'Validation and application of a radioimmunoassay for serotonin.' *Gastroenterology*, **70**, 516–522.

Köhler, C., Chan-Palay, V., Haglund, L., and Steinbusch, H. (1980). 'Immunohisto-chemical localization of serotonin nerve terminals in the lateral entorhinal cortex of the rat: demonstration of two separate patterns of innervation from the midbrain raphe.' *Anat. Embryol.*, **160**, 121–129.

Köhler, C., Chan-Palay, V., and Steinbusch, H. (1981). 'The distribution and orientation of serotonin fibers in the entorhinal and other retrohippocampal areas. An immunohistochemical study with anti-serotonin antibodies in the rat's brain.' *Anat. Embryol.*, **161**, 237–264.

Landsteiner, K. (1945). *The Specificity of Serological Reactions*. Harvard University Press, Cambridge, Mass., USA.

Lorén, I., Björklund, A., Falck, B., and Lindvall, O. (1980). 'The aluminium–form-aldehyde (ALFA) method for improved visualization of catecholamines and indolamines. I. A detailed account of the methodology for central nervous tissue using paraffin, cryostat or Vibratome sections.' *J. Neurosci. Methods*, **2**, 277–300.

Lowry, D. H., Rosebrough, N. J., Farr, A. L., and Randall, R. J. (1951). 'Protein measurement with the Folin phenol reagent.' *J. Biol. Chem.*, **193**, 265–275.

Nygren, L. G. (1976). 'On the visualization of central dopamine and noradrenaline nerve terminals in cryostat sections.' *Med. Biol.*, **54**, 278–285.

Ouchterlony, O. (1967). 'Immunodiffusion and immunoelectrophoresis.' In Weir, D. (ed.) *Handbook of Experimental Immunology*, pp. 665–706. Blackwell, Oxford.

Peskar, B. and Spector, S. (1973). 'Serotonin: radioimmunoassay.' *Science*, **179**, 1340–1341.

Pickel, V. M., Joh, T. H., and Reis, D. J. (1976). 'Monoamine-synthesizing enzymes in central dopaminergic, noradrenergic and serotoninergic neurons. Immunocyto-chemical localization by light and electronmicroscopy.' *J. Histochem. Cytochem.*, **24**, 792–806.

Ranadive, N. S. and Sehon, A. H. (1967). 'Antibodies to serotonin.' *Can. J. Biochem.*, **45**, 1701–1710.

Schipper, J., Steinbusch, H. W. M., Verhofstad, A. A. J., and Tilders, F. J. H. (1981). 'Quantitative immunofluorescence of serotonin.' *Proc. 22e Dutch Fed. Meeting*, 390.

Spector, S., Berkowitz, B., Flynn, E. J., and Peskar, B. (1973). 'Antibodies to morphine, barbiturates and serotonin.' *Pharmacol. Rev.*, **25**, 281–291.

Steinbusch, H. W. M. (1981). 'Distribution of serotonin–immunoreactivity in the central nervous system of the rat. Cell bodies and terminals.' *Neuroscience*, **6**, 557–618.

Steinbusch, H. W. M., Verhofstad, A. A. J., and Joosten, H. W. J. (1978). 'Localization of serotonin in the central nervous system by immunohistochemistry: description of a specific and sensitive technique and some applications.' *Neuroscience*, **3**, 811–819.

Steinbusch, H. W. M. and Nieuwenhuys, R. (1979). 'Serotonergic neuron systems in the brain of the lamprey (*Lampetra fluviatilis*).' *Anat. Rec.*, **193**, 693–694.

Steinbusch, H. W. M. and Verhofstad, A. A. J. (1979). 'Immunofluorescent staining of serotonin in the central nervous system.' In Simon, P. (ed.), *Adv. Pharmacol. and Ther.*, vol. 2. *Neurotransmitters*, pp. 151–160. Pergamon Press, Oxford.

Steinbusch, H. W. M., Vanderkooy, D., Verhofstad, A. A. J., and Pellegrino, A. (1980). 'Serotoninergic and non-serotonergic projections from the nucleus raphe dorsalis to the caudate-putamen complex in the rat, studied by a combined immunofluorescence and fluorescent retrograde axonal labeling technique.' *Neurosci. Lett.*, **19**, 137–142.

Steinbusch, H. W. M. and Nieuwenhuys, R. (1981). 'Localization of serotonin-like immunoreactivity in the central nervous system and pituitary of the rat, with special references to the innervation of the hypothalamus.' In Haber, B. *et al.* (eds), *Serotonin: current aspects of neurochemistry and function*. Plenum, New York, pp. 7–36.

Steinbusch, H. W. M., Nieuwenhuys, R., Verhofstad, A. A. J., and Vanderkooy, D. (1981). 'The nucleus raphe dorsalis of the rat and its projection upon the caudatoputamen. A combined cytoarchitectonic, immunohistochemical and retro-grade transport study.' *J. Physiol.*, Paris, **77**, 157–174.

Sternberger, L. A., Hardy, P. H., Jr., Cuculis, J. H., and Meyer, H. G. (1970). 'The unlabeled antibody enzyme method of immunohistochemistry. Preparation and properties of soluble antigen–antibody complex (horseradish peroxidase–antihorse-radish peroxidase) and its use in identification of spirochetes.' *J. Histochem. Cytochem.*, **18,** 315–333.

Terlou, M., Ekengren, B., and Hiemstra, K. (1978). 'Localization of monoamines in the forebrain of two salmonid species, with special reference to the hypo-thalamo–hypophysial system.' *Cell Tiss. Res.*, **190,** 417–434.

Thoenen, H. and Tranzer, J. P. (1973). 'The pharmacology of 6-hydroxydopamine.' *Ann. Rev. Pharmacol.*, **13,** 169–180.

Torre, J. C. de la and Surgeon, J. W. (1976). 'Histochemical fluorescence of tissue and brain monoamines: results in 18 minutes using the sucrose–phosphate–glyoxylic acid method.' *Neuroscience*, **1,** 451–453.

Twarog, B. M. and Page, J. H. (1953). 'Serotonin content of some mammalian tissues and urine and a method for its determination.' *J. Physiol., London*, **175,** 157–161.

Wurzburger, R. J., Kawashima, K., Miller, R. L., and Spector, S. (1976). 'Deter-mination of rat pineal gland melatonin content by a radioimmunoassay.' *Life Sci.*, **18,** 867–878.

Yamamoto, M., Chan-Palay, V., Steinbusch, H. W. M., and Palay, S. L. (1980). 'Hyperinnervation of arrested granule cells produced by the transplantation of monoamine-containing neurons into the fourth ventricle of the rat.' *Anat. Embryol.*, **159,** 1–15.

Immunohistochemistry
Edited by A. C. Cuello
© 1983 IBRO

CHAPTER 9

Preparation and Application of Monoclonal Antibodies for Immunohistochemistry and Immunocytochemistry

A. CLAUDIO CUELLO*, CÉSAR MILSTEIN†, and GIOVANNI GALFRÉ†

*Neuroanatomy/Neuropharmacology Group, Departments of Pharmacology and Human Anatomy, South Parks Road, Oxford, England

†MRC Laboratory of Molecular Biology, Cambridge, England

I INTRODUCTION

Immunohistochemistry is becoming one of the most powerful and widely used tools for the identification of transmitter specific neurons. The investigation of tissue immunoreactive sites to novel neuropeptides, neurotransmitter biosynthetic enzymes, and more recently, neurotransmitters themselves has been shown to be possible with the assistance of this methodology. These studies have been done largely with antibodies of polyclonal origin. Excellent examples of the incisiveness of this technique in the neurosciences have been provided by several laboratories. As a prominent example, at the Karolinska Institute, Hökfelt and collaborators have demonstrated in recent years the existence of a number of immunoreactive substances in unsuspected neuronal systems. More recently this group has successfully exploited the use of retrograde transport of fluorescent markers with immunofluorescence for the detection of transmitter markers (Hökfelt *et al.*, 1976, 1977; Skirboll and Hökfelt, see Chapter 18). The combination of radioautographic studies of uptake with immunocytochemistry offered one of the early examples of co-existence of putative transmitter in single neurons (Chan-Palay *et al.*, 1978; see also Chapter 20). Biosynthetic enzymes have been shown to be excellent markers for the study of aminergic systems (Hökfelt *et al.*, 1973,

1976, 1977; Pickel *et al.*, 1976; Swanson and Hartman, 1975; see also Chapters 5 and 6).

The status of GABA as a mammalian transmitter has been reinforced by the immunohistochemical identification of glutamate decarboxylase (GAD) immunoreactive sites in the CNS (Ribak *et al.*, 1981 and Wu, Chapter 7 of this book). Similarly antibodies against the acetylcholine biosynthetic enzyme choline acetyltransferase (ChAT) are being applied to demonstrate 'cholinergic' sites in the CNS (Cozzari and Hartman, 1981; Kimura *et al.*, 1980; Sofroniew *et al.*, 1982).

A new era in immunohistochemistry has also been initiated with the demonstration of immunoreactive sites for small molecular weight neurotransmitters such as serotonin (Steinbusch *et al.*, 1978; Consolazione *et al.*, 1981; see also Chapter 8).

It is expected that the introduction of the hybridoma technique for the production of monoclonal antibodies (McAb) will facilitate immunocytochemical studies by providing 'standard', well-characterized antibodies against defined and undefined nervous system antigens. This technique offers a number of advantages over conventional methods of production of antisera and novel possibilities in immunocytochemistry.

II THE HYBRID MYELOMA

The hybrid myeloma (hybridoma) technology permits the derivation of highly specific antibodies from pure or impure immunogens. The *in vitro* maintenance of hybrid myeloma cells ensures a continuous supply of large quantities of the same antibody with the same binding sites. The *in vitro* production of antibody allows the preparation of radioactive internally labelled antibodies of high specific activities.

The production of monoclonal antibodies with the hybrid myeloma technique of Köhler and Milstein (1975) consists of:

II.1 Immortalization of the Antibody-producing Cells

Spleen immunocytes from hyperimmune animals are fused with derived myeloma cells. Fusions are performed as follows: mouse × mouse, rat × mouse, rat × rat. Hybridomas with other species are currently being explored in several laboratories. The myeloma parent cell contributes to the hybridoma with its ability to grow permanently in tissue culture while the immunocytes provide the genetic information for the production of a specific antibody.

II.2 Elimination of Non-fused Parental Cells

After the cell fusion, cultures are grown in the so-called HAT (hypoxanthine, aminopterin, thymidine) selective medium (Littlefield, 1964; Szybalski *et al.*, 1962). The myeloma cell lines usually utilized are azaguanine-resistant, which is taken as an indication that the cells are lacking the enzyme hypoxanthine guanine phosphoribosyl transferase (HGPRT). These mutant cells are unable to survive in 'HAT medium'. In this medium aminopterin blocks the main biosynthetic pathway for the production of nucleic acids, and the cells are forced to use the so-called 'salvage pathway' HGPRT and thymidine kinase (Ringertz and Savage, 1976). The immunocytes from hyperimmune animals provide the genetic material for the production of a specific antibody and HGPRT, allowing the hybrids to grow in HAT medium. Non-fused parental myeloma will disappear in HAT while non-fused immunocytes are overgrown by the hybrids.

II.3   Isolation of the Desired Clone

After the elimination of parental cells the hybrids can be grown in a normal culture medium (Dulbecco's modified Eagle's medium) and antibody production tested from the spent fluid.

II.4   Production of Specific Monoclonal Antibodies

After the identification of the desired clone the hybridomas are grown *in vitro* or can be reinjected in a recipient animal and grown *in vivo* as a tumour. Figure 1 illustrates these steps.

III   PREPARATION OF MONOCLONAL ANTIBODIES (McAbs)

III.1   Raising Antibodies in Small Rodents

Cells from hyperimmune mice of the $BALB_C$ strains or rats (Wistar, DA or Lou) can be used for fusions with rat or mouse myeloma cell lines. Purified immunogens are preferred when available.

As the response to various immunogens cannot be predicted, the use of more than one protocol is recommended, i.e. variation of doses and immunization schedules. The following is a standard protocol:

The immunogen is dissolved in water to contain (generally) microgram amounts per 100 µl. Equal volumes of this solution are emulsified with complete Freund's adjuvant (Difco, East Molesey, Surrey). Emulsion can be obtained by energetically and repeatedly ejecting the suspension through the nozzle of a syringe or by vigorously shaking for minutes in a vortex. A properly prepared emulsion should not disperse when a drop of it is placed on a water surface. (For more detailed information on the preparation of emulsions see Herbert, 1978.)

A total of 200 µl of the emulsion is injected intradermally in multiple sites in

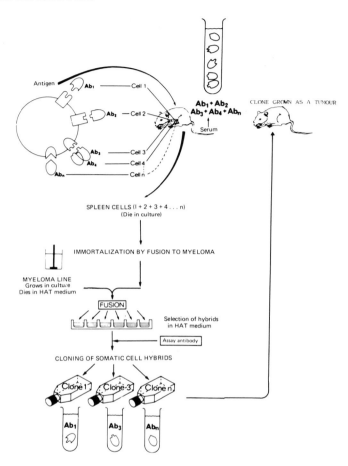

Figure 1 Scheme of the hybridoma technology as originally developed by Köhler and Milstein (1975). Animals produce highly heterogenous mixtures of antibodies (Ab_1, Ab_2, . . . Ab_n), secreted by different clones of immunocytes (Cell 1, Cell 2 . . . Cell n) and recognize different determinants from the immunogen (circle), some of them overlapping (3 and 4). Hybrids between myeloma cells and splenocytes produce monoclonal antibodies directed against simple antigenic determinants, regardless of the complexity of the antigenic stimulus. Once isolated, the hybrid clones can be grown in unlimited quantity *in vitro* or can be grown as tumours in recipient animals

the back of the animal. Fifty to 100 µl of the emulsion can be injected intraperitoneally. When intradermal injections are intended the needle has to be retrieved carefully to avoid loss of the immunogen. Larger volumes (300–600 µl) can be injected subcutaneously. Generally, injections are given at 3–5-week intervals. High-affinity antibodies for peptides have been obtained by injecting intradermally–intraperitoneally weekly for 3 weeks and with further boost injections every 3 weeks.

Bleeding to test for the presence of antibody should preferably be done 1 week after the last injection of the antigen. High-affinity antibody does not usually appear earlier than 2 months after the initiation of the immunization programme. Blood can be taken from rats and mice by cutting the end of the tail. In mice approximately 50 µl can be obtained with a glass micropipette by capillarity from the retro-ocular venous plexus.

The animals giving the best antiserum are selected for fusion. After a rest period (3–6 weeks) the same dose of antigen, dissolved in 0.2–0.4 ml of sterile saline solution, is injected intravenously; 3–4 days later the animals are sacrificed and the spleen cells used for fusion with myeloma cells.

The immunized animal should usually be of the same species as the myeloma, although interspecific fusions have been successful for the production of McAbs. Fusions with myeloma of the same species permits the easy development of tumours when hybrid myelomas are re-injected into the animal.

III.2   Cell Fusion

III.2.1   *Cell culture equipment*

The essential equipment for the production of monoclonal antibodies is common to a number of tissue culture techniques and can be summarized as follows:

—Sterile work benches.
—Incubators at 37 °C with and without CO_2 atmosphere and humidity.
—Inverted and ordinary microscopes (preferably provided with phase contrast).
—Water baths.
—Bench centrifuges.
—Storage facilities in liquid N_2.

III.2.2   *Preparation of spleen and myeloma cells for fusion*

Spleen cells
—Sacrifice the hyperimmune animal and dip the body in 70% alcohol.
—Remove the spleen under sterile conditions. Spleen can also be removed surgically from anaesthetized rodents.
—Place the spleen in a Petri dish containing about 5 ml 2.5% foetal calf serum (FCS) in Dulbecco's modified Eagle's medium (DMM) kept on ice, and wash gently.

—Transfer the spleen to a 10 ml round-bottomed tube, cutting the spleen into pieces, and add 5 ml of fresh 2.5% FCS–DMM.

—With Teflon pestle to fit (1 mm clearance) the round-bottomed plastic tubes, squash the pieces gently to make a cell suspension. A cell suspension can also be obtained by dispersing the cells out of the capsule with the tip of a needle and ejecting the liquid with a syringe.

—Allow a few minutes for clamps and pieces of spleen capsule to sediment and transfer cell suspension to a 10 ml round-bottomed plastic tube.

—Fill the tube with 2.5% FCS–DMM and centrifuge at room temperature 10 min at 400 g. Start preparing myeloma cells as indicated below.

—Resuspend pellet in 10 ml of fresh medium and centrifuge (10 min at 400 g).

—Resuspend pellet again in 10 ml of medium and count cells in a Neubaeur chamber. The suspension can also be used as a feeder layer for the culture of fused cells. The viability of these cells should be higher than 80% as assessed by phase contrast or Trypan blue exclusion test.

Myeloma cells

Approximately 10^7–6×10^7 myeloma cells from a culture in logarithmic growth are pelleted by centrifugation at room temperature for 10 min at 400 g. The pellet is resuspended in 10 μl ml of 2.5% FCS–DMM and counted.

III.2.3 *Cell fusion procedure*

(1) Parental cells are prepared as described above.

(2) 10^8 spleen cells and 10^7 (mouse) or 6×10^7 (rat) myeloma cells are mixed in a 50 ml conical tube and DMM is added to a volume of 50 ml.

(3) The cells are centrifuged at room temperature for 8 min at about 400 g.

(4) The supernatant is removed with a Pasteur pipette connected to a vacuum line. To avoid dilution of PEG remove the supernatant completely.

(5) The pellet is broken by gently tapping the bottom of the tube. The tube is placed in a 200 ml beaker containing water at 40 °C and kept there during the fusion (steps 6–12).

(6) 0.8 ml 50% PEG pre-warmed at 40 °C is added to the pellet using a 1 ml pipette, over a period of 1 min, continually stirring the cells with a pipette tip.

(7) Stirring of the cells in 50% PEG is continued for a further $1\frac{1}{2}$–2 min. Agglutination of cells must be evident at this stage.

(8) With the same pipette add 1 ml of DMM, taken from a tube containing 10 ml DMM kept at 37 °C in the hot block; stir continuously for a period of 1 min.

(9) Repeat step 8.

(10) Repeat step 8 twice but adding the medium in 30 s.

(11) Always with the same pipette and continuously stirring, add the rest of the 10 ml DMM over a period of about 2 min.

(12) With a 10 ml pipette add dropwise 12–13 ml pre-warmed DMM.

(13) Centrifuge cells at 400 g for 8 min.

(14) Discard supernatant and break the pellet by gently tapping the bottom of the tube and resuspend in 49 ml 20% FCS–DMM. (Hybridomas have also been obtained by resuspending the pellet directly in HAT medium.)

(15) Distribute the fusion suspension in the 48 wells of two Linbro plates. These may contain a feeder layer of fibroblasts.

(16) Add 1 ml of 20% FCS–DMM (step 8, spleen cells) if a fibroblast feeder is not being used. Add 10^5 spleen cells/ml.

(17) Incubate overnight at 37 °C in a CO_2 incubator.

(18) With a Pasteur pipette connected to the vacuum line remove 1 ml of culture medium from each cup. Try not to disturb the cells that have settled in the bottom.

(19) Feed the plate, adding 1 ml HAT medium to each cup. Repeat feeding with HAT medium for the next 2 or 3 days and after that once a week until vigorous growth of hybrids is observed. This should become evident under the microscope after day 10, but might take longer. At this stage the cultures become yellowish and are ready to be tested for antibody activity.

(20) Select interesting hybrids according to tests.

(21) Duplicates of the growing hybrid cultures are prepared and fed for a week with HT medium. Larger cultures can be prepared and frozen in liquid N_2. After a week in HT medium the cultures can be grown in the absence of HAT additives. Adaptation to lower concentration of serum can now be attempted.

III.2.4 *Materials for tissue culture and cell fusion*

Tissue culture grade water is used throughout. This is usually deionized and double-distilled over glass.

For the preparation of McAbs the most commonly used media are Dulbecco's Modified Eagle's Medium (DMM) and RPMI-1640.

—Limbro plates of 24 wells (Flow Labs, Cat. No. 76-033-05).

—Sterile pipettes of 1, 10, and 25 ml.

—50% solution of polyethylene glycol 1500 daltons (BDH Cat. No. 29575, UK) in sterile DMM. Add 10 g to 10 ml of DMM warmed to 37 °C. Mix by inverting tube. Adjust pH to 7.0 by leaving tube open in a sterile hood or blowing 10% CO_2/air mixture.

10× DMM Ten times concentrate solutions (10× DMM, Gibco Europe, Glasgow, Cat. No. 330-2501, or Flow Laboratories, Irvine, Cat. No. 14-330-49) are also available. About 4 litres of tissue culture grade water is autoclaved in a 6 litre glass flask and allowed to cool to room temperature. The 10× medium and other components as specified by the manufacturer are then added.

Medium can be prepared from dry powder (*Powder DMM*) (Gibco Laboratories, Grand Island, New York. Cat. No. 430-2100), following the manufacturer's instructions. This requires filter sterilizing units of 20 litres or larger.

Media prepared directly from powder gives very good results. The 1× medium is almost as good but is much more expensive and requires more 4 °C storage space. The medium prepared from the 10× concentrate is generally not as good and the batches are more variable. Concentrated medium is necessary for cloning in soft agar or agarose, and the best is to prepare 2× medium from dry powder.

HAT Medium

100× HT   136.1 mg hypoxanthine (Sigma, Poole, Dorset, England. Cat. No. H9377) and 38.75 mg thymidine (Sigma, Cat. No. T9250) are suspended in about 50 ml water and 0.1 M NaOH added dropwise until dissolved. Adjust volume to 100 ml. Store at −20 °C. Thaw at 70 °C for 10–15 min.

50× HT is made by diluting 100× HT with 1 vol. DMM. Filter sterilize and store in 25 ml aliquots at 4 °C.

1000× aminopterin. Aminopterin (Sigma Cat. No. A2255) 17.6 mg/100 ml. Proceed as for 100× HT.

50× HAT   50 ml 100× HT
5 ml 1000× aminopterin
45 ml DMM.

Filter sterilize and store in 25 ml aliquots at 4 °C.

1× HT and 1× HAT (20% FCS (foetal calf serum)).
500 ml DMM
100 ml FCS
12 ml 50× HAT or 50× HT
Antibiotics, generally penicillin.

IV   CLONING HYBRIDS

It is convenient to clone as early as possible as multiple clones in the same culture complete for growth and stability of expression. If only a few cultures are positive it is worth subdividing them by limiting dilutions. At this stage it is essential to assess the interest of the different antibodies, i.e. whether they are intended for immunocytochemistry, radioimmunoassay, agglutination tests, cytotoxicity, immunoneutralization, etc. For the selection of clones highly sensitive assay systems are required.

IV.1 Limiting Dilution Fractionation

About 3×10^5 cells are transferred to the first cup of a 24-well Linbro plate containing a feeder layer. After thorough mixing a two-fold dilution series is prepared over the first 12 cups (maximum dilution of about 600 cells in cup 12) or over all 24 cups (about one cell in cup 21 or 22 and none in cups 23 and 24). Part of the medium is changed every 4 or 5-days. Supernatants are collected and tested when the cultures approach confluence. The positive culture containing the minimum number of seeded cells can either be fractionated again as above, or cloned in semi-solid medium as soon as possible. Cloning can be attempted with this procedure assuming by dilution that, at most, only one single cell is present in each microculture well. Positive clones are selected by the presence of desired antibodies in the supernatant.

IV.2 Cloning on Semi-solid Supports

IV.2.1 *Materials*

2× DMM–20% FCS: 100 ml 2× DMM from dry powder, 40 ml FCS.

1% agar: 1 g agar (Baco Agar, Cat. No. 0140–01, Difco Laboratories) in 100 ml tissue culture grade distilled water. Autoclave for 15–20 s. Keep at 4 °C.

0.5% agar: 1 vol. 1% agar, 1 vol. 2× DMM–40% FCS. Keep at 42 °C. HAT or other additives as required.

If 10× DMM is to be used the 0.5% agar is better prepared by mixing 1 vol. 5% agar in water with 1 vol. 2× DMM–20% FCS (prepared from the 10× DMM) and 8 vol. 20% FCS–DMM (prepared from 1× DMM).

Petri dishes: 9 cm diameter plastic, tissue culture grade (Sterilin, Cat. No. 304V).

IV.2.2 *Procedure*

Pour into each Petri dish (with or without a feeder layer) about 15 ml 0.5% agar. Set for about 15 min, at room temperature. Prepare several cell suspensions containing, for instance, 100, 500, 5000, and 50,000 cells/ml. Add 1 ml 0.5% agar (at 42 °C) to 1 ml of each cell suspension (at room temperature). Mix by rotating the tube between the hands and pour immediately onto the agar base. Allow to set for at least 10 min at room temperature and incubate at 37 °C in a CO_2 incubator.

Clones can be picked at days 4–5, using a dissection microscope, or, after 7–10 days, directly, and transferred to individual cups of a 24-well Linbro plate. It may be essential to have feeder cells in the cups, especially if small clones are picked.

Positive clones can be selected by detecting specific antibodies *in situ* (Köhler and Milstein, 1975) or by replica immunoabsorption methods. Alternatively, randomly picked clones are transferred to DMM in Linbro plates for further growth and supernantant tested for antibody activity.

V TESTING ANTIBODY ACTIVITY

The choice of test for detection of antibody activity depends very much on the prospective use of the antibody. For immunocytochemical purposes it is essential to devise a test which resembles as far as possible the conditions of the antigen in tissue preparations prior or after fixation. When the localization of an antigenic site is reasonably well known a typical immunoreactive area of cell can be used as a model to detect antibodies from supernatants. The same procedure can be applied for the identification of antibodies against unknown antigens, selecting those cultures producing antibodies which bind to specific cell types or tissues.

As the concentration of antibodies in the tissue culture supernatant is very low as compared with the plasma of hyperimmune animals only highly sensitive assays should be applied.

Provided the method of choice has sufficient sensitivity to detect small amounts of antibody, a large variety of methods can be used. The description of various immunoassays which can be adopted to monitor the presence of specific antibodies in tissue culture supernatant can be found in the *Handbook of Experimental Immunology* (Weiss, 1978) or in *Practical Immunology* (Hudson and Hay, 1980). Here we will describe procedures used to detect monoclonal antibodies intended for immunocytochemical application in fixed tissue preparations. For testing monoclonal antibodies intended for unfixed tissue or tissue culture preparations see Schachner (Chapter 12 of this book). Monoclonal antibodies against substance P (coded NCl/34 HL) have been cloned by monitoring antibody activity by radioimmunoassay (Cuello *et al.*, 1979) following the protocol described below. For other substances analogous radioimmunoassay systems can be adapted. For further methodological aspects on the theory and practice of radioimmunoassay see Parker (1976).

Monoclonal antibodies against serotonin–bovine seroalbumin conjugate cultures were monitored by immunocytochemistry and haemagluttination as described below.

V.1 Radioimmunoassay

The monoclonal antibody, NCl/34 HL (anti-substance P) has been produced following the antibody activity by radioimmunoassay both in hyperimmune animals and supernatants from hybrids. The following is a radioimmunoassay procedure basically as described by Powell *et al.* (1973) and established by Kanazawa and Jessell (1976).

V.1.1   *Labelling peptides (e.g. substance P) with ^{125}I*

Materials

(1) 0.5 M sodium phosphate buffer (pH 7.4).
(2) High specific activity ^{125}I sodium iodine (Amersham) in diluted NaOH solution (pH 8.1).
(3) Sodium metabisulphate, 37 mg in 10 ml of the above buffer.
(4) Blood plasma (preferably from human blood bank).
(5) Microfine silica gel G32 (Quso) (Quartz and Co). Weight 10 mg before each iodination.
(6) Ag l-XlO, 200–400 mesh anion exchange resin in Cl⁻ form (Bio Radio).
(7) Chloramine T solution (Kodak) 26 mg in 10 ml–25 µg/20 µl) weighed out just prior to use (protect from light) and dissolved in water only at the time of labelling.
(8) Tyrosine-8 substance P (Peninsula, Beckman) 100 µg dissolved in 200 µl of 0.1 N acetic acid. Aliquot this solution into 10 µg samples and store in freezer.
(9) Solution of 20% acetone and 1% acetic acid in water.

V.1.2   *Procedure*

Iodination should be carried out in a well-protected hood and using gloves. Measure background iodination in benches, sinks, and hood before and after iodination.

(1) Take one 10 µg aliquot of tyrosine-8–substance P and add 100 µl sodium phosphate buffer and mix.
(2) Add 1 mCi of ^{125}I sodium iodine.
(3) Add 20 µl chloramine T solution while gently mixing. The reaction should continue for no more than 15 s and should then be stopped as in stage 4.
(4) To stop the reaction add 50 µl sodium metabisulphate while stirring.
(5) Add 1 ml blood plasma and mix well.
(6) Add 10 mg Quso and mix.
(7) Centrifuge at 1000 g for 5 min.
(8) Discard plasma supernatant. Keep aliquot to measure radioactivity.
(9) Add 1 ml distilled water and 0.1 ml volume Ag l-X1O resin. This can be prepared with a cut 1 ml plastic syringe.
(10) Centrifuge at 1000 g for 5 min.

(11) Discard water supernatant, take aliquot to measure radioactivity.
(12) Add 5.1 ml distilled water to wash. Mix well.
(13) Centrifuge at 1000 g for 5 min.
(14) Discard water.
(15) Add 1 ml acetone acetic acid in water to elute the peptide.
(16) Centrifuge 200 g for 10 min.
(17) Take 10 µl aliquots of the supernatant and freeze. Each aliquot should have 2.3 × 10^6 cpm/10 µl.

This basic procedure can be adopted to label other peptides. Alternatively, some radiolabelled iodinated peptides can be obtained commercially (Amersham, New England Nuclear).

V.1.3 *Materials for radioimmunoassay*

(1) Sodium barbital buffer 0.05 M (8.25 g/l), pH 8.6 (Barbiton acetate buffer for electrophoresis, Oxoid). Add blood bank plasma as 5%. Keep cool.
(2) ^{125}I-labelled (Tyr^8)-substance P. If stock tube contains 10 µl (2–3 × 10^6 cpm), add 1 ml of assay buffer and mix well. (Keep cool −0°C.) Take 0.5 ml of this and put into 10 ml of assay buffer. Use 100 µl (approximately 1–1.5 × 10^4 cpm) of this final solution for assay.
(3) Supernatant from tissue culture.
(4) Standard substance P solution or equivalent peptide. Stock tube containing 100 ng in 10 µl of 0.1 M acetic acid.
(5) Dextran-coated charcoal solution. Pre-weigh 1 g charcoal (Hopkins and Williams) and dissolve 10 ml assay buffer without plasma. Separately weight 0.1 g Dextran D500 1 (Sigma) and dissolve in 10 ml of assay buffer without plasma. Pour charcoal solution into dextran solution while stirring. Keep cool and stir continuously.

V.1.4 *Procedure for radioimmunoassay*

(1) Prepare small microbiological tubes (approximately 2 ml capacity suitable for centrifuges and γ-radiation counting) in a rack on ice. Number the tubes and add 300 µl of assay buffer to 'test tubes' and 400 µl of buffer to 2–4 tubes for blank reading (0% of binding).
(2) Add 100 µl of undiluted tissue culture supernatant. If possible prepare duplicate tubes from each hybrid. No supernatant should be added to the blank tubes. Mix well.
(3) Add 100 µl solution of iodinated peptide as indicated above and shake (Vortex).
(4) Incubate for 18–24 h at 4°C. If data are urgently needed a shorter incubation at room temperature, or 37°C, can be performed in hours.

(5) Add 200 μl of freshly made charcoal dextran solution. This solution should be continuously stirred even while pipetting. Mix well. (During the characterization of monoclonal antibodies against Leu-enkephalin the separation of free and bound antibody was done by adding bovine IgG at 0.5% and PEG, 3.000 d at 8% (final concentrations).

(6) Keep at 4 °C for 30–40 min.

(7) Centrifuge at 2000 *g* for 10 min at 4 °C.

(8) Decant in new set of tubes labelled as first set. Supernatant will indicate bound radiolabelled peptide (B) and pellet the free, radiolabelled peptide (F). When immunoglobulins and PEG is used the pellet contains the bound peptide.

(9) Measure radioactivity in a γ-counter. If the data are expressed as percentages of binding ([B/B + F] × 100) a binding of approximately 40–50% can be expected from a positive hybrid producing high-affinity antibody. Higher percentages of binding can be obtained with ammonium sulphate precipitates by concentrating immunoglobulins produced by hybrids. Figure 2a illustrates the titration of a clone producing anti-substance P antibody compared with the corresponding crude immuno-globulin fraction, and in Figure 2b the titration of a supernatant forms a hybrid clone producing anti-Leu-enkephalin monoclonal antibodies, coded NOC1.

Note the enhancement of avidity of the concentrated preparation. When positive clones have been found with this method it is advisable to test whether or not the binding is displaced by unlabelled peptide. For this, similar binding assay can be performed where 200 μl of buffer containing 50 ng of the unlabelled peptide is added to a set of tubes before starting the described procedure. This tube should have, in step 1, 100 μl of buffer as opposed to 300 μl (test samples) or 400 μl (blank samples). After step 2 of the above, the protocol tubes should be incubated for 3–5 h (or longer) at 40 °C. The procedure should then be followed up to step 9.

In most cases nanogram amounts of peptide should produce a total displacement of the binding of radiolabelled peptide, indicating that a genuine antigen–antibody binding against the peptide is present.

Likewise, the radioimmunoassay procedure can be used to further char-acterize monoclonal antibodies. For this, use constant volume and concentra-tion of antibody in all tubes (except blanks). The dilution should be about half the maximum binding capacity to allow displacement by unlabelled peptides. Decreasing concentrations of peptides diluted in 100 Nl are added in step 1 and correspondingly reducing the volume of buffer. This type of test will provide direct information on the 'intrinsic cross-reactivity' of the monoclonal in liquid phase. An example of the results of such characterization for NCl/34 monoclonal antibody is illustrated in Figure 3.

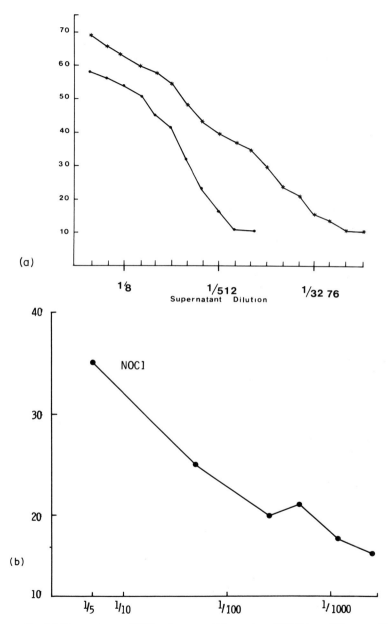

Figure 2 (a) Percentage of ^{125}I substance P bound to NCl/34 at different dilutions of (●) cell culture medium or crude Ig fraction (×). (b) Percentage of [125]I Leu-enkephalin bound to different dilutions of spent medium from a mouse hybrid myeloma (NOCl) producing anti-enkephalin monoclonal antibodies

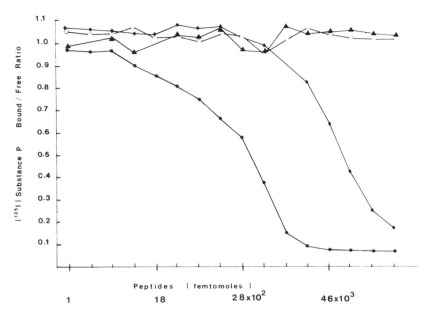

Figure 3 Characterization of the monoclonal antibody NCl/34 (anti-substance P) by radioimmunoassay. Note that femtomole amounts of substance P (●) displace the binding of NCl/34 to iodinated peptide. A partial 'intrinsic cross-reactivity' was found with the related peptide eleidosin (◆) which possesses the same tripeptide sequence as substance P in its C-terminal region. Absence of cross-reactivity was observed for β-endorphin (▲) and somatostatin (○) and other neuroactive peptides

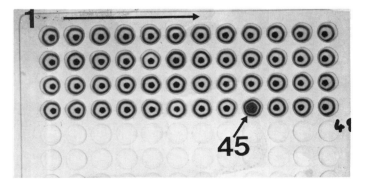

Figure 4 Screening of hybrid myelomas by haemagglutination. Sheep red blood cells were coated with serotonin–BSA immunogen and placed in wells 1 to 48. Supernatants from hybrids were added. Only well number 45 displayed characteristic agglutination, indicating the presence of specific antibodies

V.2 Haemagglutination

Haemagglutination tests have the main advantage of speed and direct visual reading of results. A disadvantage is the relative lack of precise quantitative information and low sensitivity. In some cases this technique could fail to detect positive clones. In the case of YC5/45 (anti-serotonin monoclonal antibody) this method, along with immunocytochemistry, allowed the monitoring of positive hybrids and clones together with the further characterization of the corresponding monoclonal antibodies (Consolazione *et al.*, 1981; Milstein, Wright, and Cuello, 1983). The inhibition of haemagglutination is done simply by adding excess antigen analogues to the appropriate dilutions of hybrid supernatants before the addition of antigen-coated red blood cells (RBC).

V.2.1 *Coupling antigens (proteins) to red blood cells*

Materials
—RBC, red blood cells, usually from sheep.
—Saline: 0.9% NaCl in distilled water.
—CrCl$_3$ solution: 0.5 mg/ml CrCl$_3$ in saline adjusted to about 5 pH by the addition of NaOH, taking care to avoid the formation of any precipitate.
—Protein–antigen or hapten–protein conjugates about 1 mg/ml in saline but not in PBS as phosphate inhibits the CrCl$_3$ coupling.
—PBS, phosphate buffer saline, pH 7.2.

Procedure

(1) Wash the RBC three or four times in saline.
(2) In a round-bottomed tube containing 1 volume packed RBC, add 1 volume CrCl$_3$ solution and 1 volume protein–antigen solution. The two solutions should be added simultaneously using two pipettes.
(3) Immediately resuspend the cells by inverting the tube several times and continue this for 2 min.
(4) Add at least 10 volumes PBS, mix by inversion, and spin down at 100 g for 5 min.
(5) Repeat the wash three times and resuspend the coated RBS in PBS.

Sterile-coated RBC can be stored for several weeks at 4 °C.

V.2.2 *Direct haemagglutination*

In each well of a microtitre plate (round-bottom 'U' wells) dispense 25 µl RBC:PBS (1:16 v/v). Add 25 µl of the supernatant to be tested and mix well using a plate shaker. Incubate at room temperature for 2 h. The agglutinated RBC fail to settle as a distinctive tight pellet. The plate can then be photographed. For a more accurate reading the pellet of each well can be carefully transferred on to glass slides as microscopic examination will detect very weak agglutination. Figure 4 illustrates the testing of supernatants from rat × rat fusion producing anti-serotonin antibodies.

V.2.3. *Indirect haemagglutination*

At the end of the direct agglutination test titrated amounts of anti-immunoglobulin are added to each well. The pellets are then resuspended and allowed to settle for a further 2 h. After this period results can be recorded as above. For clearer results the first antibody should be removed before the addition of anti-immunoglobulin. The second antibody must be tested before use. It must not agglutinate the coated RBC in the absence of the first antibody at the concentration used in the final test.

V.3 Immunocytochemistry

Antibodies produced by hybrid myelomas can also be tested by immunocytochemistry. In fact, this is the most relevant test to perform when the goal is to produce monoclonal antibodies as primary reagents for immunocytochemistry. For this the supernatants should be used as if they were antisera obtained by bleeding hyperimmune animals and developed according to conventional immunofluorescence or immunoenzyme techniques (see Chapters 4, 8, and 11). For known antigens it is advisable to use tissue systems where the cellular localization has been well established. As tests have to be run relatively quickly while the hybridomas are growing fast, a careful protocol should be established to allow the simultaneous immunocytochemical analysis of 100–200 supernatants. This can be simplified by pooling supernatants and individually retesting those giving a positive result. Negative cultures should be eliminated or tested with other systems in the event of the possible lack of correlation of immunoreactivities being observed in tissue preparation and liquid phase.

For unknown antigens the supernatants should be initially tested with the cellular system used as immunogen. Conditions for immunocytochemistry should resemble, as far as possible, those for the preparation used to challenge the immune system. For further details see examples in Chapter 15.

VI   DIRECT AND INDIRECT IMMUNOCYTOCHEMISTRY WITH MONOCLONAL ANTIBODIES

VI.1   Direct Immunocytochemistry with Monoclonal Antibodies

The fact that the hybridoma technique secures large quantities of specific antibodies offers a new lease of life to direct immunocytochemical techniques. Immunoglobulin fractions or purified immunoglobulin from spent medium of hybridomas producing monoclonal antibodies can be conjugated directly with a number of tags for their microscopic visualization. There are already examples of such applications, i.e. the conjugation of gold particles (see Chapter 13) and the conjugation of peroxidase to substance P monoclonal antibodies following the procedure described in Chapter 3. Figure 5

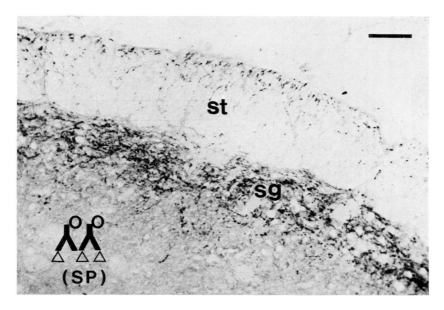

Figure 5 Direct immunoperoxidase staining of substance P immunoreactive fibres in the substantia gelatinosa of the spinal nucleus of the trigeminal nerve (sg) and spinal tract (st) of the rat. Triangles represent substance P (SP) antigenic sites recognized by monoclonal antibodies (⋀) conjugated to peroxidase (○). (Bar = 25 μm)

illustrates the direct immunoenzyme detection of substance P in the spinal nucleus of the trigeminal nerve of the rat (Boorsma *et al.*, 1982). In this case NOC1/34 monoclonal antibodies were separated by affinity chromatograph (anti-rat IgG) and conjugated by the two-step glutaraldehyde method (see Chapter 3).

VI.2   Indirect Immunocytochemistry with Monoclonal Antibodies

Following adequate characterization, monoclonal antibodies can be used in conventional indirect immunocytochemical techniques as primary antibodies. Although the tissue culture supernatants can be used directly as primary antibodies, carrier proteins from culture media can increase background. On occasions the amount of antibody molecules present may be just enough to give a positive signal. The preparation of a crude immunoglobulin fraction will suffice to overcome these limitations. For this, cells are allowed to grow to a stationary phase and the supernatant fluid is precipitated to 50% saturation by the addition of enzyme grade ammonium sulphate. The precipitate is then redissolved in approximately 1/50th of the volume of the original supernatant with phosphate buffered saline and dialysed several times in the same solution. Figure 6 illustrates immunoreactivity to substance

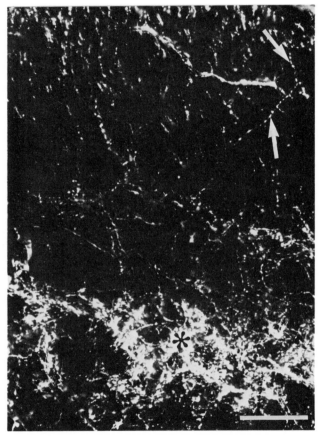

Figure 6 Indirect immunofluorescence using crude immunoglobulin fraction from NCl/34 monoclonal antibodies as primary antibodies and developed with an FITC conjugated anti-rat immunoglobulin. Fluorescent elements represent substance P immunoreactive fibres and terminal networks (asterisk) in the substantia gelatinosa of the spinal nucleus of the trigeminal nerve and tract. Arrows indicate individual axons leaving the tract in the direction of the superficial layers of the nucleus. Rat medulla oblongata, 1 μm thick cryostat section. (Bar = 20 μm)

P in the spinal trigeminal nucleus of the rat as revealed with this material diluted 1/100 (v/v) in PBS containing 0.2% Triton X-100 and developed with an anti-rat IgG immunoglobulin conjugated with FiTC (Miles-Yeda, UK).

Ascitic fluid and sera from rodents bearing hybridomas producing specific monoclonal antibodies in the peritoneal cavity or growing as solid tumours can be treated in the same manner. Figure 7 illustrates the staining of 5-HT immunoreactive sites using serum from a rat bearing hybridoma YC5/45.

Whatever the origin (supernatants, crude Ig fractions, ascitic fluid or sera) the material should be titred in order to find the optimal staining dilution according to the procedure utilized.

For fixation conditions and PAP staining with monoclonal antibodies see Chapter 11. The conditions used for indirect immunofluorescence are broadly analogous to those described by Rush and Steinbusch and collaborators (Chapters 6 and 8).

Monoclonal antibodies can also be applied as primary antibodies in electron microscopical immunocytochemistry and developed as indirect immunoperoxidase or PAP. The protocol to follow is essentially the same as for conventional immunoenzyme techniques (see Chapter 4). For typical results using NCl/34 (anti-substance P monoclonal antibody) as primary reagent in EM immunocytochemistry see Chapter 11.

At present the major difficulty in using mouse or rat monoclonal antibodies in the PAP technique is obtaining good mouse or rat PAP complexes. Sources are scanty and the material is not always reliable. For this we tend to prepare our own reagents and recently have successfully produced a rat PAP with monoclonal antibodies against peroxidase. This reagent performs as well in our hands as the best commercially available polyclonal rat PAP (Clones YC7/41 and YC7/141) (Cuello, Milstein, Wright, and Bramwell, to be published).

VII RADIOIMMUNOCYTOCHEMISTRY WITH INTERNALLY LABELLED MONOCLONAL ANTIBODIES

One of the potentially more interesting advantages of the use of monoclonal antibodies in immunohistochemistry is that they can be internally radiolabelled during their biosynthesis by incubating the antibody-producing clones in the presence of radioactive amino acids. The choice of these amino acids is based on the efficiency of their incorporation into secreted immunoglobulins in culture conditions. Lysine has been shown to be the most efficiently incorporated amino acid in these conditions and therefore most frequently used. Radioimmunocytochemistry with internally labelled monoclonal antibodies can be summarized as follows (see Figure 8):

(a) hybridomas are incubated in culture medium minus lysine (or other amino acid);

Figure 7   Indirect immunofluorescence using anti-serotonin monoconal antibodies (YC5/45) in the rat brain stem and developed FITC conjugated anti-rat immunoglobulins. Composite micrograph showing the distribution of serotonergic cell groups B7 to B9. IC, inferior colliculus; po, nucleus pontis; f1, fasciculus longitudinalis medialis; sgc, substantia grisea centralis. (Bar = 100 μm) (From Consolazione and Cuello, 1982)

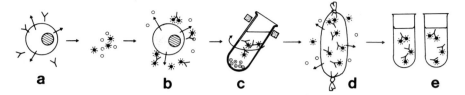

Figure 8 Flow scheme for the preparation of internally labelled monoclonal antibodies (see text)

(b) biosynthesis of monoclonal antibodies in the presence of rádioactive amino acids;
(c) separation of medium from hybrid myeloma by centrifugation;
(d) elimination of non-incorporated radioactive amino acids by column chromatography or dialysis;
(e) storage in aliquots of long-lasting, internally radiolabelled antibodies of high specific activity; and
(f) detection of tissue antigens at light and electron microscopy as illustrated in flow scheme of Figure 9 and text below.

VII.1 Preparation of Internally Labelled Monoclonal Antibodies (from Galfré and Milstein, 1981; Cuello and Milstein, 1981)

About 2×10^6 cells from an exponentially growing culture are centrifuged, resuspended in −Lys DMM and pelleted by centrifugation. They are resuspended in 1 ml incorporation medium and incubated at 37 °C in a water-saturated CO_2 incubator. Radioactive supernantant can be collected after 16–20 h incubation. Alternatively, after 8 h incubation a further 2×10^6 cells are washed as above and the pellet added to the radioactive culture (Figure 8a). The supernatant is collected after a further 10–12 h incubation (Figure 8b).

Materials
−Lys DMM: DMM without L-lysine (Gibco Bio-Cult) (DMM: Dulbecco modified medium). Dialysed FCS: foetal calf serum is dialysed against double-distilled water. After dialysis add one-ninth of 10 times balanced saline solution. [^{3}H] or [^{13}C]Lys: L, 4,5-[^{3}H]lysine monohydrochloride, 5 mCi in 5 ml (The Radiochemical Centre, Amersham, England. Cat. No. TRK 520), or L [U- ^{14}C]lysine monohydrochloride, 250 Ci in 5 ml (Cat. No. CFB 69).

Incorporation medium:
9 ml –Lys DMM   2.5 ml –Lys DMM
1 ml [^{14}C]Lys   *or*   1.8 ml [^{3}H]Lys: 0.2 DMM salts (10×)
0.5 ml dialysed FCS   0.5 ml dialysed serum

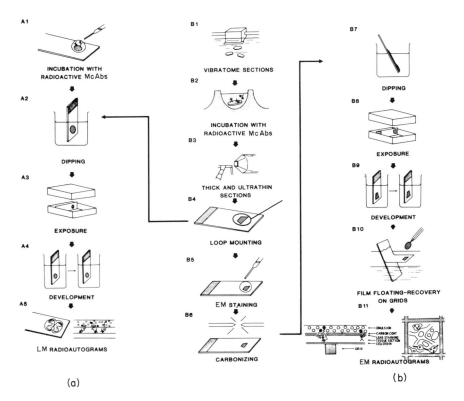

Figure 9 Flow scheme for the application of internally labelled monoclonal antibodies in light (a) and electron (b) microscopy radioimmunocytochemistry (see text)

VII.2 Characteristics of Internally Labelled Monoclonal Antibody

The radioactive supernatants of hybrid myelomas contain between 50–70%
pure monoclonal antibody which can often be used directly for electrophoretic analysis or for immunochemical and biochemical studies of the antibody
molecule itself. For example, in the case of YC5/45 HLK the sodium dodecyl
sulphate polyacrylamide (SDS) gel electrophoretic analysis of the labelled
antibody demonstrated that it was a molecule which contains a heavy chain of
a molecular weight of about 50,000 and two light chains of about 22,000

daltons. The autoradiography of the gel plate after electrophoresis revealed that one of the subclones did not synthesize the band labelled K and this was coded YC5/45 HL. In the case of the anti-substance P monoclonal antibody the radioautographic analysis of the secreted material from the clone NCl/34 HL revealed that it produced a complete immunoglobulin of the G class with a differential motility on SDS gel electrophoresis than that produced by the parental myeloma NS1 (Cuello *et al.*, 1980) and in the case of YC5/45 that one of the subclones lost the parental K light chain (Cuello and Milstein, 1981).

Internally radiolabelled monoclonal antibodies contain a number of impurities, mainly non-incorporated radioactive amino acids, which produce high background in radioimmunocytochemistry. They can be eliminated simply by extensive dialysis at 4 °C in large volumes of PBS. Other contaminants can be eliminated by passage through columns separating Ig from other radiolabelled proteins or Ig fragments. This might prove difficult when dealing with small amounts of tissue culture supernatants. In practice, pre-absorption of the diluted preparation in the presence of rat brain powder suffices to eliminate unwanted radiolabelled molecules which can unspecifically bind to tissue preparations.

The incubation dilution of internally labelled monoclonal antibodies will depend on the 'strength' of the preparation resulting from antibody affinity and its specific activity. Antibody affinity can be assessed from the titre (maximum working dilution) using the corresponding unlabelled monoclonal antibody and the second will depend on the amount of radioactive amino acids effectively incorporated in the immunoglobulin secreted by the hybridoma. In our experience with radiolabelled monoclonal antibodies NC1/34, YC5/45 and NOC1 this varies from 1:1 to 1:50 (spent medium:diluent).

VII.3 Light Microscopy

At present the experience gathered in our laboratory is centred on the use of 10 μm thick cyrostat sections and 1 μm thick plastic embedded sections and it can be summarized as below (see also flow scheme of Figure 9).

Cryostat sections (This protocol can also be applied to paraffin-embedded sections).

—10 μm thick cryostat sections obtained at −20 °C are recovered in chromalum subbed glass slides.
—Sections are pre-incubated for approximately 15 min in PBS containing 0.1 or 0.2% Triton X-100 and incubated in appropriate dilutions in PBS of tissue culture supernatant containing radiolabelled monoclonal antibodies pre-absorbed with nanogram amounts of rat brain powder per millilitre of solution. The period of incubation depends on the nature of the experiment. Short incubations (30–60 min) at 37 °C in a humid chamber give

satisfactory results with internally labelled monoclonal antibodies of high titre. More economically, larger dilutions can be used in overnight incubations at 4 °C in humid chambers.

—Wash the preparations several times in PBS containing Triton X-100.

—In a dark room provided with a safelight Ilford 'S' (or the Wratten No. 2 filter of Kodak emulsions are preferred), warm up the photographic emulsion to 40–42 °C for some minutes before dipping the sections. We use Ilford K-5 diluted 1:1 (v/v) emulsion/water when a large grain is desired and Ilford L-4 for small grains (1:3 or 1:4 v/v) (Ilford Ltd, Ilford Essex, UK). Leave the sections to 'just dry' and dip into emulsion for approximately 10 s. Let the section drip for a few seconds and wipe surface opposite to section with tissue paper. Stand slides to dry on a rack for approximately 20 min (safe lights off).

—Place sections on black lightproof box containing drierite or similar desiccant and tape the box joint all round with a dark plastic tape. Date, identify, and store at 4 °C in a refrigerator. Exposure time varies according to density of immunoreactive sites of the tissue under study, the titre, and specific activity of radioactive monoclonal antibodies. Good radioautographs can be obtained with internally radiolabelled monoclonal antibodies of high specific activity after exposures as short as 2 or 3 days. It is recommended that several slides be dipped simultaneously and then exposed for different periods to find the optimal exposure time.

—After various intervals (average 1 week) develop latent image in the following freshly prepared solution: Kodak D19 (as instructed by the manufacturers) for Ilford K2 and K5 and DK 170 for Ilford L4. This solution is prepared as follows: 20 ml DK 170 developer stock (DK 170 Stock = anhydrous Na-sulphate 25 g, potassium bromide 1 g and distilled water 200 ml. Add 0.45 g of Amidol (2-4 diaminophenol hydrochloride). Gently dissolve Amidol and bring solution to 20 °C. As fixative use a solution of 25% sodium thiosulphate adjusted to 20 °C. Independently of the developer used, prepare the following series of beakers: developer, wash in water, fixative, three final washes in water. Standard developing time should be 3–5 min, first wash in water approximately 30 s, fixation 5 min, and final washes 2 min each. A thorough final washing is essential to prevent the late removal of silver grains by sodium thiosulphate remaining absorbed in the tissue. Let slides dry standing on a rack. Add mounting media and coverslip. Cryostat sections can be conveniently counterstained with neutral red. Cryostat or paraffin-embedded slides are best analysed with bright field. Thick plastic-embedded sections should preferably be examined under phase contrast for fine details and dark field for overall survey of the preparation.

Figure 10A illustrates results obtained for the light microscopic localization

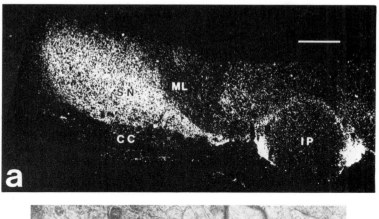

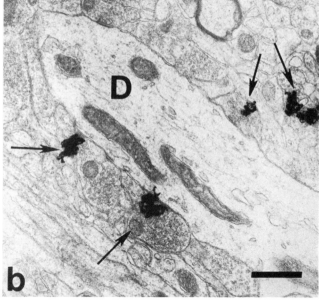

Figure 10 (a) Light microscopic radioautograph (dark field) of rat brain stem showing the binding of ^{3}H-NCl/34 (radiolabelled anti-substance P antibody); SN, substantia nigra; IP, nucleus interpeduncularis; CC, crus cerebri; ML, medial lemniscus. (Bar = 100 μm) (b) Radioimmunocytochemical preparation of the electron microscopic level of the rat substantia nigra (pars reticulata) with ^{3}H-NCl/34. Clusters of silver grains are seen over nerve terminal profiles (arrows) in the neuropile. Three of these nerve terminals are establishing axo-dendritic synapses with a typical large dendrite (D) of this region of the brain. (Bar = 1 μm.) (From Cuello *et al.*, 1982a)

of substance P immunoreactive sites with an internally labelled monoclonal antibody (3H-NC1) in the ventral mesencephalon of the rat brain stem.

VII.4 Electron Microscopy

Although many different treatments of tissue preparations are compatible with high-resolution radioimmunocytochemistry, we will refer to a single procedure here (for flow diagram see Figure 9). For researchers interested in other approaches we suggest consultation of the manuals by Rogers (1979) and Williams (1980).

VII.4.1 *Fixation of the tissue*

As for immunoenzyme technique (for details see Chapter 11) a compromise has to be found between good ultrastructure and preservation antigenicity of the substance under investigation. For most tissue and neural antigens the combination of 4% paraformaldehyde and 0.5% glutaraldehyde seems most adequate.

VII.4.2 *Tissue sectioning*

Good results have been obtained by the use of 40–200 μm thick Vibratome (Oxford) sections of previously fixed blocks of nervous tissue. Thin sections facilitate the penetration of radiolabelled antibodies but they have a tendency to curl up during further processing. The choice of thickness depends on the characteristics of the material under study. Thus, homogeneous material can be cut thinly while areas of the CNS requiring orientation should be cut relatively thickly (up to 200 μm) to facilitate flat embedding and recognition of nuclear or subnuclear organization.

VII.4.3 *Incubation with radiolabelled antibodies*

For electron microscopy the Vibratome sections are incubated at 4 °C for up to 24 h in wells containing the corresponding dilutions of radiolabelled monoclonal antibody/PBS, without Triton X-100 (see Chapter 11). A short pre-incubation (up to 1 h) of the Vibratome slice in PBS containing 0.1% Triton X-100 improves penetration without much damage to tissue preservation. After incubation the tissue slices are washed several times in PBS. Post-fixation in glutaraldehyde can now be attempted if necessary. The tissue is now processed as detailed in Chapter 11.

VII.4.4 *Thick sections*

Before furthering the preparation of the experimental material for high-resolution radioautography, it is advisable to analyse the success of the incubation with radiolabelled monoclonal antibodies by obtaining 1 μm thick tissue sections of the plastic-embedded tissue. This will also allow the recognition of tissue landmarks at light microscopy level and will allow for further trimming of the blocks. The ultramicrotome 1 μm 'thick' sections can be cut using a dry glass knife and can be collected on glass slides with the aid of fine forceps. Properly labelled, frosted glass slides should be used. Place a few drops of distilled water on the slide and without touching the knife edge, collect sections (or section) and deposit them in the drop (or drops) of distilled water. The section should float on the drop and be dried in an oven at 80 °C for 2–3 min. The slides can now be treated as for light microscopic radioautography (see preceding section and flow diagrams of Figure 9).

VII.4.5 Ultrathin sections

It is expected that the electron microscopic demonstration of the binding sites of internally labelled antibodies can be demonstrated with various procedures. So far, adaptation of the dipping procedure of Salpeter and Bachman (1964) has been applied. After light microscopic analysis the selected areas of the blocks are trimmed for ultrathin sectioning. For this, ribbons of ultrathin sections displaying silver–gold interference are mounted with a loop on celloidin coated glass slides (Figure 9). At least two or three slides per block (each containing a couple of ribbons) should be prepared. Coated glass slides should be prepared in advance and stored in dust-free boxes. Acid–alcohol cleaned, dry frosted and glass slides (not the frosted end) are dipped in celloidin solution for about 2–3 s. The celloidin solution is prepared as follows: 720 mg of good-quality celloidin is dissolved in a disposable beaker containing 90 ml 0.8% amylacetate. Cover the beaker and stir continuously either overnight or for several hours. Let amylacetate evaporate by standing the glass slides on racks. After a couple of days check that the film can be effectively detached by floating as described below.

—Stain sections with uranylacetate, lead citrate, or both as for conventional electron microscopy routine on glass Petri dishes with the bottom filled with dental wax or paraffin. Staining solutions should be placed gently with a Pasteur pipette over the ultrathin sections. If lead citrate is carried out place a few pellets of sodium hydroxide to absorb the environmental CO_2. Washes should be performed very gently with a Pasteur pipette or wash bottle. Let the preparation dry and keep covered and free from dust.
—A thin layer of carbon (approximately 5 nm thick) is needed to prevent chemography. Follow equivalent instructions and check whether or not the

carbon coat interferes with excessive electron opacity. As a general rule, carbonizing a piece of white porcelain with a drop of oil allows discrimination when an effective layer of carbon has been deposited. The carbonizing should be completed when a contrast is just observed between the surface under the drop of oil and the rest of the porcelain.

—A solution of 1:5.5 (emulsion:water (v/v)) should be prepared in advance in the dark room and brought to 50 °C. (It is convenient to have separate aliquots so that the emulsion need not be melted more than once.) Dip slides slowly and keep in the emulsion for a few seconds before draining. Do not wipe the back of the slide. In order to obtain a constant thickness of emulsion coating, 'dipping' devices can be constructed for a more controlled withdrawal of the slide. A simple model has been described by Dr Parry at Oxford and has been reproduced in various manuals (Rogers, 1979; Williams, 1980). Allow the slides to drain on a rack for 30 min to 1 h at room temperature and in constant darkness. Once dried the slides are transferred to properly labelled light-tight boxes containing drierite and sealed with black tape.

—Expose the radioautograms for 1 month or more at 4 °C. The approximate time of exposure is four times that obtained for the same material at light microscopy. Take one slide of the series at a time.

—If using Ilford L-5, develop with Kodak D19B, freshly made as follows: To 100 ml distilled water add, while stirring: Elon 220 mg; anhydrous sodium sulphate 7.2 g; hydroquinone 880 mg; anhydrous sodium carbonate 4.8 g; potassium bromide 400 mg. Filter with Whatman paper No. 1. For development, follow the same scheme as for light microscopy, but the slides should remain in the developer for only 2 min. When opening the box, remove the tape slowly. After developing allow the tissue sections to dry for a few minutes.

—For floating the celloidine (see Figure 9, B10) with the developed ultrathin section, prepare a very clean, large glass container filled to capacity with distilled water. Remove floating particles by wiping the surface with a lens paper. With a glass slide and using a new corner per side, scratch a square of approximately 2 or 3 cm around the ultrathin sections. Breathe gently on to the square and dip the slide slowly at an angle into the water allowing a side of the square to touch the surface simultaneously along the whole extent of the scratch. The square should detach at that point and float while while the slide is being progressively immersed. Move the glass slide carefully sideways to complete detachment. If the emulsion–celloidin layer does not detach easily we have found that freezing the scratched glass slides facilitates the posterior detachment of the celloidin. Once floating the celloidin can be stretched and flattened with the heat of a lamp.

—Collect the sections on conventional EM grids, shiny side down. Holding with fine forceps, lower one edge carefully until one end of the ribbon is touched and then allow it to drop towards the other end. Place wet filter paper on the surface of a suction device. The suction should hold the paper firmly in position. With a fast parallel movement, lower the device to the celloidin and grids which should stick to the filter paper. Remove the device from the water and place (filter paper and grids upwards) on a Petri dish to dry in an oven at 60°C. After drying, sections are ready to be examined under the electron microscope.

VIII   POTENTIAL APPLICATIONS OF MONOCLONAL ANTIBODIES IN NEUROIMMUNOCYTOCHEMISTRY

VIII.1   Monoclonal Antibodies and Specificity of Staining

When polyclonal antibodies are applied in immunocytochemistry higher concentrations of the antisera are usually required than for radioimmuno-assay, a system conventionally used for sera characterization and for quantitative analysis of immunoreactive substances. As an individual population of antibodies recognizes different determinants with different affinities it is frequently the case that the antibodies which are expressed in immunocytochemistry are not the same as those expressed in radioimmunoassay. This, of course, does not occur when applying monoclonal antibodies, as the same population of antibodies with a single combining site are present in the incubation medium regardless of the concentration of immunoglobulins used in the assay system. The characterization of the antibody-combining sites done with radioimmunoassay will therefore apply to immunocytochemistry when using the same monoclonal antibody. Nevertheless the immune reaction will not necessarily establish the chemical nature of tissue substances recognized by monoclonal antibodies. It is therefore advisable to retain the term 'immunoreactivity' even when dealing with monoclonal antibodies as primary reagents (see Section X, Chapter 1).

An advantage of monoclonal antibodies as primary reagents for immunocytochemistry is that they immortalize difficult or rare antibodies. An example of such antibodies is given by the rat hybrid line coded YC5/45 which secretes monoclonal antibodies to serotonin. When this antibody is tested by indirect immunofluorescence it detects serotonin-containing cell bodies and terminals in the central (Consolazione *et al.*, 1981; Consolazione and Cuello, 1982) peripheral nervous systems. Competition experiments demonstrated that this antibody displayed strong cross-reactivity with dopamine, tryptamine, and 5-methoxytryptamine in liquid media (Consolazione *et al.*, 1981). This provides an example of antibody cross-reactivity resulting from multi-recognition by a single molecular species, i.e. the 'intrinsic cross-reactivity' of the monoclonal antibody (Milstein *et al.*, 1980). Such cross-reactivity is of a more specific nature than the cross-reactivity associated with ordinary polyclonal antisera. Polyclonal antisera are complex mixtures of monoclonal antibodies and their cross-reactivities might result from cross-reaction of individual antibody molecular species. The intrinsic cross-reactivity to dopamine and other amines of this monoclonal antibody is more apparent than real, as the antibody shows a much higher affinity for the serotonin–bovine seroalbumin conjugate, but does not recognize bovine seroalbumin alone. Formaldehyde also shifts the cross-reaction towards serotonin in haemagglutination tests. When the antibody was tested in tissue preparations it completely failed to reveal dopamine sites in areas of the brain where the presence of this amine is well documented, namely the zona compacta of the substantia nigra and ventro-tegemtnal groups. It does appear that with paraformaldhyde fixation, YC5/45 does not reveal the dopamine antigenic sites in brain tissue preparations. On further studies using tissue model systems we have established that the formaldehyde fixation is essential for the generation of 'serotonin' immunoreactive sites (Milstein, Wright, and Cuello, 1983). The results thus emphasize the relevance of the method used for detection. When performing immunocytochemical studies, specificity can be introduced by the antibody interactions ('antibody specificity' of both primary and secondary antibodies) and also by the conditions of the incubations, and preparation of the tissue ('method specificity') (see Chapter 1). Here again monoclonal antibodies can be invaluable tools to explore 'methods specificity' as there is no risk that different antibody molecular species can be expressed under different experimental circumstances. Thus, in the case of YC5/45 experimental evidence showed that the antibody sees only serotonin sites in fixed brain-stem tissue by the pretreatment with drugs which affect the monoamine content in the brain. Thus α-methyl-*p*-tyrosine in conditions which produce a very drastic depletion of the catecholamine content in neurones of the central nervous system did not affect the immunofluorescence, while depletors of 5-HT such as the tryptophan hydroxylase inhibitor *p*-chlorophenylalanine resulted in a marked diminution of the binding of YC5/45 to neurones in the raphe nuclei system (see Figure 11).

The use of monoclonal antibodies as primary reagents tends to improve the quality of the immunostain as unwanted antibodies or carrier immunoglobulins are eliminated. This results in a better signal to noise ratio which can be critical when dealing with small numbers of antigenic sites. Background is, in these cases, dependent upon the quality of secondary antibodies used to

------

Figure 11 (**A**) Control preparation showing immunofluorescent cell bodies and processes in the nucleus raphe dorsalis of the rat incubated with YC5/45 HL. (**B**) Nucleus raphe dorsalis incubated with YC5/45 HL. Pargyline-pretreated rat displaying some enhancement of immunofluorescent reaction. (**C**) Nucleus raphe dorsalis incubated with YC5/45 HL. Note the almost total disappearance of immunofluorescence in the same area in rats pretreated with the tryptophan hydroxylase inhibitor

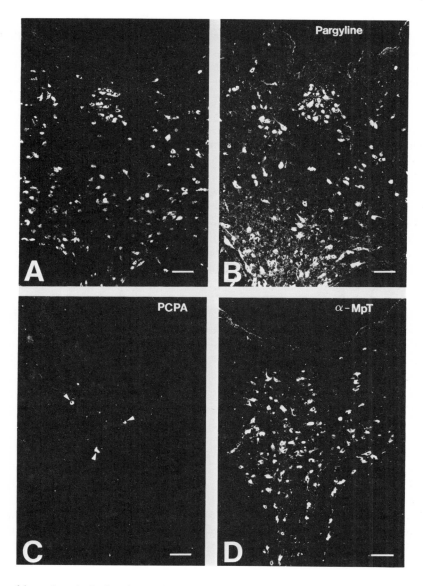

parachlorophenyl-alanine (PCPA). Some remaining weak fluorescent cell bodies are indicated with arrowheads. (**D**) Nucleus raphe dorsalis incubated with YC5/45 HL. Immune reaction equivalent to control in a rat pretreated with the tyrosine hydroxylase inhibitor α-methyl paratyrosine (α-MpT). (Bars = 100 μm.) Reprinted by permission of the publisher from 'Immunocytochemical detection of serotonin with monoclonal antibodies', by Consolazione *et al.*, *J. Histochem. Cytochem.*, **29,** 1425–1430. Copyright 1981 by The Histochemical Society Inc.

demonstrate the antibody binding in tissue. The first demonstration of such applications for an intracellular antigen was provided by the anti-substance P monoclonal antibody coded NC1/34 (Cuello *et al.*, 1979). For NC1/34 radioimmunoassay was used to analyse the 'intrinsic cross-reactivity' of this monoclonal antibody. NC1/34 showed no cross-reactivity with a number of brain peptides while cross-reacting completely with small C-terminal fragments of the peptide and by 5% with the related eleidosin. The good correlation of this particular monoclonal antibody in radioimmunoassay and immunohistochemistry can be explained as follows: in both cases the NC1/34 recognizes the C-terminal portion of the peptide and this part of the molecule is seemingly not affected by the aldehyde fixation which most probably affects the N-terminal portion of the molecule. In opposition to this case an anti-Leu-enkephalin antibody coded NOC1 has been derived from a mouse × mouse hybridoma which shows greater affinity for 'enkephalines' antigenic sites in fixed tissue preparation than in radioimmunoassay systems. It is therefore necessary to extensively characterize monoclonal antibodies and test in various systems in order to have a better understanding of tissue antigenic sites prior and after fixation.

The fact that monoclonal antibodies can be produced in large amounts is of some relevance as immunohistochemistry requires larger amounts of antibody molecules than radioimmunoassay. This aspect is also of practical importance as interesting monoclonal antibodies for research or histopathological diagnoses can be widely distributed to compare results among different laboratories or to be used as 'standards'.

VIII.2   Monoclonal Antibodies as Developing Antibodies

VIII.2.1   *Direct immunocytochemistry*

In the direct immunocytochemical technique the primary antibody itself constitutes a developing antibody. In this method the primary antibody is bound to a suitable tag which allows the microscopical detection of the antigen–antibody complexes in tissue preparations. The lack of amplification of this procedure and the loss of immunoglobulins during the isolation of specific antibodies made the technique a non-appealing alternative and it was therefore abandoned. The advent of monoclonal antibodies can radically change this situation as the hybridoma secretes only the desired antibody molecules, thus avoiding the use of affinity columns for the purification of specific antibodies. With monoclonal antibodies the simple separation of the immunoglobulins should suffice for the efficient coupling of specific antibodies to a marker molecule. This has been shown to be possible with direct conjugation of HRP to the anti-substance P monoclonal antibody (see Figure 5). For this, rabbit immunoglobulin against rat IgG (Dako, Denmark) was coupled to CNBr activated Sepharose beads (Pharmacia, Sweden) and the eluate, presumably pure monoclonal antibody NC1/34, was conjugated to horseradish peroxidase by a two-step method (Boorsma *et al.*, 1982). This resulted in a 400,000 dalton preparation with 1:1 monoclonal antibody/horseradish peroxidase and approximately 100% of the monoclonal antibody was effectively conjugated in contrast to the usually low yield obtained when polyclonal antibodies are used. The large molecular weight of the HRP–McAb conjugate was similar to that of the PAP (peroxidase–antiperoxidase) complex. The immunohistochemical application of this enzyme monoclonal antibody complex resulted in a very clean immunostain in areas known to contain the peptide in the rat CNS. Very fast immunocytochemical results can be obtained with this procedure. Direct immunocytochemistry with monoclonal antibodies could prove to be of relevance for diagnostic applications of biopsy material.

The introduction of various sizes of gold particles as antibody markers might also offer new possibilities to direct immunohistochemical techniques with monoclonal antibodies (see Chapter 13). It is conceivable that different monoclonal antibodies could be tagged to different sizes of gold particles. This, and the combined use of immunoenzyme techniques, should allow the simultaneous detection of various antigenic sites at light and electron microscope levels. Direct immunocytochemistry with monoclonal antibodies using enzymic or metal markers (or other tags) should expand the possibilities of simultaneous detection of various antigenic sites both at light and electron microscopic level.

VIII.2.2 *Indirect immunocytochemistry*

Monoclonal antibodies have not been used extensively so far as developing reagents in immunocytochemistry. Nevertheless they might very well replace conventional antibodies as standard reagents for indirect immunocytochemical techniques. In our laboratory we have successfully used a mouse monoclonal anti-rabbit IgG antibody as a bridge antibody for rabbit-based PAP techniques (McMillan, Sofroniew, Sidebottom, and Cuello, in preparation). Our preliminary results would indicate that unspecific background staining diminishes considerably when using this monoclonal antibody, while there is no substantial difference in the magnitude of the signal even when non-concentrated supernatant from tissue culture medium is utilized.

Rat-based PAP technique can also be performed with a rat antiperoxidase monoclonal antibody provisionally coded YC6 (Milstein, Cuello, Wright and Bramwell, to be published). Similar positive results have also been obtained by Mason and collaborators (personal communication) with a mouse anti-peroxidase monoclonal antibody.

These positive results using monoclonal antibodies as developing reagents are somewhat surprising, as one might expect that polyclonal antibodies could be more effective in amplifying the signal given by a primary antibody as different antibodies of the mix could recognize different determinants of a single immunoglobulin. It is possible that the success of the application of monoclonal antibodies as developing antibodies depends both on their association constant and on the possible recognition of repetitive determinants.

VIII.3   Immunocytochemical Applications of Internally Labelled Monoclonal Antibodies

The high specific activity (50–2000 Ci/mmol for 3H-NC1/34 HL) obtained by the internal labelling of monoclonal antibodies results in enhanced sensitivity of this procedure as compared with conventional immunocytochemistry. At the light microscopic level successful radioautographs were obtained 72 h following incubation. It is hoped that the use of internally labelled monoclonal antibodies at light microscopic level will allow the quantification of the immunohistochemical reaction. Preliminary observations would indicate that this is feasible (Cuello *et al.*, 1982a). This method may offer a meaningful alternative for quantification in immunocytochemistry. Previous attempts have been based on the use of fluorescent markers, or, more recently, on the intensity of peroxidase reaction following the chain of antibodies required for the PAP techniques. In all these cases the final signal of the immune reaction is distant to the primary antibody binding while with radioimmunocytochemistry the signal should be directly related to the binding of the primary antibody. The validity of these assumptions can only be tested experimentally.

Another potential application of 'radioimmunocytochemistry' is the detection of minute amounts of antigenic material which happen to occur in highly localized areas. This again is possible due to the high specific activity of internally labelled monoclonal antibodies. An example of this is provided by the reaction of 3H-YC5/45 on cryostat sections. Vertebrate retina is suspected of containing only traces of an indolamine, probably serotonin. The application of 3H-YC5/45 demonstrated clearly a binding of this antibody in amacrine cell bodies and their processes in the internal plexiform layer of the frog retina (Osborne *et al.*, 1981).

Internally labelled monoclonal antibodies do not require developing antibodies for the detection of antigenic sites. Therefore this compromise is less costly in terms of tissue preservation in electron microscopy where the use of conventional immunoenzyme techniques result in a compromise between good ultrastructural preservation and penetration of high molecular weight antibody complexes. A potential advantage of 'radioimmunocytochemistry' is the elimination of the electron-dense products resulting from the application of immunoenzyme techniques which on occasions obscure the fine ultra-structural details of immunoreactive sites. The main disadvantage of fine resolution radioautography with monoclonal antibodies resides in the need for high technical expertise and the long exposure times.

Radioimmunocytochemistry can be combined with immunoenzyme techniques for the simultaneous detection of two antigenic sites at light and electron microscopical levels (Cuello *et al.*, 1982a; Priestley and Cuello, 1982). Encouraging results have been obtained for the simultaneous detection of two intracellular antigens: substance P and serotonin, in the raphe nuclei (see Figure 12) and substance P and Leu-enkephalin in the substantia gelatinosa of the spinal nucleus of the trigeminal nerve. The combined use of radioimmunocytochemistry and immunoenzyme techniques might find wider applications in fields unrelated to neurobiology.

VIII.4 Monoclonal Antibodies in Histopathology

Immunohistochemistry began with research related to histopathology. Nowadays, a number of diagnoses are based on immunohistochemical analysis of tissue preparations. The methodology is nevertheless restricted to those researchers having access to limited sources of relevant antibodies. Therefore, up to now, the application of this technique has been restricted to major medical institutions. It is possible that monoclonal antibodies will change this situation.

An example of the potential use of monoclonal antibodies in histopathology is given by the application of YC5/45 to detect serotonin immunoreactive sites in normal and pathological specimens. At present the microscopic diagnosis of serotonin-producing carcinoid tumours is based on the morphological pattern and only occasionally confirmed by silver staining for the argyrophilic or argentaffinic reaction, or by electron microscopic analysis. All these procedures are either erratic or do not substantially add to the diagnostic analysis. For example, non-reactive tumours to silver salts are often found which are otherwise considered carcinoid tumours by the microscopic pattern and biochemical data. Immunocytochemistry offers a more reliable approach towards the microscopic diagnosis of carcinoids. The monoclonal antibody YC5/45 has demonstrated that a close correlation exists for immunohistochemistry of 5-HT immunoreactive sites and the clinical and biochemical data (Cuello *et al.*, 1982b).

Up to the present few neuropathological studies have been done using immunocytochemistry for neurotransmitter substances, despite the fact that this technique can accurately demonstrate the presence or absence of neuroactive substances in cell groups or tracts in defined nuclear areas. The restricted use of this technique is partially due to the inaccessibility of relevant antibodies. The main reason for this is simply that scanning immunoreactive

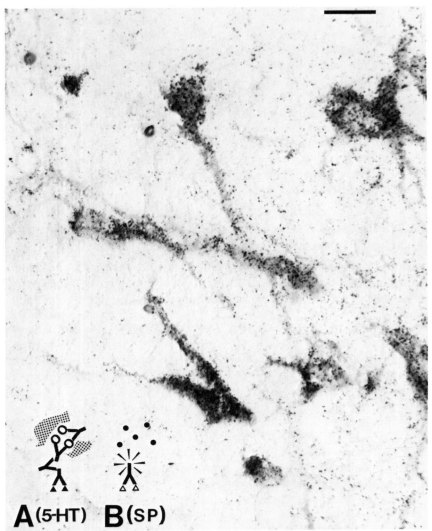

Figure 12 Combined radioimmunocytochemistry and PAP immunocytochemistry; cryostat sections (10 μm thick) of raphe magnus of the rat medullar oblongata. Antigenic sites A (5-HT serotonin, ▲) were demonstrated by using anti-serotonin monoclonal antibodies (YC5/45) and developed according to the peroxidase–antiperoxidase technique, producing a homogeneous brownish enzyme reaction product over cell bodies and dendrites of raphe magnus neurones. Antigenic sites B (SP, substance P) (△) were demonstrated by radioimmunocytochemistry using anti-substance P internally labelled monoclonal antibody (3H-NCl/34) producing characteristic silver grains in emulsion. Note that cells in the field contain both neuroactive substances.
(Bar = 20 μm) (From Cuello *et al.*, 1982a)

sites in human brain requires a considerable amount of specific antibodies due to the size and number of microscopic preparations. As monoclonal antibodies can be produced in large amounts such scanning will be more practical in the future. As an example of the histopathological application, NC1/34 has shown that while large concentrations of substance P immunoreactive terminals were present in the substantia gelatinosa of the spinal cord of control human nervous systems, there was an almost complete absence of such terminals from this region in all patients suffering from familial dysautonomia, a neurological condition associated with specific neuronal losses and with diminished pain sensitivity (Pearson *et al.*, 1982).

VIII.5 Monoclonal Antibodies to Unknown Antigens

When an animal is immunized with a given immunogen multiple antibodies are likely to be produced against many determinants. All these antibodies will be mixed in the polyclonal serum. The isolation of a single molecular species of immunoglobulin produced by a given clone facilitates the immunological dissection of those determinants. This virtue of the hybridoma technique is being used extensively in neurobiology for the identification of molecular components or cell types. For many of these studies the resulting monoclonal antibodies are being used as primary antibodies in immunocytochemistry.

Examples of such applications are the recognition of defined neuronal cell groups in the nervous system of the leech by monoclonal antibodies originating from immunizing animals with the entire leech nerve cord (Zipser and McKay, 1981). Similarly the immunization with cultured cells has allowed the preparation of monoclonal antibodies which in conventional immunocytochemistry recognize determinants present only in central (Cohen and Selvendran, 1981) or peripheral (Vulliamy *et al.*, 1981) mammalian nervous systems. Schachner and collaborators (1981) (see also Chapter 15) have shown that glial cells can be classified convincingly by using various sets of monoclonal antibodies against unknown surface determinants, followed by immunofluorescence or immunoenzyme techniques. In the rat retina monoclonal antibodies have been reported to recognize different cell types (Barnstable, 1980) or determinants distributed with a characteristic topographic gradient (Trisler *et al.*, 1981). Along the same lines, we have recently isolated an antibody which binds preferentially to a given synaptic area: the substantia gelatinosa of the spinal cord (Cuello, Galfré and Milstein, in preparation). All these .applications of monoclonal antibodies will not only give a new impetus to immunocytochemistry but will also help our understanding of a large number of basic problems in the neurobiology of cell to cell recognition, differentiation and establishment of synapses, and the nature of their molecular components.

Even though monoclonal antibodies are powerful tools which can be of enormous assistance in neurobiological research they are limited in their powers. Thus the single combining sites of a monoclonal antibody can cross-react to a variable degree with more than one determinant (see introduction of Section VIII.1, and Chapter 1, Section X). Therefore the determinants recognized by them are not necessarily equivalent to a given amino acid sequence or molecular conformation.

ACKNOWLEDGEMENTS

We would like to thank Eric Sidebottom, John Priestley, Bruce Wright, Frances MacMillan, Adriana Consolazione, and John Jarvis for their collaborative efforts in the work mentioned here. The technical assistance of Steven Bramwell, Brian Archer, and Julia Lloyd together with the secretarial help of Mrs Ella Iles is also much appreciated. Grants from the Wellcome Trust (UK) and financial assistance from the E. P. Abraham Cephalosporin Trust is also acknowledged.

REFERENCES

Barnstable, C. J. (1980). 'Monoclonal antibodies which recognise different cell types in the rat retina.' *Nature*, **286**, 231–235.

Boorsma, D. M., Cuello, A. C., and Van Leuwen, F. W. (1982). 'Direct immunocytochemistry with a horseradish peroxidase conjugated monoclonal antibody against substance P.' *J. Histochem. Cytochem.* (submitted).

Chan-Palay, V., Jonsson, G., and Palay, S. L. (1978). 'Serotonin and substance P co-exist in neurons of the rat's central nervous system.' *Proc. Natl. Acad. Sci. USA*, **75**, 1582–1586.

Cohen J. and Selvendran, S. Y. (1981). 'A neuronal cell-surface antigen is found in the CNS but not in peripheral neurones.' *Nature*, **291**, 421–423.

Consolazione, A. and Cuello, A. C. (1982). 'CNS serotonin pathways.' In Osborne, N. N. (ed.), *Biology of Serotonergic Transmission*, pp. 29–61. J. Wiley & Sons, Chichester, England.

Consolazione, A., Milstein, C., Wright, B., and Cuello, A. C. (1981). 'Immunocytochemical detection of serotonin with monoclonal antibodies.' *J. Histochem. Cytochem.*, **29**, 1425–1430.

Cotten, J. and Selvendran, S. (1981). 'A rat central nervous system specific neuronal cell-surface antigen defined by a monoclonal antibody.' *Nature*, **241**, 421–423.

Cozzari, C. and Hartman, B. K. (1981). 'Preparation of antibodies specific to choline acetyltransferase from bovine brain.' *J. Neurochem.*, **20**, 1075–1081.

Cuello, A. C., Galfré, G., and Milstein, C. (1979). 'Detection of substance P in the central nervous system by a monoclonal antibody.' *Proc. Natl. Acad. Sci. USA*, **76**, 3532–3536.

Cuello, A. C., Galfré, G., and Milstein, C. (1980). 'Development of a monoclonal antibody against a neuroactive peptide. Immunocytochemical applications.' In Pepeu, G., Kuhar, M. J., and Enna, S. J. (eds), *Receptors for Neurotransmitters and Peptide Hormones*, pp. 349–363. Raven Press, New York.

Cuello, A. C. and Milstein, C. (1981). 'Use of internally labelled monoclonal antibodies.' In Bizollon, Ch. A. (ed.), *Physiological Peptides and New Trends in*

Radioimmunology, pp. 293–305. Elsevier–North Holland, Amsterdam.

Cuello, A. C., Priestley, J. V., and Milstein, C. (1982a). 'Immunocytochemistry with internally labelled monoclonal antibodies.' *Proc. Natl. Acad. Sci. USA*, **79**, 665–669.

Cuello, A. C., Wells, C., Chaplin, A. J., and Milstein, C. (1982b). 'Serotonin-immunoreactivity in carcinoid tumours demonstrated by a monoclonal antibody.' *Lancet*, **i**, 771–773.

Galfré, G. and Milstein, C. (1981). 'Preparation of monoclonal antibodies—strategies and procedures.' *Methods in Enzymology*, **73**, 3–46.

Herbert, W. J. (1978). 'Mineral-oil adjuvants and the immunisation of laboratory animals.' In Weir, D. M. (ed.), *Handbook of Experimental Immunology*, 3rd Edition, pp. A3.1–A3.14. Blackwell, Oxford.

Hökfelt, T., Fuxe, K., Goldstein, M., and Joh, T. H. (1973). 'Immunohistochemical localisation of three catecholamine synthesising enzymes: aspect on methodology.' *Histochemie*, **33**, 231–254.

Hökfelt, T., Johansson, O., Fuxe, K., Goldstein, M., and Park, D. (1976). 'Immuno-histochemical studies on the localisation and distribution of monoamine neuron systems in the rat brain. I. Tyrosine hydroxylase in the mes- and diencephalon.' *Med. Biol.*, **54**, 427–453.

Hökfelt, T., Johansson, O., Fuxe, K., Goldstein, M., and Park, D. (1977). 'Immuno-histochemical studies on the localisation and distribution of monoamine neuron systems in the rat brain. II. Tyrosine hydroxylase in the telencephalon.' *Med. Biol.*, **55**, 21–40.

Hudson, L. and Hay, F. C. (1980). *Practical Immunology* (2nd edition). Blackwell, Oxford.

Kanazawa, I. and Jessell, T. (1976). 'Post-mortem changes and regional distribution of substance P in the rat and mouse nervous system.' *Brain Res.*, **117**, 362–367.

Kimura, H., McGeer, P. L., Peng, J. H., and McGeer, E. G. (1980). 'Choline acetyltransferase containing neurons in rodent brain by immunohistochemistry.' *Science*, **208**, 1057–1059.

Köhler, G. and Milstein, C. (1975). 'Continuous culture of fused cells secreting antibody of pre-defined specificity.' *Nature*, **256**, 495–497.

Littlefield, J. W. (1964). 'Selection of hybrids from mating of fibroblasts *in vitro* and their presumed recombinants.' *Science*, **145**, 709–716.

Milstein, C., Clark, M. R., Galfré, G., and Cuello, A. C. (1980). 'Monoclonal antibodies from hybrid myelomas.' In Fougerau, M., and Dausset, J. (eds), *Progress in Immunology*, pp. 17–33. Academic Press, New York and London.

Milstein, C., Wright, B., and Cuello, A. C. (1983). 'The discrepancy between the cross reactivity of a monoclonal antibody to serotonin and its immunohistochemical specificity.' *J. Mol. Immunol.*, **20**, 113–123.

Osborne, N. N., Nesselhut, T., Nicholas, D. A., and Cuello, A. C. (1981). 'Serotonin: a transmitter candidate in the vertebrate retina.' *Neurochem. Int.*, **3**, 171–176.

Parker, C. W. (1976). *Radioimmunoassay of Biologically Active Compounds*. Prentice Hall, Englewood Cliffs, New Jersey.

Pearson, J., Brandeis, L., and Cuello, A. C. (1982). 'Depletion of axons containing substance P in the substantia gelatinosa of patients with diminished pain sensitivity.' *Nature*, **275**, 61–63.

Pickel, V. M., Joh, T. H., and Reis, D. J. (1976). 'Monoamine-synthesising enzymes in central dopaminergic, noradrenergic and serotonergic neurons: immunocytoche-mical localisation by light and electron microscopy.' *J. Histochem. Cytochem.*, **24**, 792–806.

Powell, D., Leeman, S., Tregear, G. W., Niall, H. D., and Potts, J. T. (1973). 'Radioimmunoassay for substance P.' *Nature New Biol.*, **241**, 252–254.

Priestley, J. V. and Cuello, A. C. (1982). 'Co-existence of neuroactive substances as revealed by immunohistochemistry with monoclonal antibodies.' In Cuello, A. C. (ed.), *Co-transmission*. Macmillan, New York and London, pp. 165–188.

Ribak, C. E., Vaughn, J. E., and Barber, R. P. (1981). 'Immunocytochemical localisation of GABA-ergic neurones at the electron microscopical level.' *Histochem. J.*, **13**, 555–582.

Ringertz, N. R. and Savage, R. E. (1976). *Cell Hybrids*. Academic Press, New York and London.

Rogers, A. W. (1979). *Techniques of Autoradiography*. Elsevier–North Holland, Amsterdam, New York, and Oxford.

Salpeter, M. M. and Bachman, L. (1964). 'Autoradiography with the electron microscope.' *J. Cell Biol.*, **22**, 469–477.

Schachner, M., Kim, S. K., and Zehnle, R. (1981). 'Developmental expression in central and peripheral nervous system of oligondendrocyte cell surface antigens (O-antigens), recognised by monoclonal antibodies.' *Dev. Biol.*, **83**, 328–338.

Sofroniew, M. V., Eckenstein, F., Thoener, H. and Cuello, A. C. (1982). 'Topography of choline acetyltransferase-containing neurons in the forebrain of the rat.' *Neurosci. Lett.*, **33**, 7–12.

Steinbusch, H. W. N., Verhofstad, A. A. J., and Joosten, H. W. J. (1978). 'Localisation of serotonin in the central nervous system by immunohistochemistry: description of a specific and sensitive technique and some applications.' *Neuroscience*, **3**, 811–819.

Swanson, L. W. and Hartman, B. K. (1975). 'The central adrenergic system: an immunofluorescent study of the location of cell bodies and their efferent connections in the rat utilising dopamine-β-hydroxylase as a marker.' *J. Comp. Neurol.*, **163**, 467–505.

Szybalski, W., Szybalska, E. H., and Kagni, G. (1962). 'Genetic studies with human cell lines.' *Natl. Cancer Inst. Monogr.*, **7**, 75–89.

Trisler, G. D., Schneider, M. D., and Nirenberg, N. (1981). 'A topographic gradient of molecules in retina can be used to identify neurone position 11.' *Proc. Natl. Acad. Sci. USA*, **78**, 2145–2149.

Vulliamy, T., Rattray, S., and Mirsky, R. (1981). 'Cell surface antigen distinguishes sensory and autonomic peripheral neurones from central neurones.' *Nature*, **291**, 418–420.

Weiss, D. M. (ed.) (1978). *Handbook of Experimental Immunology*. Blackwell, Oxford.

Williams, M. A. (1980). *Autoradiography and Immunocytochemistry*. In Glauert, A. M. (series ed.), series *Practical Methods in Electron Microscopy*. Elsevier–North-Holland, Amsterdam, New York, and Oxford.

Zipser, B. and McKay, R. (1981). 'Monoclonal antibodies distinguish identifiable neurones in the leech.' *Nature*, **289**, 549–554.

Immunohistochemistry
Edited by A. C. Cuello
© 1983 IBRO

CHAPTER 10

Immunohistochemical Double Staining Techniques

F. VANDESANDE

Zoölogical Institute, K.U. Leuven, Belgium

I   INTRODUCTION

In immunocytochemical studies it is sometimes desirable to demonstrate more than one antigen, in the same cell. For cell bodies this can sometimes be realized by sequential immunocytochemical staining of adjacent semi-thin serial sections. Indeed, using semi-thin sections it is possible to identify a same cell in several adjacent serial sections (Van Leeuwen *et al.*, 1979).

Nerve cell processes or subcellular particles such as secretory granules, however, cannot be identified in adjacent sections and the simultaneous visualization of more than one antigen in such structures has to be done on single tissue sections. For demonstration of two or more different antigens in the same tissue section several methods are available. One of them consists of a double autoradiographic stripping technique using two different radio-isotopes (Van Rooijen, 1972). Other methods are a combination of auto-radiography and one of the available immunofluorescence or immunoenzyme techniques (Henderson and Smithyman, 1974; Van Rooijen and Streefkerk, 1976).

This chapter deals only with the purely immunocytochemical methods.

II CRITICAL REVIEW OF THE EXISTING METHODS

II.1 Double Staining using the Direct Immunofluorescence Method

Double staining using the direct immunofluorescence method is a very simple and rapid technique which is usually performed by incubating a tissue section with a mixture of two specific antisera, each labelled with a different fluorochrome. The most widely used fluorochromes are fluorescein isothiocyanate (FITC) giving a green, and rhodamine B isothiocyanate (RITC) giving an orange-red fluorescence. Two antigens in the same cell are detected by intermediate colours.

This method has all the advantages and shortcomings of the direct immunofluorescence technique and is the least sensitive of all the immuno-cytochemical methods (Vandesamde, 1979).

II.2 Sequential Immunofluorescent Staining

In this method (Pernis, 1968; Nash *et al.*, 1969) the different antigens in a tissue section are detected by sequential applications of the corresponding fluorescein-labelled antibodies. After incubation with the first antiserum the section is washed, mounted in buffered saline, and the coverslips sealed with nail polish. Selected fields are photographed and their position in the section are recorded with the aid of the vernier calibrations on the object guide of the microscope.

The fluorescence of the positively reacting cells is then destroyed by photochemical destruction of the fluorochrome groups by ultraviolet light. This is accomplished by exposure of each field to the full beam of ultraviolet light for a period of 10–20 min, depending on the intensity of the initial fluorescence.

After verification of the completeness of the photochemical destruction, the coverslips are gently removed by immersion of the slide in a buffer solution. The tissue section is then incubated with the second fluorochrome-labelled antiserum and so on. Photographs of the selected fields are taken after each incubation with a new antiserum.

To facilitate the identification of individual cells within a sequence of photographs, the final prints can be made by projecting the negative image through a lattice of coordinates obtained by stretching silk thread across the masking frame holding the photographic paper, and aligning the image from each series of photographs in the same way (Nash *et al.*, 1969). With this method elegant studies have been performed but it shows the shortcomings of the direct immunofluorescence technique. Another problem with this technique is that beyond a certain dose of ultraviolet light the photochemical damage to the tissue is detrimental to further immunohistochemical staining.

If the label is removed more than twice, the results tend to become unsatisfactory. One can prevent this photochemical damage by omitting the ultraviolet irradiation before each new incubation and basing the analysis of the pictures on the gradual appearance of new fluorescent objects. But even then a progressive weakening of the cellular fluorescence with repeated photography of the same field has to be taken into account. This is not only due to the cumulative photochemical damage to the fluorochrome by repeated photography of the same area, but also to the increased staining of the background, resulting in a decreasing signal to noise ratio. As these techniques only have a historical value, no detailed methodological description of them is provided. More recently two antigenic sites (serotonin and substance P) could be demonstrated by sequential immunofluorescence using primary antibodies raised in different species (rat and rabbit) and developed with the corresponding FITC and RITC-labelled anti-IgG (Priestley and Cuello, 1982).

II.3   Multiple Staining using the Peroxidase-labelled Antibody Method

In 1968 Nakane adapted the peroxidase-labelled antibody method to localize multiple antigens in a single tissue section. In the peroxidase-labelled antibody method (Sternberger, 1979; Vandesande, 1979) the sites of antibody–antigen reaction are marked by histochemical localization of the enzymes. One of the best and most widely used enzymes for this purpose is horseradish peroxidase.

Since a number of stable reaction products of peroxidase with different colours are available and the reaction products are not an integral part of the antibody, Nakane postulated that if the antibody could be selectively eluted from the tissue section without removing the reaction products, and if the antigens to be localized subsequently were not denatured by the elution process, the method could be used for the simultaneous localization of multiple tissue antigens by repeating the elution and the indirect histochemical procedure each time with a different substrate of peroxidase.

Nakane could obtain three different colours by employing following substrates of peroxidase:

(a) 3,3'-diaminobenzidine (free base) resulting in yellowish-brown reaction products;
(b) α-naphthol followed by pyronin staining resulting in reddish-pink reaction products; and
(c) 4-Cl-1-naphthol resulting in greyish-blue reaction products.

For the selective and total elution of antibodies from tissue section, Nakane obtained the best results with solutions of low pH, glycine–hydrochloric acid buffer, and unbuffered hydrochloric acid. The ability of these solutions to dissociate antigen–antibody complexes varied considerably from one antigen to another. This selective and total elution of all antibodies used in a preceding staining step is absolutely necessary to prevent:

(a) an immunological reaction between the primary antiserum used during the preceding staining step and the peroxidase-labelled antibodies applied during the subsequent staining step; and
(b) a histochemical reaction between the peroxidase-labelled antibodies applied during the preceding staining step and the substrate of peroxidase used during the subsequent staining step.

As we shall see later, the elution method of Nakane is sometimes unsatisfactory.

The sequence in which the substrates are used is also important. The optimal sequence of substrates as determined by Nakane is: 3,3'-diaminobenzidine, α-naphthol-pyronin, 4-Cl-1-naphthol. Multiple staining using the peroxidase-labelled antibody method has the same advantages and shortcomings as the other enzyme-labelled antibody methods (Vandesande, 1979). Most of these shortcomings can be attributed to the labelling process itself.

The covalent binding between the peroxidase and antibody diminishes the efficiency of the method because it partly destroys the antibody activity and it gives rise to an unseparable mixture of conjugated and non-conjugated antibody. This leads to a mutual competition for the antigen. Conjugation may also diminish the specificity of the method because conjugates tend to adsorb to polar groups present in the tissue preparation (protein–protein interaction) (see also Chapter 3). Until now all this makes unlabelled antibody enzyme methods preferable. However, the quality of the conjugates has been significantly improved during recent years. This was mainly due to the use of pure antibodies and extensive purification of the prepared conjugates. In this connection, the work of Boorsma and Streefkerk (1978) needs to be mentioned. These workers have developed a method for rapid and large-scale purification of conjugates prepared with the two-step glutaraldehyde method (Avrameas and Ternynck, 1971) (see Chapter 3). In this method the conjugate reaction mixture is applied to protein-A–Sepharose which has affinity for IgG (coupled or uncoupled with peroxidase) and not for peroxidase. Subsequently the appropriate fractions are applied to Concanavalin A–Sepharose which has affinity for peroxidase (coupled with IgG) and not for uncoupled IgG. The quality of enzyme-labelled antibodies will certainly further improve when extremely pure monoclonal antiperoxidase antibodies become available. At that point, a re-evaluation of the enzyme-labelled antibody methods might be justified.

II.4 Simultaneous Immunoperoxidase–Immunofluorescence Staining

Canese and Bussolati (1977) and Lechago *et al.* (1979) have shown that it is possible to sequentially combine immunoperoxidase and immunofluorescence techniques to demonstrate two different antigens in the same tissue section. In this technique the first antigen is localized with one of the available immunoperoxidase techniques and the second antigen is localized by the indirect immunofluorescence technique. With the simultaneous use of incident immunofluorescence and transmitted bright field microscopy (Lechago *et al.*, 1979) it is possible to visualize and to photograph both antigens together. As the secondary antisera, used in both staining sequences, are directed against rabbit IgG, and as after the first staining sequence no elution of antibodies is performed, one would expect an immunological reaction between the rabbit antibody used in the first staining sequence and the FITC-labelled antibody used in the second staining sequence, and between free binding sites of the secondary antibody used in the first staining sequence and the primary rabbit antibody used in the second staining sequence. It appears, however, that these reactions, which would render the method worthless, can be prevented by the deposition of polymeric DAB oxidation product formed during the first staining sequence, if at least this deposition is sufficiently strong (Sternberger and Joseph, 1979). Indeed Sternberger *et al.*, (1970) have shown that the DAB polymeric reaction product creeps along the molecular surface at which it is liberated. Therefore it is possible that, if the DAB concentration is high and the reaction time long enough, sufficient DAB polymeric reaction product will be formed to mask all the antigenic and catalytic sites of the immunological reagents used in the first staining sequence, resulting in the prevention of interactions with reagents of the second sequence. This interpretation is in accordance with the observation of Sternberger and Joseph (1979), that progressive dilution of the DAB reagent used in the first staining sequence results in a progressive decrease of the blocking effect due to the deposition of polymeric DAB reaction product.

The consequences of this observation for the simultaneous immunoperoxidase–immunofluorescence staining technique are twofold: When two antigens are in separate cells or fibres the method will work only if a sufficiently strong DAB reaction is used. When, however, the two antigens are in the same cells or fibres, or if the two antigens are part of a molecular complex (as in the case of the posterior lobe hormones and their carrier proteins the neurophysins) the method becomes unreliable. Indeed Lechago *et al.* (1979) have observed that when the brown DAB precipitate is strong its blocking effect becomes non-specific and the demonstration of two different antigens inside the same cell is no longer feasible. Theoretically the non-specific blocking effect can be eliminated without affecting the specific blocking effect by progressive decrease of the DAB reaction. In practice, however, this is very difficult because one can never be sure that a positive fluorescence obtained in such circumstances is due to a specific immunological localization of the second antigen and not to an immunological or catalytic interaction between the reagents of the first and second staining sequence. Lechago *et al.* (1979) tried to avoid these problems by elution of all antibodies after the first staining sequence. For this purpose they used the method described by Tramu *et al.* (1978). This elution improved the fluorescence somewhat, but it detracted significantly from the demonstration of the peroxidase reaction.

II.5   Double Staining using the Unlabelled Antibody Method with Elution of the First Sequence Antibodies and Peroxidase

To avoid the shortcomings of the indirect peroxidase-labelled antibody method, Vandesande and Dierickx (1975) and Vandesande *et al.* (1977) adapted the PAP technique to localize two different antigens in a single tissue section. After localization of the first antigen, the antibodies and the peroxidase are selectively eluted from the tissue section without removing the coloured reaction product identifying the antigenic sites. As the antigen to be localized subsequently is not denatured by the elution process, this second antigen is localized in a similar way as for the first antigen, using a substrate that develops a reaction product of different colour.

For brown reaction products 3,3′-diaminobenzidine and for greyish-blue reaction products 4-Cl-1-naphthol are used. This method has all the advantages (high sensitivity and method specificity) of the original PAP method of Sternberger *et al.* (1970) and results in clear and low background pictures. The elution process is the most critical step of the staining procedure. This elution must be complete, selective, and may not denature the antigen to be localized in the subsequent staining sequence. The PAP complex and the GAR (goat anti-rabbit) antibodies are easily removed by simple incubation of the tissue section in a 0.2 M glycine buffer, pH 2.3, containing 0.5 M sodium chloride. Some primary antibodies of low affinity can also be eluted in the same way. If, however, antibodies of high affinity are used, selective and complete elution of the antibodies is obtained by electrophoresis at 20 V/cm in 0.05 M glycine buffer (pH 2.2) containing 30% dimethylformamide. With the use of an appropriate electrophoresis apparatus the method is simple and easy. However, every time that a new unknown primary antiserum is used the completeness of the elution must be checked.

This can be done by performing the first staining sequence omitting the DAB reaction, followed by the electrophoresis step and a second application of the first staining sequence but now omitting the primary antiserum. If this results in a negative staining one can be sure that the elution is complete. It cannot be proved that the method will work with all antibodies, but until now we could not find one antiserum that could not be eluted with this method. Moreover, after fixation in Bouin-Hollande + 10% of a saturated watery solution of sublimate, the method did not alter the antigenic reactivity of a lot of antigens, such as: oxytocin, mesotocin, vasopressin, vasotocin, isotocin, neurophysin I, neurophysin II, somatostatin, CCK, LHRF, and ACTH.

Because a denaturation during the elution process cannot, however, be excluded *a priori*, the ability of the antigens to withstand elution of antibody must be determined for each system.

II.6 Double Staining using the Unlabelled Antibody Method without Elution of the First Sequence Antibodies and Peroxidase

If the double staining technique is performed without elution of the first sequence antisera and peroxidase before application of the second staining sequence one should expect colour mixing due to the following possible interactions:

(a) immunological interaction between the GAR serum of the second sequence and the primary antibody of the first sequence;
(b) immunological interaction between the GAR serum of the second sequence and the PAP of the first sequence;
(c) immunological interaction between the primary antiserum of the second sequence and the GAR of the first sequence;
(d) immunological interaction between the PAP of the second sequence and the GAR of the first sequence;
(e) catalytic interaction between the PAP of the first sequence and the 4-Cl-1-naphthol of the second sequence,

The double staining method applied under our standard conditions (see Section III.2.3) without elution of the first sequence antibodies and peroxidase always results in colour mixing, as can be expected from the possible interactions between the reagents of the first and second staining sequence.

Sternberger and Joseph (1979) have, however, observed that none of these reactions took place when their own standard conditions were used. Colour mixing did, however, occur upon dilution of the DAB used in the first sequence reaction.

How may these apparently contradictory results be explained? One of the important differences between our standard conditions and those of Sternberger and Joseph is the DAB reaction. Our DAB solution contains 0.0125% DAB and 0.003% H_2O_2 in 0.05 M Tris-HCl, pH 7.6 and is applied at room temperatue (20 °C) for a period of 3–5 min. In the Sternberger and Joseph standard conditions a DAB solution containing 0.05% DAB and 0.01% H_2O_2 in Tris-saline pH 7.6 is used for 8 min. This means that under the Sternberger–Joseph standard conditions a much stronger DAB reaction is performed than under our standard conditions.

These observations suggest that the failure of colour mixing in the Sternberger–Joseph conditions may be due to blocking of the possible catalytic and immunological interactions between reagents of the first and second staining sequence by the polymeric DAB oxidation product. These authors also suggest that it is equally possible that the use of the first sequence link antiserum in excess, which selects for high-affinity antibodies, blocks all antigen sites of the primary antibody, and that in turn the use of the first set PAP in excess blocks all free antibody-combining sites of the link antibody.

Our results indicate, however, that this cannot be the case because in our standard procedure we always use an excess first link antiserum and an excess first sequence PAP. As already mentioned this always results in colour mixing. These results strongly suggest that the blocking effect observed by Sternberger and Joseph, and by Lechago *et al.* (1979) has to be imputed to the polymeric DAB oxidation product. This is not so surprising because Sternberger *et al.* (1970) had previously shown that the DAB reaction product creeps along the molecular surface at which it is liberated. Making use of this blocking effect Sternberger and Joseph have developed a double PAP staining technique without elution of the first sequence antibodies and peroxidase before application of the second sequence. It is clear that this method can only work if, during the first staining sequence, a very strong DAB reaction is performed.

When the two antigens are localized in different cells or fibres the method is reliable. A disadvantage of the method is, however, that the strong DAB reaction needed for optimalization of the blocking effect, results in a relatively high background staining, rendering colour interpretation difficult. Therefore the authors found it necessary to use controls for pure brown and pure blue. As control for pure brown, a complete double staining in which the second sequence primary antiserum is replaced by buffer can be used. When the first sequence primary antiserum is replaced by buffer in the otherwise complete staining sequence, only blue stain occurs and the resulting colour can be used as a control for pure blue. A staining with two antisera known to reveal constituents in different locations can also be used as brown and blue controls. Sternberger and Joseph have shown that the first sequence primary antiserum, if used at saturating concentrations, blocks reaction of the second sequence primary antiserum, when the two different antigenic determinants are either on the same molecule or in close proximity. In that case the location of the second antigen remains undetected.

Progressive dilution of the first sequence primary antiserum will, however, reveal the second antigen by mixed colour staining. This is a second disadvantage of the method because progressive dilution of the first sequence primary antiserum beyond saturating concentration decreases the sensitivity of the method.

II.7 Double PAP Staining with Elution *versus* Double PAP Staining without Elution

As already mentioned the double PAP staining with elution of the first staining sequence antibodies and peroxidase by means of electrophoresis is a very simple method resulting in clear and low background pictures. The method is reliable even when the two antigens are localized in the same molecular complex. The double PAP staining without elution of the first sequence antibodies and peroxidase needs a very strong DAB reaction during the first staining sequence to be reliable. This results in a relatively high background staining, rendering colour interpretation difficult so that colour controls for pure brown and pure blue are needed.

When the two antigens are localized in the same molecular complex, or in close proximity, not only a strong DAB reaction but also a progressive dilution series of the first sequence primary antiserum is needed to reveal the second antigen. This dilution decreases the sensitivity of the method, and is time-consuming. Therefore, at least in our opinion, the double PAP staining with elution by electrophoresis is the method of choice. In exceptional cases in which total elution of the first sequence antibodies might not be obtained by electrophoresis, then the double PAP staining without elution could possibly be useful. On the other hand, if electrophoresis fails, one can also try the elution method described by Tramu *et al.* (1978).

III PROTOCOLS

III.1 Multiple Staining using the Peroxidase-labelled Antibody Method
(see also Nakane, 1968)

III.1.1 *Materials*

Appropriately fixed paraffin sections, paper tissue, rotating–shaking apparatus, moist chamber, plain glass trays with removable slide racks.

III.1.2   *Reagents*

—Lugol solution: 10 mg/ml KI and 5 mg/ml I_2
—$NaHSO_3$ solution: 5 g $NaHSO_3$ in 100 ml H_2O
   Lugol and $NaHSO_3$ solutions are only needed if the fixative contained
   sublimate
—Buffered saline: 0.01 M Tris/HCl pH 7.6 in 0.9% NaCl
—Pre-immune goat serum diluted 1/5 in buffered saline
—Specific rabbit primary antisera optimally diluted in buffered saline
—Peroxidase-labelled goat anti-rabbit IgG serum diluted in buffered saline
   (try to find the dilution where staining is optimal and background minimal)
—DAB solution: Dissolve 25 mg 3,3'-diaminobenzidine in 200 ml 0.05 M
   Tris-HCl buffer. Filter and add 2 ml 0.3% freshly prepared H_2O_2
   This results in a final DAB concentration of 0.0125% and H_2O_2 concentra-
   tion of 0.003% (prepare just before use)
—α-naphthol solution: solve 10 g α-naphthol in 100 ml 40% alcohol; filter and
   add 2 ml 30% H_2O_2
—Pyronin solution: solve 0.1 g in 96 ml 40% alcohol and add 4 ml aniline oil
—4-Cl-1-naphthol solution: disolve 100 mg 4-Cl-1-naphthol in 10 ml alcohol,
   add 190 ml 0.05 M Tris-HCl pH 7.6; filter and add 5 ml 0.3% freshly
   prepared H_2O_2
—Glycine–HCl buffer 0.2 M pH 2.2
—Chrome–glycerin jelly: suspend 10 g gelatin (granulated or sheets) in 80 ml
   H_2O. Allow to soak 1–2 h, then dissolve by warming. Add to this solution
   70 ml glycerol, 0.25 g phenol crystals and mix well. This mixture must be
   melted before use since it gels at room temperature. For easy heating it can
   be stored in a small Erlenmeyer flask

III.1.3   *Procedure*

Before performing a multiple staining:
(a) Determine the optimal dilution of the primary antisera and of the
    peroxidase-labelled goat anti-rabbit IgG serum.
(b) Control the ability of the antigen to withstand elution of antibody by
    incubating a tissue section first in the glycine–HCl buffer pH 2.2 for 1 h,
    followed by a wash in buffered saline and the normal staining procedure.
    Compare with a normal stained section.
(c) Control the efficiency of elution of antibodies from their antigen with
    glycine–HCl buffer pH 2.2. The efficiency of elution can be tested in the
    following manner. Incubate a section with the primary antiserum fol-
    lowed by peroxidase-labelled goat anti-rabbit IgG but do not stain. Elute
    the antibodies by immersion in 0.2 M glycine–HCl buffer pH 2.2 for 1 h on
    the rotating–shaking apparatus. Incubate again with peroxidase-labelled
    goat anti-rabbit IgG and stain for peroxidase.

If either the primary antiserum or the peroxidase-labelled goat anti-rabbit IgG remains on the section, the antigenic sites will stain. If both antisera were removed completely no staining will occur. If the elution with glycine–HCl is incomplete try elution by electrophoresis (see Section III.2.3).

Steps for staining procedure
1—xylene (2 × 5 min)
2—dry ethanol (2 × 2 min)
3—wash by immersion in H_2O
4—Lugol solution (2 min)   ⎱ only if sublimate was present in the
5—NaHSO₃ solution (2 min)   ⎰ fixative
6—wash by immersion in H_2O
7—wash by immersion in buffered saline
8—incubate with pre-immune goat serum 1/5 (moist chamber, 15 min)
9—jet-wash with buffered saline
10—wash on a rotating–shaking apparatus with buffered saline (5 min) and blot with tissue paper
11—incubate overnight in the moist chamber at room temperature with the appropriate dilution of the first primary antiserum (250 µl per slide)
12—jet-wash with buffered saline
13—wash on the rotating–shaking apparatus (5 min) and blot
14—incubate with optimal dilution of peroxidase conjugated goat anti-rabbit IgG (250 µl per slide, 25 min)
15—jet-wash with buffered saline
16—wash on the rotating–shaking apparatus (5 min)
17—immerse the slides in 0.05 M Tris-HCl, pH 7.6
18—stain for 3–5 min in freshly prepared DAB solution at 20 °C on the rotating–shaking apparatus
19—control the staining under the microscope
20—wash with buffered saline
21—immerse the slides in glycine–HCl buffer pH 2.2 on the rotating–shaking apparatus for 1 h at room temperature
22—immerse the slides in 0.05 M Tris-HCl buffer pH 7.6
23—jet-wash with buffered saline
24—repeat steps 8 to 17 but now using in step 11 the appropriate dilution of the second primary antiserum
25—immerse for 24 h in a freshly prepared α-naphthol–H_2O_2 solution
26—wash in buffered saline
27—stain for 3–24 h in pyronin solution
28—rinse in alcohol
29—control the staining under the microscope
30—wash in buffered saline

31—immerse the slides in glycine–HCl buffer pH 2.2 on the rotating–shaking apparatus for 1 h at room temperature

32—immerse the slides in 0.05 M Tris–HCl buffer pH 7.6

33—jet-wash with buffered saline

34—repeat steps 8 to 17 but now using in step 11 the appropriate dilution of the third primary antiserum

35—stain for 3–5 min in 4-Cl-1-naphthol solution at 20 °C on the rotating–shaking apparatus

36—control the staining under the microscope

37—rinse in distilled H_2O

38—mount in chrome–glycerin jelly

III.2 Double Staining using the Unlabelled Antibody Method with Elution of the First Sequence Antibodies and Peroxidase

III.2.1 *Materials*

The same materials are used as in III.1.1, but in addition an appropriate electrophoresis apparatus is needed. Such an apparatus can be home made in Perspex or PVC. The scheme of such an apparatus is reproduced in Figure 1.

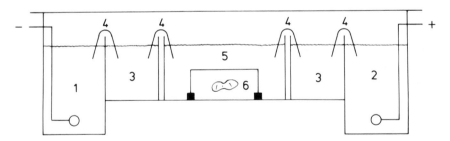

Figure 1 (1) cathode chamber, (2) anode chamber, (3) buffer chamber, (4) paper bridges, (5) electrophoresis chamber, (6) tissue section. The paper bridges are made from Gelman absorbent sheets (part no. 51290). Compartments 1, 2, and 3 are filled with a solution of 0.2 M glycine–HCl buffer pH 2,2 containing 0.5 M NaCl to decrease resistance. Compartment 5 is filled with a mixture of 25 ml 0.2 M glycine-HCl buffer pH 2.2 + 50 ml dimethylformamide + 100 ml bidest. The electrophoresis chamber is constructed in such a way that up to ten tissue sections can be processed together

III.2.2 *Reagents*

All reagents mentioned in Section III.1.2 are needed except the peroxidase-labelled goat anti-rabbit IgG serum, the α-naphthol and the pyronin solution. In addition one needs:

—GAR (goat anti-rabbit IgG serum) diluted 1/20;
—PAP (peroxidase–antiperoxidase complex) diluted 1/300 (this dilution depends on the bath PAP).

III.2.3 Procedure

Before performing a double staining:
—Search the optimal dilutions of the primary antisera
—Control the ability of the antigens to withstand elution of antibody by electrophoresis at 20 V/cm (this potential difference has to be measured over the tissue section). This control can be done by performing first an electrophoresis followed by a normal PAP staining and comparing the result with a normal PAP-stained adjacent section
—Control the efficiency of the elution of antibodies from their antigens by electrophoresis at 20 V/cm
    Proceed therefore as follows: perform on a section a normal PAP staining but omit the DAB reaction step. Elute the antibodies by electrophoresis and wash in buffered saline. Perform a second normal PAP staining but now omitting the primary antiserum. If no staining is obtained the elution was complete

Steps for staining procedure
1—xylene (2 × 5 min)
2—dry ethanol (2 × 2 min)
3—wash by immersion in H_2O
4—Lugol solution (2 min)   ⎱ only if sublimate was present in the
5—$NaHSO_3$ solution (2 min) ⎰ fixative
6—wash by immersion in H_2O
7—wash by immersion in buffered saline
8—incubate with pre-immune goat serum 1/5 (moist chamber, 15 min)
9—jet-wash with buffered saline
10—wash on a rotating–shaking apparatus with buffered saline (5 min) and blot with tissue paper
11—incubate overnight in the moist chamber at room temperature with the appropriate dilution of the first primary antiserum (250 μl per slide)
12—jet-wash with buffered saline
13—wash on the rotating–shaking apparatus with buffered saline (5 min) and blot
14—incubate with GAR 1/20 (moist chamber, 25 min)
15—jet-wash with buffered saline
16—wash on the rotating–shaking apparatus (5 min) and blot
17—incubate with PAP 1/300 (moist chamber, 25 min)
18—jet-wash with buffered saline

19—wash on the rotating–shaking apparatus with buffered saline (5 min) and blot
20—equilibrate the slides in 0.05 M Tris-HCl buffer pH 7.6
21—stain for 3–5 min in freshly prepared DAB solution at 20 °C in the rotating–shaking apparatus
22—wash with buffered saline
23—control the staining under the microscope
24—elute all antibodies by electrophoresis at 20 V/cm for 1–2 h
25—wash in buffered saline
26—repeat steps 8 to 20 but now using in step 11 the appropriate dilution of the second primary antiserum
27—stain for 3–5 min in freshly prepared 4-Cl-1-naphthol solution at 20 °C on the rotating–shaking apparatus
28—wash with buffered saline
29—control the staining under the microscope
30—rinse in distilled H_2O
31—mount in chrome–glycerin jelly.

Remarks
(a) be sure that GAR and PAP are used in excess;
(b) if the elution of all antibodies at 20 V/cm is incomplete, a higher voltage can be used, but then cooling becomes necessary;
(c) the reaction product of 4-Cl-1-naphthol is soluble in organic solvents and is light-sensitive.

III.3 Double Staining using the Unlabelled Antibody Method without Antibody Removal

III.3.1 *Materials*

The same materials are needed as Section III.2.1, except the electrophoresis apparatus.

III.3.2 *Reagents*

The same reagents as Section III.2.2 are used except that the DAB solution must be more concentrated.
—DAB solution: disolve 100 mg diaminobenzidine tetrahydrochloride in 200 ml buffered saline pH 7.6. Filter and add 0.01% hydrogen peroxide. Prepare just before use.

III.3.3 *Procedure*

Before performing a double staining:

(a) search the optimal dilutions of the primary antisera;
(b) prepare a control for pure blue by staining a section with the complete staining sequence but in which the first sequence primary antiserum has been replaced by buffer;
(c) prepare a control for pure brown by staining a section with the complete staining sequence but in which the second sequence primary antiserum has been replaced by buffer.

Staining

Use the same staining sequence as Section III.2.3, using in step 21 the 0.05% DAB solution containing 0.01% hydrogen peroxide. Stain for 8 min. Omit steps 24 and 25.

Remark

To find out if the two antigenic determinants are present in the same cell, nerve cell process, or molecular complex, it is necessary to use a progressive dilution series (beyond the optimal dilution) of the first sequence primary antiserum. If the two antigenic determinants are known to be present in different cells this dilution series can be omitted.

IV SUPPLIERS

—Horseradish peroxidase-conjugated goat anti-rabbit IgG Nordic, Immuno-logical Netherlands.
—Peroxidase–rabbit antiperoxidase complex (PAP): UCB–Christiaens, Bioproducts-peptide Department, Rue Berkendael, 68, B-1060 Brussels, Belgium.
   Dealer for Canada: Bio-Ria, 10900 rue Hamon, Montreal, PQ, Canada H3M 3A2.
   Dealer for USA: Bio-Ria, 9809 Merioneth Drive, Louisville, Kentucky, USA 40299.
—Rotating–shaking apparatus: Taumler typ 54131, Heidolph-Elektro KG, C842, Kelheim, Germany.

REFERENCES

Avrameas, S. and Ternynck, T. (1971). 'Peroxidase labelled antibody on Fab conjugates with enhanced intracellular penetration.' *Immunochemistry*, **8**, 1175–1179.
Boorsma, D. M. and Streefkerk, J. G. (1978). 'Improved method for separation of peroxidase conjugates.' In Knapp, W., Holubar, K., and Wick, G. (eds), *Immunof-*

luorescence and Related Staining Techniques, pp. 225–235. Elsevier–North Holland Biomedical Press, Amsterdam.

Canese, M. G. and Bussolati, G. (1977). 'Immuno-electroncytochemical localization of the somatostatin cells in the human antral mucosa.' *J. Histochem. Cytochem.*, **25**, 1111.

Henderson, D. C. and Smithyman, A. M. (1974). 'The simultaneous detection of two protein antigens in lymphoid tissues by combining immunofluorescence and autoradiography.' *J. Immunol. Methods*, **6**, 115–120.

Lechago, J., Sun, N. C. J., and Weinstein, W. M. (1979). 'Simultaneous visualisation of two antigens in the same tissue section by combining immunoperoxidase with immunofluorescence techniques.' *J. Histochem. Cytochem.*, **27**, 1221–1225.

Nakane, P. K. (1968). 'Simultaneous localization of multiple tissue antigens using the peroxidase-labelled antibody method: A study on pituitary glands of the rat.' *J. Histochem. Cytochem.*, **16**, 557–560.

Nash, D. R., Crabbé, P. A., and Heremans, J. F. (1969). 'Sequential immunofluorescent staining: a simple and useful technique.' *Immunology*, **16**, 785–790.

Pernis, B. (1968). 'Relationships between the heterogeneity of immunoglobulins and the different plasma cells.' *Cold Spring Harbor Symp. Quant. Biol.*, **32**, 333.

Priestley, J. V. and Cuello, A. C. (1982). In *Co-Transmission*. Macmillan, New York and London. (Ed. A. C. Cuello) pp. 165–188. 'Co-existence of neuroactive substances as revealed by immunohistochemistry with monoclonal antibodies.'

Sternberger, L. A. (1979). *Immunocytochemistry*. John Wiley & Sons, New York, Chichester, Brisbane, Toronto.

Sternberger, L. A. and Joseph, S. A. (1979). 'The unlabeled antibody method.' *J. Histochem. Cytochem.*, **27**, 1424–1429.

Sternberger, L. A., Hardy, P. H. Jr., Cuculis, J. J., and Meyer, H. G. (1970). 'The unlabeled antibody–enzyme method of immunohistochemistry. Preparation and properties of soluble antigen–antibody complex (horseradish peroxidase–antihorseradish peroxidase) and its use in the identification of spirochetes.' *J. Histochem. Cytochem.*, **18**, 315–333.

Tramu, G., Pillez, A., and Leonardelli, J. (1978). 'An efficient method of antibody elution for the successive or simultaneous localization of two antigens by immunocytochemistry.' *J. Histochem. Cytochem.*, **26**, 322–324.

Vandesande, F. (1979). 'A critical review of immunocytochemical methods for light microscopy.' *J. Neurosci. Methods*, **1**, 3–23.

Vandesande, F. and Dierickx, K. (1975). 'Identification of the vasopressin producing and of the oxytocin producing neurons in the hypothalamic magnocellular neurosecretory system of the rat.' *Cell Tissue Res.*, **164**, 153–162.

Vandesande, F., Dierickx, K., and De Mey, J. (1977). 'The origin of the vasopressinergic and oxytocinergic fibers of the external region of the median eminence of the rat hypophysis.' *Cell Tissue Res.*, **180**, 443–452.

Van Leeuwen, F. W., De Raay, C., Swaab, D. F., and Fisser, B. (1979). 'The localization of oxytocin, vasopressin, somatostatin and luteinizing hormone releasing hormone in the rat neurohypophysis.' *Cell Tissue Res.*, **202**, 189–201.

Van Rooijen, N. (1972). 'A method for the separate detection of two labelled antigens in lymphoid tissues, using two different radioisotopes and a double autoradiographic stripping technique.' *J. Immunol. Methods*, **2**, 197–207.

Van Rooijen, N. and Streefkerk, J. G. (1976). 'Autoradiography and immunohistoperoxidase techniques applied to the same tissue section.' *J. Immunol. Methods*, **10**, 379–383.

Immunohistochemistry
Edited by A. C. Cuello
© 1983 IBRO

CHAPTER 11

Electron Microscopic Immunocytochemistry for CNS Transmitters and Transmitter Markers

J. V. PRIESTLEY and A. C. CUELLO

Neuroanatomy–Neuropharmacology Group, University Departments of Pharmacology and Human Anatomy, South Parks Road, Oxford

I INTRODUCTION

This chapter concerns the use of immunocytochemistry for the ultrastructural localization of central nervous system transmitters and transmitter markers. The methodology which has been most widely used for such studies is the peroxidase–antiperoxidase (PAP) pre-embedding procedure (Pickel, 1981; Ribak *et al.*, 1981) and this will be considered in detail. A protocol for the related technique of PAP post-embedding staining will also be presented (Appendix 1), although this approach has so far been confined mainly to neuroendocrine studies (Moriarty, 1976; Van Leeuwen, 1980b). However, a large number of other ultrastructural immunocytochemical procedures are potentially applicable to the CNS. In Section I the various techniques available will be listed and compared. Various other chapters in this volume cover material also relevant to a general review of electron microscopic (EM) immunocytochemical techniques, notably those on the use of peroxidase conjugated antibodies (Chapter 3) and of protein A–colloidal gold complexes (Chapter 12) and immunoglobulin–gold conjugates (Chapter 13).

II   ULTRASTRUCTURAL IMMUNOCYTOCHEMICAL TECHNIQUES

II.1   Ferritin-labelled Antibody Methods

For the study of certain membrane surface markers it is possible to identify in the electron microscope unlabelled antibodies (de Petris, 1978); however, for the localization of intracellular antigens it is normally necessary to label the antibody in some way with an electron-opaque marker (Sternberger, 1967). Over 20 years ago Singer (1959) introduced a method for doing this when he showed that immunoglobulins can be conjugated to the iron-rich macromolecule ferritin. The ferritin can be conjugated either directly to the relevant antibody (direct labelled technique) or to a second antibody which is directed against the first (indirect labelled technique, Figure 1). Both these

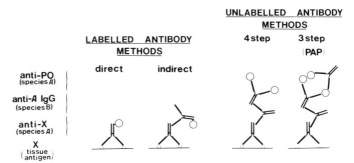

Figure 1   Diagrammatic representation of four different immunocytochemical procedures employing peroxidase (PO) as final marker. Circles represent peroxidase. In the labelled methods peroxidase is conjugated to an immunoglobulin, either directly to the primary antibody (anti-X) or to a second antibody (anti-A IgG) which binds to the primary antibody. In the unlabelled methods the peroxidase is bound by an anti-peroxidase antibody (anti-PO). Analogous staining procedures employing ferritin as final marker are possible. See text for further details

techniques have been used and have been applied particularly successfully for the ultrastructural localization of surface antigens (Sternberger, 1979; de Petris, 1978). Various methods of labelling antibodies with heavy metals were developed at about the same time as the ferritin-labelled techniques (Sternberger, 1967), with perhaps the most useful being those employing uranium as a label (Sternberger *et al.*, 1965). However, none of these was particularly successful because of the difficulty of introducing sufficient heavy metal atoms into an antibody to confer electron-opacity while still retaining the antibody activity. The ferritin-labelled techniques have themselves not been widely used for the localization of intracellular antigens because of the difficulty of obtaining adequate penetration of labelled antibodies into fixed tissue. This is a problem which is faced by all pre-embedding staining procedures and will be discussed fully in Section III. However, the solution which has often been adopted, namely to carry out staining on ultra-thin sections (post-embedding staining, Figure 2), proved to be unsatisfactory for

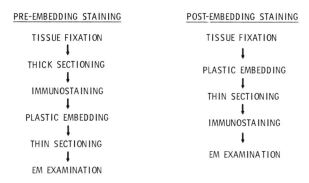

ULTRASTRUCTURAL IMMUNOCYTOCHEMICAL TECHNIQUES

PRE-EMBEDDING STAINING	POST-EMBEDDING STAINING
TISSUE FIXATION	TISSUE FIXATION
THICK SECTIONING	PLASTIC EMBEDDING
IMMUNOSTAINING	THIN SECTIONING
PLASTIC EMBEDDING	IMMUNOSTAINING
THIN SECTIONING	EM EXAMINATION
EM EXAMINATION	

Figure 2 Schematic of the different stages involved in either pre- or post-embedding staining

the ferritin-labelled methods because of initial problems of non-specific adsorption of labelled antibodies to the EM embedding medium (Striker *et al.*, 1966). More recently this problem has been partly overcome, and successful post-embedding staining has been carried out on sections embedded in cross-linked bovine serum albumin (BSA) (Kraehenbuhl and Jamieson, 1973) on water-soluble methacrylate-embedded sections (Shahrabadi and Yamamoto, 1971), and on ultra-thin, frozen sections (Singer *et al.*, 1973). This latter procedure seems particularly promising and has now been applied in combination with an iron–dextran antibody conjugate (Dutton *et al.*, 1979) and with protein A–colloidal gold complexes (Geuze and Slot, 1980) to allow the simultaneous ultrastructural localization of two different antigens. In addition, methods based on ferritin and colloidal gold allow particle counting and an approach to quantification not possible with enzymic labels (Williams, 1977). However, despite these recent advances in the ferritin-labelled techniques, they are not yet generally suitable for studies of small intracellular antigens, and other methods must be used.

II.2   Enzyme-labelled Antibody Methods

In theory enzymic markers should be more sensitive than labels using heavy metals or structured electron opacity (ferritin). This is because it should be possible to produce a cytochemical intensification of the antibody–antigen binding simply by increasing the substrate incubation time during the enzymic reaction (Sternberger, 1979). The possibility of using enzymic labels for immunocytochemistry was opened up in 1966 with the introduction of methods for conjugating enzymes to antibodies (Nakane and Pierce, 1966; Avrameas and Uriel, 1966). Several different enzymes are available which could be used as labels (Avrameas, 1970) but horseradish peroxidase has a number of properties which make it particularly suitable. Thus there are easy cytochemical methods for its detection, the pure enzyme is available commercially, there are relatively low endogenous levels of peroxidase in biological tissue, and the peroxidase molecule is probably smaller than other possible labels such as acid phosphatase (Sternberger, 1979). Various methods have been introduced to improve the efficiency and specificity of the conjugation reaction while retaining antibody and enzyme activity. These methods include the two-stage conjugation procedure employing glutaraldehyde introduced by Avrameas and Ternynck (1971) and the use of periodate for conjugation via peroxidase carbohydrate residues (Nakane and Kawaoi, 1974). Relatively easy and reproducible preparation of peroxidase-labelled antibodies is now possible and these reagents have been used widely for both light and electron microscopic immunocytochemistry (Kuhlmann, 1977; Avrameas, 1970; Nakane, 1973) (for critical appraisal and protocols see Chapter 3). However, as with the ferritin-labelled techniques for electron microscopy, it has generally been necessary to carry out pre-embedding staining with all the associated difficulties of poor antibody penetration into tissue sections.

In an effort to facilitate diffusion into sections Kraehenbuhl and Jamiesen (1974) have prepared a very small enzyme-labelled immuno-reagent with a molecular weight of only 70,000 as compared to about 200,000 for traditional peroxidase-conjugated IgG. This reagent consists of a haem-bearing octapeptide isolated from cytochrome c which is conjugated to a Fab (antigen binding) fragment, but so far little work has been reported using it. Substantial progress has also been made with post-embedding staining for peroxidase-labelled antibodies and it has been possible to decrease the non-specific adsorption of reagents to plastic embedded sections by using various alternative embedding media. These include methyl-butyl methacrylate (Kawari and Nakane, 1970) and a procedure developed by Mazurkiewicz and Nakane (1972) which involves the staining of thick polyethylene glycol-embedded sections followed by re-embedding in Epon for ultramicrotomy. Staining has also been carried out successfully on Epon-embedded sections following etching with H_2O_2 (Nakane, 1971). However, despite the wide application of these various techniques for the study of both intra- and extracellular antigens, they have not generally proved useful for CNS studies outside the neuroendocrine system. The ultrastructural localization of transmitters and transmitter markers has required the use of the more sensitive unlabelled antibody techniques described next.

II.3 Unlabelled Antibody Methods

Some of the problems of the ferritin- and enzyme-labelled antibody methods derive from the need to covalently link the label to an antibody with the inevitable resultant loss of both antibody and enzyme activity. A way round this difficulty was provided in 1969 when Mason *et al.* (1969) and Sternberger and Cuculis (1969) independently introduced unlabelled enzyme methods which did not depend on a covalent linkage in order to bind antibody and enzyme. With these methods an antibody directed against peroxidase binds the enzyme, and use is made of the divalent characteristic of IgG to bind the antiperoxidase antibody to the anti-tissue antigen antibody via an intermediate link antibody (Figure 1). Initially, a four-step staining procedure was used in which the three antibodies and the peroxidase enzyme were added separately and sequentially. Subsequently, Sternberger and colleagues (1970) developed a three-step staining procedure in which peroxidase enzyme and antiperoxidase were added in a single stage already bound together. The peroxidase and antiperoxidase form a soluble complex consisting of three enzyme molecules bound to two antibody molecules and referred to as the PAP (peroxidase–antiperoxidase) complex (protocol for preparation of PAP complex in Chapter 4.III). Use of the PAP complex overcomes problems of antiperoxidase purification and of loss of weakly bound enzyme which were inherent in the original four-step procedure (Sternberger, 1979). Various workers have compared the sensitivity of the PAP procedure with that of the two-step labelled and the four-step unlabelled methods. Using as criterion the maximum dilution of primary antibody which could be used while still achieving successful immunostaining, the PAP procedure was found to be from 20 to 250 times more sensitive than the other methods. It also appears to be more specific than other available methods, possibly due to the specific binding properties of the link antibody (Sternberger, 1979). Two techniques

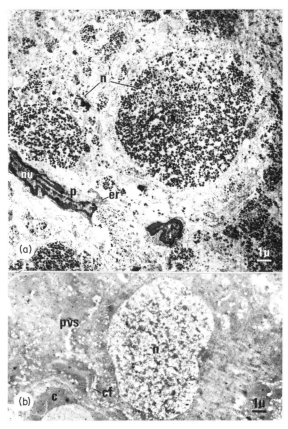

Figure 3   Post-embedding staining for vasopressin in formalin fixed rat neurohypophysis (Reproduced by permission of Springer-Verlag from van Leeuwen and Swaab,
1977): (a) anti-vasopressin plasma (1:800); (b) control, pre-immune plasma (1:800).
n = neurosecretory granules, p = perivascular cell with nucleus (nu) and endoplasmic
   reticulum (er), cf = collagen fibres in perivascular space (pvs), c = capillary

related to that of PAP have also been developed; namely phosphatase–anti-
phosphatase (Mason and Sammons, 1978) and ferritin–antiferritin (Marucci
et al., 1974), but these have not so far found wide application. Because of its
high sensitivity the PAP procedure has become the method of choice for
ultrastructural studies of CNS transmitter-related antigens. Post-embedding
PAP staining can be carried out both with and without prior etching of plastic,
and this has been applied extensively in neuroendocrine studies for the
localization of hormones, releasing factors, and neurophysins in the hypo-
thalamo–hypophyseal system (Moriarty, 1973; Silverman, 1976; Van
Leeuwen, 1980b). Figure 3, taken from the work of Van Leeuwen, shows an

example of post-embedding staining for the localization of vasopressin. Pre-embedding PAP staining was introduced by Pickel and colleagues (1975) and has been used mainly for the ultrastructural localization of neuropeptides, transmitter-synthesizing enzymes, and transmitters (Pickel, 1981; Ribak *et al.*, 1981). Figure 4 shows pre-embedding staining for tryptophan hydroxylase as originally applied in Pickel's group.

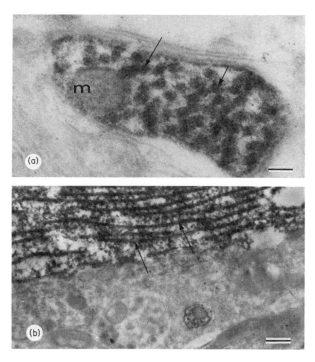

Figure 4 Pre-embedding staining as originally employed by V. Pickel and colleagues. Tryptophan hydroxylase in nucleus locus coeruleus: (a) reaction product within type I process is associated with subcellular organelles (arrows). Mitochondrion (m) is unstained (reproduced by permission of Elsevier/North Holland from Pickel *et al.*, 1977b). (Bar = 0.01 μm.) (b) Staining of microtubules (arrows) in an axon cut in longitudinal section

The different staining sequences involved in pre- and post-embedding staining are indicated in Figure 2. As already mentioned, the major advantage of post-embedding staining is that the immunoreagents are applied directly to the surface of the ultrathin sections thus avoiding problems of penetration into the tissue. In general this means that stronger fixatives can be used (see Section III.1) and internal staining of organelles which have been cut open by sectioning is possible. In addition the staining sequences are relatively quick and it is possible to carry out staining of serial EM sections for different antigens (e.g. Van Leeuwen and Swaab, 1977; Moriarty, 1976). Figure 5 shows such serial staining for pituitary glycoprotein hormones, carried out by Childs (formerly Moriarty). Unfortunately the trans-mitter-related antigens generally do not retain sufficient antigenicity following-

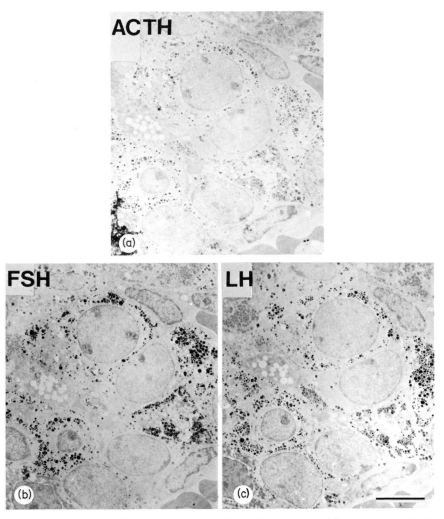

Figure 5 Post-embedding staining of serial sections provided by Dr G. V. Childs (formerly Moriarty). Triple sections of a field from the pituitary of a 6-day-old male rat stained with (a) 1:10,000 anti-ACTH (17–39); (b) 1:8000 anti-FSH(β); and (c) 1:10,000 anti-bovine LH(β). Cells stain for FSH and LH but not for ACTH (unpublished micrographs). (Bar = 10 μm.)

ing dehydration and plastic embedding to allow detection with post-embedding staining even using the sensitive PAP method (e.g. Buijs and Swaab, 1979). Goldsmith and Ganong (1975), for example, showed that for hypothalamic LHRH fixation did not significantly change the levels of immuno-assayable material but dehydration and embedding removed 98% of it. Hence pre-embedding staining has been widely adopted for transmitter localization. However, Pelletier and colleagues (e.g. Pelletier and Leclerc, 1979; Pelletier *et al.*, 1981) and Beauvillain and colleagues (Beauvillain and Tramu, 1980; Beauvillain *et al.*, 1980) have described successful post-embedding staining for several small neuropeptides, so post-embedding staining should not be discounted altogether for CNS studies. Pre-embedding staining brings all the problems of antibody penetration already referred to; problems that ought to be more acute than with the labelled antibody methods because of the large molecular size of the PAP complex (400,000 daltons). In the next section the various factors involved in the development of successful pre-embedding PAP staining will be considered in detail, and then followed in Section IV by a detailed experimental protocol as used in our laboratory. Information relating to post-embedding staining is also included at various points of Section III, and a representative protocol is provided in Appendix 1.

III   VARIABLES IN PAP ULTRASTRUCTURAL IMMUNOCYTOCHEMISTRY

III.1   Tissue Fixation

III.1.1   *Aldehyde fixatives*

Fixation of tissue prior to immunostaining has two major functions; namely to retain antigens *in situ* and to preserve tissue structure. At the same time, fixation should not seriously interfere with the ability of antibodies to interact with tissue antigens. However, the preservation of both good ultrastructure and antigenicity is not easy, since antigenicity depends on portions of intact primary and tertiary protein structure, the very structure which is disturbed by the intra- and intermolecular protein cross-links formed by the commonly used EM fixatives (Pearse, 1968). Thus it is normally necessary to adopt a compromise in which antigenicity and ultrastructure are preserved adequately if not optimally. The fixatives which have been most widely used for EM immunocytochemistry are the aldehydes: formaldehyde, its redissolved solid polymer, paraformaldehyde, and glutaraldehyde. Generally, glutaraldehyde seems to give an ultrastructure superior to that of the formaldehydes but with greater loss of antigenicity. With pre-embedding staining there is the added complication of antibody tissue penetration, and failure to immunostain may

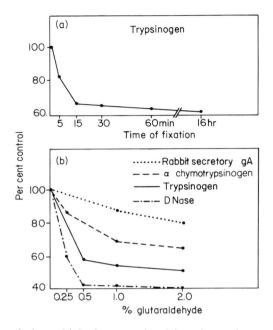

Figure 6 Effect of glutaraldehyde on antigenicity of proteins attached to agarose beads (reproduced by permission of Elsevier/North Holland from Kraehenbuhl and Jamieson, 1973). (a) Time course of effect of 0.5% glutaraldehyde on antigenicity of bovine trypsinogen. (b) Effect of glutaraldehyde at various concentrations on antigenicity of several insolubilized antigens. The antigens were exposed to each concentration of glutaraldehyde for 16 h

be due either to a loss of antigenic sites or of a failure of antibodies to reach those sites. Kraehenbuhl and Jamieson (1974) have examined this problem by looking at the effect of glutaraldehyde on antigens covalently linked to agarose beads. A similar preparation has been used by Larsson and colleagues (1979) to select tissue treatments which favour preservation of particular antigens. The results of Kraehenbuhl and Jamieson are shown in Figure 6. They found that up to a concentration of 0.5% glutaraldehyde loss of antigenicity was proportional to the concentration of fixative, but with different antigens differing greatly in their sensitivity. This emphasizes the importance of testing different concentrations of fixative for each antigen and also each tissue under study. In practice, most workers have used a mixture of paraformaldehyde and glutaraldehyde. Recently, the importance of the pH of the fixative has also been emphasized (Berod *et al.*, 1981). In their original pre-embedding staining protocol Pickel and colleagues used 1% glutaraldehyde, 1% paraformaldehyde in 0.1 M sodium cacodylate buffer (pH 7.2) to successfully localize the enzymes tyrosine hydroxylase, dopamine-β-hydroxylase, tryptophan hydroxylase (Pickel *et al.*, 1976) and the peptide substance P (Pickel *et al.*, 1977a). Figure 4 shows the localization of tryptophan hydroxylase using this fixative. A similar mixture has been used by Buijs and Swaab (1979) for the localization of vasopressin and oxytocin. More recently several research groups have used 4% paraformaldehyde with between 0.05 and 0.4% glutaraldehyde depending on the particular antigen and tissue (Pickel, 1981; Ribak *et al.*, 1981; Cuello *et al.*, 1980). Using such a mixture we have localized the transmitter 5-HT and the peptides substance P and enkephalin (see Figures 11, 13, and 19: also Cuello *et al.*, 1980; Priestley, 1981; Priestley *et al.*, 1982; Somogyi *et al.*, 1982). Various other groups have used similar conditions for identification of other transmitter-related antigens including tyrosine hydroxylase (Pickel *et al.*, 1979; Halasz *et al.*, 1977), glutamic acid decarboxylase (Ribak *et al.*, 1981; see also Chapter 7) and TRH (Johansson *et al.*, 1980). Figure 7 shows the effect of different fixation and tissue sectioning schedules on substance P immunostaining. Methods of sectioning are discussed in Section III.2. The figure shows the decrease in staining intensity observed as conditions are altered in order to improve ultrastructure. Figure 8 shows GAD immunostaining in axon terminals and presynaptic dendrites obtained by Ribak and colleagues (Ribak *et al.*, 1976, 1977) using a 4% paraformaldehyde–0.4% glutaraldehyde mixture. When higher concentrations of glutaraldehyde were used (1 and 5%) non-specific staining was seen. Figure 9 shows an example of staining for the peptide enkephalin in a neuronal perikarya from recent work by Pickel and co-workers (1980). Perfusion fixation through the left ventricle or descending aorta is necessary for preservation of both good ultrastructure and antigenicity, preferably with manually assisted respiration and some form of variable pressure perfusion device (Vaughn *et al.*, 1981; Gonzalez Aguilar and De Robertis, 1963). Following perfusion we leave the brain in the same fixative for a further 2 hours, although longer periods in fixative are reported, apparently without deleterious results (Vaughn *et al.*, 1981; Kraehenbuhl and Jamieson, 1974).

Post-embedding procedure

For post-embedding staining satisfactory results have been described using simple immersion fixation (e.g. Weber *et al.*, 1978; Bugnon *et al.*, 1977) and much higher concentrations of glutaraldehyde. Thus, Van Leeuwen reported little difference in preservation of antigenicity between 4% formalin, and 2.5% glutaraldehyde + 1% paraformaldehyde (Van Leeuwen, 1977). In some studies it has also been possible to stain OsO_4 fixed material (Beauvillain and Tramu, 1980; Rodning *et al.*, 1978; Pelletier *et al.*, 1981). However, although OsO_4 fixation gives very good preservation of ultrastructure it has generally been considered incompatible with immunocytochemical techniques (e.g. Pelletier and Leclerc, 1979). Another fixative of interest is the perio-

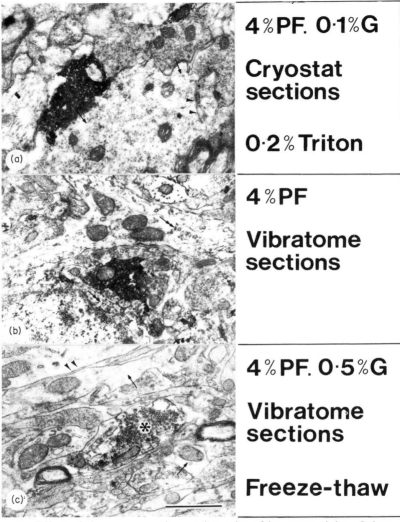

Figure 7 Effect of tissue preparation on intensity of immunostaining. Substance P immunoreactive terminals as revealed by rat monoclonal antibodies in the spinal trigeminal nucleus examined using different tissue fixation and tissue sectioning/ incubation conditions. As the concentration of glutaraldehyde in the fixative is increased, and procedures such as Triton treatment and cryostat sectioning are avoided, the ultrastructure is improved, although the intensity of immunostaining is decreased. In (c) asterisk indicates the lightly stained terminal. Arrowheads indicate membranes, sharp and intact in (c) but fuzzy and broken in (a). In (b), which had no glutaraldehyde in the fixative, there is some indication of presumably non-specific staining in a dendrite and in neuronal cytoplasm (double arrows). Arrows indicate direction of visible synaptic contacts. (Bar = 1 μm)

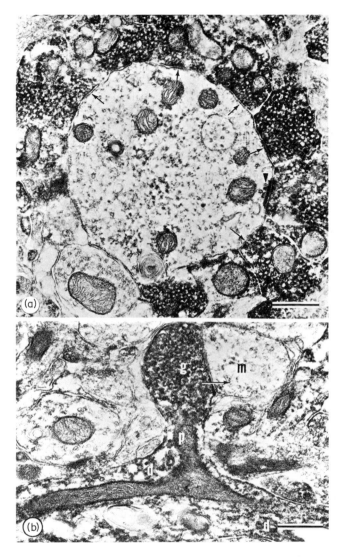

Figure 8 Pre-embedding staining for glutamate decarboxylase (GAD) as obtained by Ribak and colleagues following tissue fixation with 4% paraformaldehyde, 0.4% glutaraldehyde. (a) GAD positive terminals in the substantia nigra making synaptic contacts (arrows) with a transversely sectioned dendrite. Arrowhead indicates a subjunctional dense body. Bar = 0.5 μm (from Ribak *et al.*, 1976). (b) GAD positive presynaptic dendrite in the external plexiform layer of the rat olfactory bulb (Ribak *et al.*, 1977). Notice the association of reaction product with various membranes within a granule cell gemmule (g), dendrite (d) and pedicle (p). A mitral cell dendrite (m) is unlabelled. (Bar = 0.5 μm.) Reproduced by permission of Elsevier/North Holland

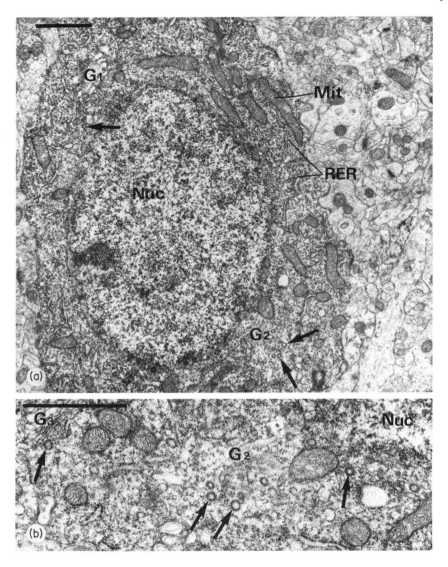

Figure 9   Enkephalin-like immunoreactivity within a neuronal perikaryon in the rat neostriatum (reproduced by permissioon of Alan R. Liss, Inc., from Pickel *et al.*, 1980). Notice granular reaction product throughout nucleus and cytoplasm. Arrows indicate 'alveolate' vesicles. 4% paraformaldehyde, 0.2% glutaraldehyde fixation. (Bar = 1 μm)

date–lysine–paraformaldehyde fixative developed by McLean and Nakane (1974) especially for EM immunocytochemistry and directed against the lipid and carbohydrate components of cell structure. This has been used both for pre-embedding (Hunt *et al.*, 1980; see also Chapter 7) and post-embedding (McLean and Nakane, 1974) staining. Finally, buffered picric acid paraform-aldehyde (Zamboni and de Martino, 1967) has also been widely used (e.g. Weber *et al.*, 1978; Beauvillain *et al.*, 1980; Tougard *et al.*, 1979). Thus, for any EM immunocytochemical study although 4% paraformaldehyde + about 0.1% glutaraldehyde can be recommended to begin with, these other fixatives should be tried if there is no initial success. For post-embedding staining it is possible to avoid primary fixatives altogether by using the techniques of freeze-substitution and of freeze-drying, but so far only a few reports have been published using these methods (Silverman and Zimmerman, 1975; Coulter and Terracio, 1977).

III.2   Tissue Sectioning Methods for Pre-embedding Staining

A number of methods are available for sectioning un-embedded fixed material prior to immunostaining, and include use of McIlwain and Sorvall tissue choppers, the Vibratome, and frozen tissue procedures based on the cryostat or the freezing microtome. We routinely use a Vibratome (Oxford Instruments), in which sections are cut by a vibrating razor blade which advances at variable speed and amplitude through a stationary tissue block immersed in buffer (Hökfelt and Ljungdahl, 1972). This instrument produces minimal tissue damage, easily cuts sections from 10 to 100 µm in thickness, and has the advantage compared with tissue choppers of being able to handle tissue blocks of quite large surface areas (Smith, 1970; Vaughn *et al.*, 1981; Pickel, 1981). As will be described below in the section on processing for electron microscopy (Section III.4), this staining of large 40 µm Vibratome sections allows light and electron microscopic correlations to be performed. However, penetration of immunoreagents into such fixed sections is poor, and in the past the various cryosectioning methods have often been used because they provide greater antibody penetration due to the tissue disrup-tion caused by the freezing and cutting process (Sternberger, 1979). Figure 10 shows the degree of penetration typically seen for immunoreagents into a Vibratome cut slice.

In our experience the disruption of ultrastructure caused by cryostat sectioning is great, and a more satisfactory way of increasing penetration of immunoreagents is to rapidly freeze and thaw cryoprotected tissue prior to Vibratome sectioning. Figure 7 shows the sort of ultrastructural preservation which can be obtained using these two different approaches. Infiltration of tissue blocks with 30% sucrose is adequate for cryoprotection, and for rapid freezing Vaughn and colleagues recommend the use of liquid Freon or

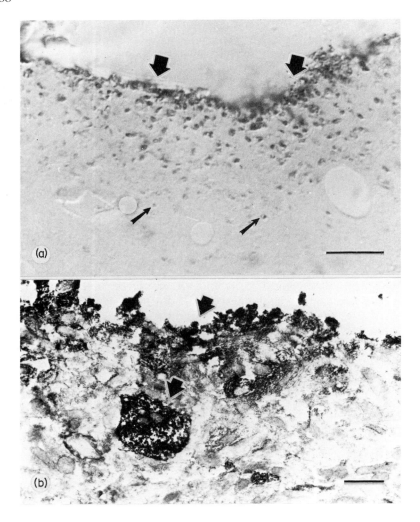

Figure 10　Penetration of immunoreagents into 40 μm thick Vibratome sections. PAP immunostaining was carried out but whole serum was used for the primary antibody, giving strong non-specific staining. Following embedding sections were cut on the ultramicrotome transverse to the plane of Vibratome sectioning. This allows the depth of staining away from the tissue surface to be examined. (a) 2 μm semi-thin section photographed using interference contrast illumination. Heavy staining is seen on the surface of the section (arrowheads) with intensity of staining decreasing away from the surface. Occasional sites of immunoreaction can be seen deeper in the tissue (arrows). (Bar = 10 μm.) (b) Electron micrograph showing the surface of the tissue section. The heavy surface staining (arrow heads) is seen to correspond to an area of extensive disruption of ultrastructure. (Bar = 1 μm)

propane cooled by liquid nitrogen (Vaughn *et al.*, 1981; Barber *et al.*, 1978), although we have found direct immersion of tissue in liquid nitrogen to be satisfactory. In our procedure, at the same time as thawing, the material is given a considerable osmotic shock which probably produces microfractures in the tissue. This increases penetration of immunoreagents but does not produce the ultrastructural damage seen with cryosectioning, and seems to be preferable to the use of detergents to increase penetration (described below, Section III.3). The handling of material for post-embedding staining is dealt with in the section on processing for EM (Section III.4).

III.3 PAP Immunostaining

The principles of PAP staining have been covered briefly already (Section II.3) and are described fully elsewhere (Sternberger, 1979), so only those features peculiar to EM immunostaining will be considered here. Problems related to antibody purity are dealt with in Chapter 1. However, it should be noted that before a particular antibody is applied at the ultrastructural level the characteristics of its staining at light microscopic level should be examined so that this information can be applied for the preparation of an EM protocol. As a general rule, if immunostaining is difficult for a particular antibody at light microscopic level it will be more difficult at the electron microscopic level. What follows refers mainly to pre-embedding staining, and as with tissue fixation and sectioning the aim is to strike a balance between conditions optimal for immunostaining and those optimal for ultrastructural preservation.

III.3.1 *Reagent penetration*

For light microscopic work it is normal to make up reagents in buffer containing a detergent such as Triton X-100 which increases antibody penetration and is also reported to reduce non-specific staining, possibly by decreasing hydrophobic interactions (Van Leeuwen, 1980b; Hartman, 1973). However, such detergents dissolve membranes and should be avoided in EM work if possible (see Figure 7). Apparently certain antigens such as the membrane-bound enzymes DBH and TH require exposure to detergent for successful immunostaining and in their case Pickel (1981) recommends 0.25% Triton for just 15 min prior to immunostaining. Penetration can also be enhanced by increasing the ionic strength of the reagent buffer solutions (Pickel, 1981), a procedure which in addition reduces non-specific ionic interactions (Van Leeuwen, 1980b). We have found phosphate buffered saline (PBS) to be quite suitable for making up all reagent solutions (see Appendix 2). An alternative approach sometimes adopted for increasing immunoreagent penetration is to use antibody fragments rather than the complete IgG (Kraehenbuhl and Jamieson, 1974). Thus, Barber and colleagues use a Fab (antigen-binding) fragment in the PAP complex in all their work (Barber *et al.*, 1978, 1979; Vaughn *et al.*, 1981), although the wisdom of this procedure has been questioned by Sternberger (1979).

III.3.2 *Method specificity* (see Chapter 1)

Background non-specific staining is often not as serious a problem in the ultra-thin EM sections as it is in the thick sections used for light microscopy (Vaughn *et al.*, 1981), but still all efforts should be made to keep such staining to a minimum. It is normal to pre-incubate sections and make up all immunoreagents in non-immune serum of the species which provides the link antibody (Sternberger, 1979), although other sources of protein can be used instead (Vaughn *et al.*, 1981; Sofroniew *et al.*, 1979). This procedure has the effect of saturating non-specific binding sites in the tissue which might otherwise bind antibodies. Non-specific binding can apparently also be caused by the presence of excess fixative, especially the bifunctional reagent glutaraldehyde, and Vaughn and colleagues (1981) emphasize the importance of washing sections thoroughly before starting the immunostaining. Free aldehyde groups can also be blocked by pre-incubation of sections in sodium borohydride (Lillie and Pizzolato, 1972). However, pretreatment of sections with chemical reagents, including those frequently used for abolishing endogenous peroxidase and pseudoperoxidase activity (e.g. Straus, 1971; Weir *et al.*, 1974) is not recommended for EM immunocytochemistry unless their effect on preservation of both ultrastructure and of antigenicity is clearly known.

III.3.3 *Serum specificity* (see Chapter 1)

The causes of non-specific staining discussed so far all come under the category of 'method specificity' (Vandesande, 1979; Van Leeuwen, 1980b); that is they arise from mechanisms other than that of the interaction of antibody and tissue antigen. For ultrastructural immunocytochemistry it is important that non-specific staining due to impurities in the primary antisera, categorized as 'serum specificity'· be kept to a minimum also. Thus, it is recommended that purified antibodies be used, prepared by techniques such as salt fractionation, column chromatography and immunoabsorption (Weir, 1978). However, none of these methods are ideal since preparation of immunoabsorbents requires the use of relatively large amounts of pure antigen, frequently only low and medium affinity antibodies are selected for, and in addition such purified sera still consist of an undefined range of antibodies directed against a range of different antigenic determinants (Swaab *et al.*, 1977; Sternberger, 1979; see also Chapter 1). Because of these various difficulties we have adopted instead the use of monoclonal antibodies (Köhler and Milstein, 1975) produced by hybrid myeloma cells grown in tissue culture. This approach allows the continuous production of well-characterized high-affinity antibodies directed against a single antigenic determinant and these are ideal reagents for both light and electron microscopic immunocytochemistry (Cuello *et al.*, 1979, 1980; for production and application of monoclonal antibodies see Chapter 9). We have so far successfully developed monoclonal antibodies directed against the neuropeptide substance P (Cuello *et al.*, 1979) and against the indoleamine transmitter 5-HT (Consolazione *et al.*, 1981). With these reagents we have obtained exceptionally 'clean' immunostaining with negligible background and therefore avoided some of the interpretative problems found with ultrastructural immunocytochemistry (see Section V). However, if such highly specific primary reagents are not available various other steps should be taken to minimize the effect of contaminants in the traditional antisera. Staining by low-affinity cross-reacting antibodies can be abolished by use of antisera at high dilution (Van Leeuwen and Swaab, 1977), and much non-specific staining can be prevented by pre-incubation of sera with acetone-extracted tissue powders (Vaughn *et al.*, 1981).

Optimal staining is generally obtained by the use of long incubations in high dilution primary antisera and for pre-embedding staining we have found overnight incubations at 4 °C to be most suitable. Very long incubation times should be avoided because of the gradual ultrastructural deterioration which occurs in buffer solutions, and for the remaining antibodies in the PAP sequence 1 h incubations are adequate. The best dilution of primary antibody should always be determined individually for each different serum, but the link antibody and the PAP complex can normally be used at 1/10 and 1/50 dilution respectively. For post-embedding staining some workers have used very much shorter incubation times for the primary antibody (Van Leeuwen *et al.*, 1976; Moriarty and Halmi, 1972) and 5–10 min incubations in PAP are frequently used (Sternberger, 1979).

III.4   Processing for Electron Microscopy

III.4.1   *Localization of peroxidase*

Peroxidase in the bound PAP complex is localized by addition of its substrate, hydrogen peroxide, and an electron donor which on oxidation produces a coloured reaction product. Although several such electron donors are available which can be used at light microscopic level (e.g. La Vail, 1978; Nakane, 1968), their reaction products are either soluble or not electron dense, and therefore not suitable for electron microscopy. For ultrastructural immunocytochemistry the only electron donor which has been widely used is

3,3'-diaminobenzidine (DAB) and on oxidation this forms an insoluble polymer which is able to chelate with osmium tetroxide, thus becoming electron-opaque. Alternative substrates have been developed such as *o*-toluidine stabilized with sodium nitroprusside (e.g. Somogyi *et al.*, 1979) and *p*-phenylene-diamine with pyrocatechol (Hanker *et al.*, 1977; Hanker, 1979) although their use in ultrastructural immunocytochemistry has not so far been very successful (Pickel, 1981). We have tested the first of these substrates and found it to be too sensitive for routine use since it detects the slightest presence of non-specific background staining. Diaminobenzidine is though to be carcinogenic and must be handled with extreme care. All excess reagent and contaminated staining equipment should be neutralized in bleach. DAB is normally made up in 0.05 M Tris pH 7.6 (Graham *et al.*, 1966) although phosphate buffer may be used instead (La Vail and La Vail, 1974), and sections pre-incubated in the DAB solution (0.03–0.05%) for 5–10 min before addition of H_2O_2 (to give 0.001–0.01% H_2O_2). Use of old solutions and of buffers with lower pH increases non-specific staining, although several groups prefer to work at pH 5.5 which is nearer to the optimum for the enzyme (La Vail, 1978; Vacca *et al.*, 1980). During staining the progress of the reaction should be followed using a dissecting microscope and the reaction terminated by transfer of sections to fresh buffer before non-specific staining becomes significant (after about 10 min). After washing, sections are osmicated, dehydrated, and embedded in plastic as for routine EM processing. Heavy-metal staining should be used sparingly because the DAB reaction deposit is difficult to locate in well contrasted specimens; for this reason we normally avoid procedures such as en bloc staining with uranyl acetate. However, for pre-embedding staining OsO_4 cannot be omitted altogether since it chelates with the DAB reaction deposit rendering it stable and electron-dense enough for EM localization. For post-embedding staining osmium is generally omitted prior to resin embedding (see Section III.1) but can be applied after the immunostaining has been carried out (e.g. Moriarty and Halmi, 1972; Van Leeuwen *et al.*, 1976).

III.4.2   *Embedding and EM sectioning procedures*

Although any standard embedding procedure can be used for pre-embedding staining, we have found it helpful to use a two-stage flat embedding technique originally developed for Golgi EM studies (Stell, 1965; Somogyi, 1978). Sections are examined flat embedded on glass slides and then re-embedded for ultramicrotomy. This procedure allows light microscopic examination of EM processed material, thus giving a direct light EM correlation. It facilitates identification and thin sectioning of sparsely stained material, and it provides easy handling of large sections with minimum loss of potentially valuable material. Figure 11 shows the application of this tech-

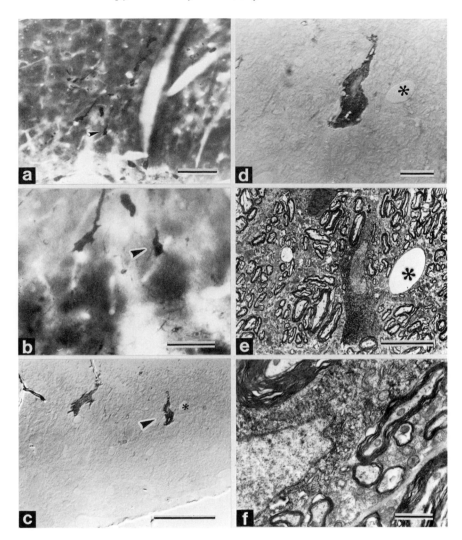

Figure 11 Localization of 5-HT immunostained neurons in nucleus reticularis paragigantocellularis. Use of a two-stage embedding procedure allows a single cell (arrow) situated close to a blood vessel (asterisk) to be examined at both light and electron microscopic level. (a,b) Immunostained cells in the 40 μm thick sections plastic-embedded on glass slides. (Bars = 100 μm (a) and 50 μm (b).) c,d. The same cells as they appear in the 2 μm semi-thin section cut on the ultramicrotome following re-embedding in capsules. Interference contrast illumination. (Bars = 50 μm (c) and 10 μm (d).) (e,f) One of the cells photographed in the electron microscope. Diffuse reaction product fills the cytoplasm and there is heavy staining of membranes. (Bars = 10 μm (e) and 1 μm (f))

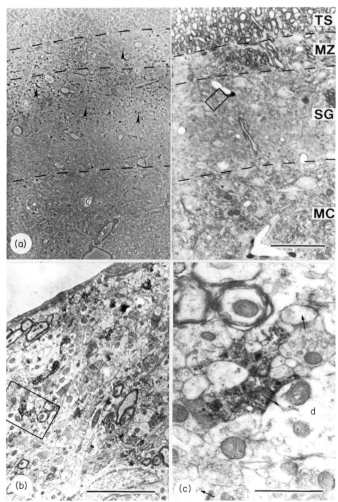

Figure 12 Use of serial semi-thin (2 μm) and ultra-thin sections to allow the precise localization of immunostained profiles. Substance P terminals in the substantia gelatinosa (SG) of the spinal trigeminal nucleus. (a) Light micrographs. Two serial semi-thin sections. One is observed under phase contrast to reveal immunostained structures (arrowheads). The other is stained (Azur II–toluidine blue/tetraborate) to reveal general cytoarchitecture. TS = spinal tract, MZ = marginal zone, SG = substantia gelatinosa, MC = magnocellularis subnucleus. (Bar = 50 μm.) (b,c) Electron micrographs. (b) Low-power micrograph corresponding in area to the square in (a) (Bar = 5 μm)
(c) High-power micrograph corresponding in area to the square in (b). A group of immunostained terminals can be seen, one of which makes synaptic contact onto an unstained dendrite (d). Arrows indicate direction of various synapses visible in the section. (Bar = 1 μm)

nique for the localization of 5-HT containing neurons in the brainstem. Following re-embedding we also routinely take a couple of thin (2 μm) sections immediately before commencing ultra-thin sectioning. One of these thin sections is stained (Azur II–toluidine blue/tetraborate), thus allowing the localization of all EM examined profiles in relationship to the general neuronal groupings in the section. This is particularly important, for instance, if the distribution and appearance of stained profiles in a morphologically complex tissue is being described. In Figure 12 this approach has been used to allow the exact localization of a group of substance P containing terminals in the substantia gelatinosa of the spinal trigeminal nucleus. Whatever embedding procedure is adopted great care should be taken during sectioning because of the very limited depth of tissue suitable for examination. Because of the immunoreagent penetration problems already discussed (Sections III.2 and 3), the centre of each slice normally shows good ultrastructure with no immunostaining while the surfaces show poor structure and heavy staining (Figure 10). Sections for EM examination must be taken from an intermediate region where both structure and immunostaining are acceptable. It is recommended also that serial sections are taken using membrane-coated single-slot grids and one or two grids in a series contrasted with heavy metals (uranyl acetate and lead citrate). Interesting features of a stained profile can then be examined in serial sections even if obscured in places by the reaction deposit, while more information about ultrastructure can be obtained from the corresponding contrasted grids (Figure 13). In grids which have not been stained with heavy metals, contrast can be increased by using low voltage and small-aperture microscope settings. An alternative approach to assist localization of the tissue area which has optimum structure and staining is to section the specimen in a plane perpendicular to the face of the tissue slice that was exposed to the immunoreagents (Vaughn *et al.*, 1981). In this way the entire tissue slice thickness is visible in the EM sections and the optimum area can be selected for photography. However, the disadvantage with this approach is that in any series of sections only a small area of tissue is suitable for examination and a lot of potentially valuable material can be lost during trimming of the block.

Post-embedding staining For post-embedding staining various specialized embedding procedures may need to be adopted. It may be necessary to test a number of alternative dehydration and resin-embedding schedules to see which gives maximum retention of antigenicity for the particular compound under study (e.g. Van Leeuwen, 1977; Moriarty and Halmi, 1972). Occasionally embedding media other than the epoxy resins may need to be tried, such as the water-soluble methacrylates (Shahrabadi and Yamamoto, 1971) or cross-linked BSA (Kraehenbuhl and Jamieson, 1973). These methods are discussed briefly in the sections on labelled antibodies (II.1 and 2) and

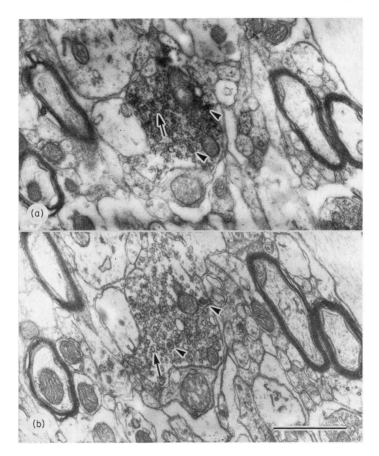

Figure 13 Use of heavy metal counter-staining of serial ultra-thin sections. A terminal lightly immunostained for substance P is shown at the centre of each field and contains both large dense core vesicles (arrowheads) and small agranular round vesicles (arrows). In (a) low voltage small aperture microscope settings have been used and no heavy metal counterstaining has been employed. Some immunostaining of the terminal is visible. In the serial section (b) counter-staining has been used. The immunostaining is less evident but more details of the ultrastructure can be seen. (Bar = 1 μm)

embedding procedures based on freeze-substitution and freeze-drying are referred to in Section III.1. However, using the PAP procedure it is normally possible to carry out staining on epoxy resin embedded material, and Sternberger (1979) has suggested that protein denaturation with consequent loss of antigenicity is in fact less likely with such resins than with water-soluble embedding media. Of the resins routinely available Van Leeuwen (1977) found no difference with respect to retention of immunoreactivity between Araldite 6005 and Epon 812. Immunostaining may be possible directly on the embedded sections (Moriarty and Halmi, 1972) but is increased following etching of the plastic using 5% H_2O_2 (Sternberger, 1979) or alcoholic sodium hydroxide (Van Leeuwen, 1980b).

IV PROTOCOL FOR PAP PRE-EMBEDDING ULTRASTRUCTURAL IMMUNOCYTOCHEMISTRY

The detailed protocol given below has been used successfully by the authors for the localization of the neuropeptides substance P and enkephalin and for the transmitter 5-HT. The general procedure to be followed is shown in Figure 14. It has so far been applied in the brain stem raphe and trigeminal nuclei, the substantia nigra, and the caudate-putamen of the rat (Cuello *et al.*, 1980, 1981; Priestley, 1981; Priestley *et al.*, 1982; Somogyi *et al.*, 1982). However, before attempting this procedure the reader should consult Section III for full details of possible variations in approach. Information on suppliers of equipment and reagents, and on preparation of fixative and buffer solutions, can be found in Appendix 2.

Day 1: Early in the morning a rat is anaesthetized with 0.5–0.7 ml Equithesin and perfused via the descending aorta. The cannulation procedure is described in detail by Gonzalez Aguilar and De Robertis (1963) and involves exposure of the abdominal aorta just below the left kidney and introduction of a cannula in the cephalic direction (Figure 15). The inferior portion of the aorta is ligated and the vena cava cut to allow drainage of venous blood. With this procedure the animal continues breathing during the first stages of the perfusion. Perfusion is begun with 15 ml 0.1 M phosphate buffer pH 7.4 containing a few mg heparin, followed by the fixative. 100 ml of 4% paraformaldehyde 0.1% glutaraldehyde in 0.1 M phosphate buffer is delivered automatically over a period of 30 min using a syringe pump (Sage Instruments). Subsequently the brain is dissected out and left in the same fixative for a further $2\frac{1}{2}$ h. Blocks a few mm thick are then cut from the brain area of interest and transferred to 0.1 M phosphate 30% sucrose until completely infiltrated, indicated by the fact that the tissue blocks sink to the bottom of the container (6–8 h). Perfusion and initial infiltration takes place at room temperature, but if the length of time in sucrose buffer is to be extended the tissue blocks are transferred to a cold-room (4 °C).

Following sucrose infiltration (normally the evening of day 1) the tissue blocks are transferred to a plastic cup and rapidly frozen by being plunged into liquid nitrogen. Blocks should not be larger than a few mm³ or else they are liable to fracture. The frozen tissue is then thawed by being dropped into warm (25 °C) 0.1 M phosphate buffer and 40 μm sections subsequently cut on

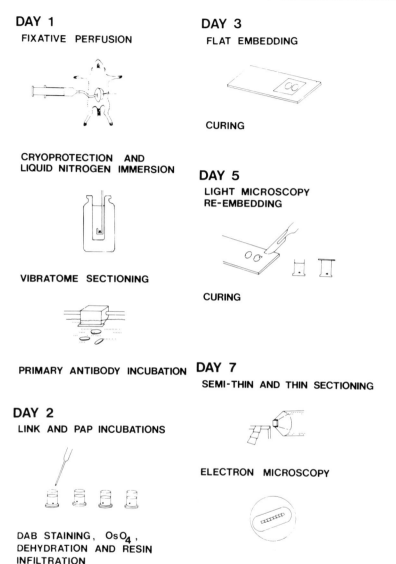

DAY 1

FIXATIVE PERFUSION

CRYOPROTECTION AND
LIQUID NITROGEN IMMERSION

VIBRATOME SECTIONING

PRIMARY ANTIBODY INCUBATION

DAY 2

LINK AND PAP INCUBATIONS

DAB STAINING, OsO$_4$,
DEHYDRATION AND RESIN
INFILTRATION

DAY 3

FLAT EMBEDDING

CURING

DAY 5

LIGHT MICROSCOPY
RE-EMBEDDING

CURING

DAY 7

SEMI-THIN AND THIN SECTIONING

ELECTRON MICROSCOPY

Figure 14 Protocol for pre-embedding staining. See Section IV for full details

a Vibratome (Oxford). Tissue blocks for cutting should be no more than 4–5 mm in thickness but can be 25–50 mm^2 surface area, and are cut in phosphate buffer cooled to 4 °C by a refrigerated circulating bath (Neslab). Following sectioning the 40 μm slices are transferred to phosphate buffered

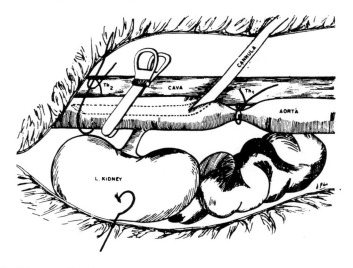

Figure 15 Diagram showing operation to introduce the perfusion cannula into the abdominal aorta (from Gonzalez Aguilar and De Robertis, 1963). The inferior portion of the aorta is ligated with thread Th_1 and a clamp placed on the upper portion of the aorta above the kidney arteries. A slit is made in the aorta above Th_1 and the cannula introduced in the cephalic direction. The clamp is opened to permit the passage of the cannula but maintains pressure on it, ligature Th_2 is then tightened and the clamp removed. Reproduced by permission of Harcourt Brace Jovanavich Inc.

saline (PBS) and if necessary are dissected by hand into smaller areas ready for the immunostaining. A couple of hours may need to be allowed for the sectioning and microdissecting stages.

Immunostaining is begun with 30 min in 10% normal serum from the species in which the link antibody was raised (probably goat if rabbit-raised primary antibodies are used, and rabbit if rat or mouse monoclonal antibodies are applied), followed by 15 min wash and then incubation in the primary antiserum. Unless otherwise stated incubations are carried out at room temperature and PBS is used for washes. Antisera in the PAP sequence are made up in 1% normal serum of the link antibody species. For incubations we have found it convenient to use the flat ends of cut-off EM embedding capsules (TAAB) since these allow sections of quite large surface area to be incubated in small volumes (100–150 µl) of reagents. Incubation solutions are removed using a 2.5 ml syringe fitted with a blunt needle and a rubber teat instead of a plunger (Figure 16) and sections are stirred regularly using puffs of air from a Pasteur pipette.

After 1 h in the primary antiserum at room temperature, the sections are transferred to a cold-room and incubation continued overnight (10–12 h) at 4 °C.

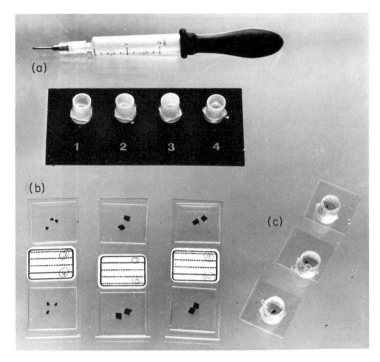

Figure 16   Apparatus used for immunoreagent incubation and for flat embedding. (a) Cut-off EM capsules used for antibody incubation, and suction syringe used for removing incubation solutions from capsules. (b) Immunostained osmicated sections flat-embedded in Durcupan on glass slides. (c) Sections re-embedded in EM capsules ready for ultra-microtomy

Day 2:   Sections are removed from the cold-room and incubation continued at room temperature:

—1 h primary antiserum (e.g. rabbit)
—45 min PBS (wash)
—1 h link antibody (e.g. IgG fraction of goat anti-rabbit IgG)
—45 min PBS (wash)
—1½ h PAP (e.g. rabbit PAP).

Using a fine brush, sections are then transferred to glass bottles (e.g. scintillation vials) for a 45-min PBS wash ready for incubation in 3,3′diamino-benzidine (DAB). DAB should be treated with great care. Disposable gloves should be worn, incubations should be carried out in a fume cupboard, and all excess reagent and contaminated apparatus neutralized with bleach. DAB solutions are made up fresh and incubation carried out in the dark. Staining sequences continue as follows:

—10 min 0.06% DAB in 0.05 M Tris HCl pH 7.6 (e.g. 1.2 mg DAB in 2 ml)
—add H_2O_2 to give 0.01% H_2O_2 (e.g. 20 µl 1% H_2O_2 to 2 ml of DAB Tris).

The progress of the reaction is followed using a low-power microscope and terminated by replacing the reagents by fresh buffer (0.1 M phsophate) before non-specific background staining becomes unacceptable (after about 10 min).

After DAB staining EM processing begins. Any standard schedule can be used. We have found the following procedure convenient since it allows sections to reach the resin stage by the end of day 2.

—45 min 0.1 M phosphate buffer (wash)
—1½ h 1% OsO_4 in 0.1 M phsophate (all these stages in a fume cupboard)
—10 min buffer
—10 min 50% ethanol
—10 min 70% ethanol (or 30 min in 70% ethanol plus 1% uranyl acetate)
—10 min 90% ethanol
—2 × 15 min absolute ethanol
—2 × 15 min propylene oxide
—Durcupan (Fluka) overnight.

Day 3: Tissue is embedded in Durcupan. As described in Section III.4, we have adopted a two-stage flat embedding procedure which allows easier handling of material and correlative microscopic analysis.

Tissue slices are placed on glass slides in a drop of resin and covered using a plastic coverslip (Bel-Art, USA). This procedure is carried out on a warm plate and just enough resin is used so as to fill the space between slide and coverslip. Sections are then left to cure for two days at 56 °C (see Figure 16).

Day 5: The coverslip is removed from the cured specimens by scoring the edge with a sharp point and lifting carefully. Sections are then examined in a light microscope using bright field illumination, and the areas of interest are photographed. We have used a Leitz Dialux 20 for all light microscopy fitted with a Vario-Orthomat automatic photographic system, and Ilford Pan F fine-grain film.

The resin-embedded sections can be kept indefinitely and then re-embedded for EM analysis when needed. The slide-mounted specimen is warmed slightly to soften the resin and the area of interest cut out using a pointed piece of razor blade and with the aid of a dissecting microscope. The piece of tissue in its thin slice of resin is then flat-embedded in the base of a TAAB capsule using more Durcupan and with the relevant immunostained surface downwards. The top of the capsule is cut parallel to the base, the capsule filled to the brim with resin and then topped with a glass coverslip. This assembly is then incubated at 56 °C for two days to cure.

Day 7: When the re-embedded sections have cured, the glass coverslip is removed leaving a smooth resin surface. This allows the block-embedded sections to be examined in a light microscope and the approach to the specimen surface during cutting with the ultramicrotome to be closely monitored. As soon as the desired area is reached two semi-thin sections are taken, followed by a series of ultra-thin sections which are mounted on formvar-coated single-slot grids. Details on serial sectioning can be found in any standard EM text (Reid, 1975). One of the semi-thin (2 µm) sections is toluidine stained (see Appendix 2) and both semi-thins then examined using bright-field, phase, or interference contrast (Leitz ICT) illumination. Ultra-thin sections are examined both with and without lead citrate contrasting. For examination of uncontrasted sections we have used a Philips 201 electron microscope at the following settings: high tension 40 kV, condenser lens aperture 100 µm, object lens aperture 20 µm.

Trouble shooting: If problems are encountered in obtaining specific staining using the procedure above, the following points should be checked carefully:

(a) Do the fixation and incubation conditions being used give staining at light microscopic level on cryostat cut sections? If not, try using 4% paraform-aldehyde fixative without glutaraldehyde and make up immunoreagents in Triton X-100 (e.g. 0.2%). If staining now occurs reduce Triton concentration (or use 30 min pre-incubation in PBS 0.2% Triton prior to antibody incubations), and increase the glutaraldehyde content of the fixative until just sufficient staining remains to allow location in the electron microscope. If staining cannot be detected at light microscopic level on cryostat sections, almost certainly something is wrong with the immunoreagents.

(b) Test a wide range of primary antibody dilutions on cryostat sections. Lack of specific staining generally indicates that the primary antibody is ineffective or has lost activity. All stock immunoreagents should be kept frozen in small aliquots at relatively high concentration (e.g. ×10). Repeated freezing and thawing, or storage for long periods unfrozen, will destroy specific activity. High background staining indicates that the link sera and PAP have lost specificity. PAP should not be stored once an aliquot has been thawed and diluted. Although such solutions may retain sufficient activity for over a year to be used at light microscopic level, optimum activity declines after only a couple of weeks.

V INTERPRETATION OF STAINING RESULTS

As with any experimental technique, the real usefulness of EM immuno-cytochemistry depends as much on the correct interpretation of results as it does on achieving results. Many questions of interpretation are common to both light and electron microscopic immunocytochemistry and so will be only briefly referred to here since they are covered in Chapter 1. These include problems of possible cross-reactivity in the primary antisera (serum specificity) and the presence of anomalous staining due to problems in methodology (Van Leeuwen, 1980b; Vandesande, 1979). False-negative staining may occur if antisera are used at either too low or too high a dilution (Bigbee *et al.*, 1977; see also Chapter 4), or, of course, simply if the antigen is present in too low a concentration to be detected using immunocytochemistry. In this latter case it may be possible to increase tissue antigen levels with some pharmacological manipulation (e.g. Hökfelt *et al.*, 1978; Lidov *et al.*, 1980). False-positive staining may result from the use of antisera at too high a concentration (Van Leeuwen, 1980a), and from non-specific adsorption of immunoreagents to sections. Such staining can be reduced by the use of aggregate-free antisera at high dilution, by preadsorption of antisera with acetone extracted tissue powders, and by treatment of sections with normal serum of the link antibody species in the PAP staining sequence (see Section III.3 and Chapter 4). Buijs and Swaab (1979) have described false-positive post-embedding staining of dense core vesicles for vasopressin following the use of increased incubation times in the primary antiserum and in DAB. It is proposed by this group that specificity of staining should be checked by attempting staining in a tissue which is known to lack the relevant antigen (Swaab *et al.*, 1977).

There are, however, problems of interpretation which are peculiar to EM immunocytochemistry. The major difficulty with the pre-embedding staining procedure is probably the fact that the immunoreagents must diffuse through tissue structures in order to obtain access to antigenic sites. An adequate or uneven reagent penetration may mean a failure to reveal certain tissue antigens or may cause an anomalous staining pattern. Thus, in a study on a relatively homogeneous preparation of viral antigens Wendelschafer-Crabb and colleagues (1976) observed a gradient of specific staining away from the site of reagent access, while post-embedding staining of similarly fixed tissue showed uniform staining. Detection of such a 'penetration artefact' in a complex tissue such as neuropil would be very difficult. With pre-embedding staining Wendelschafer-Crabb *et al.* (1976) also showed that migration of electron-dense reaction product away from sites of attached PAP complex may occur. Novikoff and colleagues (1972) have shown that DAB reaction product may diffuse from sites of its oxidation and then be absorbed by adjoining membranes such as those of mitochondria and endoplasmic reticulum. Workers using pre-embedding staining to localize neuropeptides in nerve terminals frequently describe staining of dense core vesicles and of adjoining membranes of small vesicles and mitochondria (Hunt *et al.*, 1980; Cuello *et al.*, 1977; Barber *et al.*, 1979; Chan-Palay and Palay, 1977). However, in other reports such membrane-associated staining has not been described (Johansson *et al.*, 1980; Pickel *et al.*, 1977a) and so the question of whether the neuropeptides are localized in small agranular synaptic vesicles as well as in large dense-core vesicles must remain for the, present unanswered. Figure 17 shows how the pattern of staining for substance P in a nerve terminal may vary in different experiments. Interestingly, in a comparison between pre- and post-embedding staining for enkephalin in the median eminence, Beauvillain and colleagues (1980) obtained small vesicle membrane staining in pre-embedding but not in their post-embedding protocol. However, although this could be due to the pre-embedding DAB diffusion described above, it could also be due to simple failure of post-embedding staining.

A further serious problem with both pre- and post-embedding staining is the possible diffusion and re-location of antigen during the tissue fixation stages. At the light microscopic level such a re-location is generally inconsequential but for EM immunocytochemistry may lead to serious misinterpretation concerning the ultrastructural antigen localization. In poorly fixed tissue showing extensive disruption of organelles, interpretation clearly must be cautious (Novikoff, 1980), but even in well-preserved ultrastructure the localization may be artefactual. This question of re-location has been considered in some detail for enzyme cytochemistry (e.g. Hayat, 1973) and similar principles will apply for the immunocytochemical localization of enzymes and neuropeptides. Kraehenbuhl and Jamieson (1974) have described the possible re-localization of calcitonin from storage granules into the general cytoplasmic matrix, and there has been discussion about the real significance of cytoplasmic staining for neurohypophysial hormones and carrier proteins (Silverman, 1976). Similarly, diffuse staining throughout cytoplasm and nucleus has been described for enkephalin neurons (see Figure 9 of this chapter, reproduced from Pickel *et al.*, 1980). Using antisera directed against 5-HT several groups have described at light microscopic level general staining of somata including nuclei and proximal dendrites (Hökfelt *et al.*, 1978; Lidov *et al.*, 1980; Consolazione *et al.*, 1981), and our EM studies have shown immunoreactivity diffusely localized in cytoplasm and associated with a number of membranous structures (Figure 11). This may well represent re-location, as the extreme lability of the catecholamines and indoleamines has already been well documented in the context of the formaldehyde condensation fluorescence methods (e.g. Falck, 1962). In contrast, the cytoplasmic enzyme glutamic acid decarboxylase frequently appears as membrane-bound in immunocytochemical micrographs (e.g. Wood *et al.*, 1976; see also Figure 8b of this chapter). The occasional small vesicle staining for neuropeptides discussed above may also represent artefactual relocation.

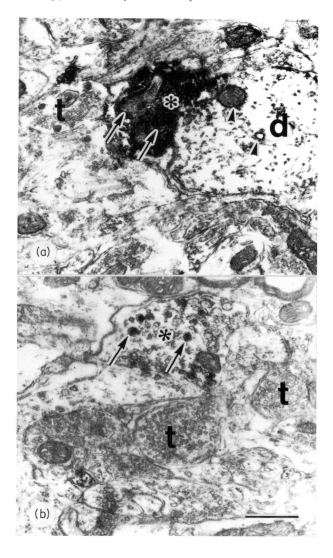

Figure 17 Effect of tissue preparation on apparent antigen localization. (a) and (b) both represent substance P immunostained terminals (asterisks) in the spinal trigeminal; (t) marks unstained terminals. In (a) mild fixation conditions have been used which preserve antigenicity and do not seriously restrict immunoreagent access. A nerve terminal is filled with reaction product which covers membranes of mitochondria and agranular vesicles (arrows). There is also some (non-specific) staining in an adjoining dendrite (d) (arrowheads). In contrast stronger fixation conditions have been used in (b) and now reaction product appears to be localized mainly over dense core vesicles (arrows). (Bar = 0.5 μm)

There are no simple controls that can be adopted to test for re-location, and the examples cited here are intended to serve simply as a warning. Before detailed interpretations of localization are made based on EM immunocyto-chemistry, all other available information from biochemical studies and from cytochemical studies using other fixation schedules should be considered.

VI   FUTURE DEVELOPMENTS IN ULTRASTRUCTURAL IMMUNOCYTOCHEMISTRY

In recent years many new neuroanatomical research techniques have been developed which aim to go beyond the simple description of the morpho-logical appearance and relative position of structure, and allow workers to begin to describe neuronal connectivity (e.g. Robertson, 1978; Jones and Hartman, 1978). At the same time biochemical and physiological studies have been relating gross physiology to the activity of specific neurotransmitters and to particular neurons (e.g. Dray, 1979). Probably one of the major contribu-tions of EM immunocytochemistry in the next few years will be as a link between these two different approaches, identifying the neuroactive com-pounds involved in specific neuronal networks and providing a firm basis for the interpretation of physiological results. Some of this work can be done using existing immunocytochemical techniques, but new methods will also need to be developed. At the same time the study of specific cell surface markers may give more direct information about neuronal development and function. In this final section we will attempt to sketch some of the developments in these various areas which can be expected in the near future from ultrastructural immunocytochemistry.

EM immunocytochemical techniques for the localization of CNS transmit-ters and transmitter markers are quite a new development and there is therefore still much that can be done simply by applying the existing methodology. Thus, for many of the neuropeptides only very preliminary reports on their EM localization have been published and most of these refer to localization in nerve terminals rather than in cell somata. For the newly developed transmitter-directed antibodies (Steinbusch *et al.*, 1978; Verhof-stad *et al.*, 1980; Consolazione *et al.*, 1981) at the time of writing this review no research papers have reported their EM localization. In the striatum and substantia nigra detailed studies have described the transmitter content of various types of nerve terminals and cell bodies (Pickel *et al.*, 1980; Ribak *et al.*, 1976, 1979; Cuello *et al.*, 1981; Somogyi *et al.*, 1982), but many other areas of the brain remain unexplored. Few workers have attempted to quantify numbers of immunoreactive terminals in a given neuropil (Pickel *et al.*, 1980; Johansson *et al.*, 1980) or to carry out correlative light and electron microscopy (Chan-Palay and Palay, 1977). Thus there is still much useful work that can be done simply by detailed description of the EM appearance and distribution of transmitter characterised neuronal structures.

This chapter has been concerned primarily with PAP immunocytochemistry and only passing reference has been made to other immunocytochemical techniques (see Section II). However, with several of these procedures significant advances have been made in recent years which may make them more useful for CNS studies. Particularly interesting are recent improved procedures for the production of ultra-thin frozen sections (Tokuyasu, 1978) and their labelling using ferritin (Tokuyasu and Singer, 1976) or iron–dextran (Dutton *et al.*, 1979) labelled antibodies. Such particulate labels are claimed to allow higher resolution, obscure less ultrastructure than the enzyme-based labels, and offer the possibility of quantitation of the immunoreaction. Another interesting and recently developed particulate label is colloidal gold (see Chapters 12 and 13). Such gold sols can be stabilized using antibodies and then used for immunocytochemistry (Horisberger and Rosset, 1977) and are apparently quicker to prepare and easier to visualize than the ferritin-labelled antibodies. Alternatively, the particles can be stabilized with protein A and the colloidal gold protein A complex used as a general indirect label (e.g. Slot, 1980; see also Chapter 12). There seems to be great potential for its use in a variety of unlabelled staining techniques instead of using anti-IgG antibodies (Notani *et al.*, 1979; Roth *et al.*, 1980; Slot, 1980). Figure 18 (kindly supplied by Dr Van Leeuwen) shows the difference between PAP and protein A/gold when applied for post-embedding staining of vasopressin. Another protein which has recently been used in immunocytochemistry, instead of using a link antibody, is avidin, an extract from egg white, which specifically binds the vitamin biotin (Melamed and Green, 1963). Gold or HRP–avidin conjugates can be prepared, and will then bind a biotin-tagged anti-IgG antibody (e.g. Hsu *et al.*, 1981). Apart from the various advantages already mentioned, these different techniques can all potentially be used to localize at EM level more than one antigen in a single section. Although several techniques exist for the localization of multiple antigens in single sections at the light microscopic level (e.g. Nakane, 1968), most of these are inapplicable to EM work because they depend either on the localization of a fluorophore or of peroxidase electron donors which cannot be used for EM (see Section III.4). The development of a simple procedure for the EM localization of multiple antigens would greatly facilitate the analysis of the relationship between nerve terminals containing different transmitters. At present this can only be done by comparing the results of separately performed studies, which is extremely difficult in a complex neuropil and requires analysis of large numbers of EM pictures before firm conclusions can be drawn. An alternative approach would be to stain serial EM sections for different antigens using post-embedding staining, but so far such staining of nerve terminals in the CNS has been largely unsuccessful.

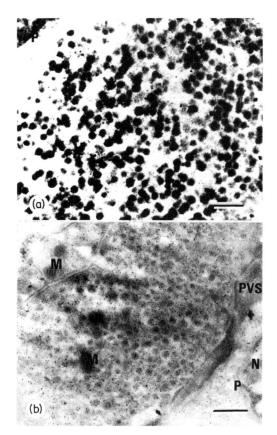

Figure 18 Comparison of PAP and protein A–colloid gold staining techniques. Post-embedding staining for vasopressin of 4% formalin-fixed rat neural lobe. In (a) the PAP method was used, in (b) protein A–gold particles of 5 nm were applied followed by uranyl acetate counterstaining. Note that structures both within the nerve fibre such as mitochondria (M) and outside the fibre such as a pituicyte (P) and the perivascular space (PVS) show negligible labelling. N = nucleus of pituicyte. Unpublished micrographs supplied by Dr Van Leeuwen. (Bar = 0.5 μm)

Most of the potential dual staining procedures mentioned above have the disadvantage of only being applicable to post-embedding staining because of the large molecular size of the various labels, and also many require difficult ultracryo-sectioning techniques. We are therefore currently exploring an alternative approach which involves tagging the primary antibody with a radioactive label and then visualizing its distribution using autoradiography (Cuello and Milstein, 1981). Radioactively labelled antibodies have been developed before, and indeed have been used successfully in conjunction with peroxidase-labelled antibodies for the ultrastructural localization of two different antigens (Gonatas *et al.*, 1974), but have not been widely used because of the difficulty of preparing radioactive covalently labelled antibodies. However, using the monoclonal antibody technique (Köhler and Milstein, 1975) it is possible to radioactively label the monoclonal antibody simply by growing the hybrid myeloma cells in the presence of ^{3}H-amino acids (see Chapter 9). These reagents have several advantages over more traditional immunostaining techniques and in addition can be used in conjunction with PAP pre-embedding immunocytochemistry for the EM localization of more than one antigen (Cuello *et al.*, 1982).

In addition to the development of procedures for the localization of multiple antigens, an interesting area for the possible future development of ultrastructural immunocytochemistry is its use in combination with other transmitter labelling techniques. Thus, several recent papers have described the use of immunocytochemistry at the light microscopic level in combination with fluorescence histochemistry (e.g. Johnson *et al.*, 1980; Sladek and McNeill, 1980), with receptor autoradiography (e.g. Sar and Stumpf, 1979) and with transmitter uptake autoradiography (e.g. Beaudet *et al.*, 1980; Chan-Palay, 1979b; see Chapter 17). The development of any of these procedures at the ultrastructural level would be a very useful additional tool for the study of interactions between transmitter-characterized neuronal structures.

Immunocytochemical techniques are usually only used to describe the distribution of transmitter-related antigens, but it is possible at the light microscopic level to map particular transmitter pathways also. This can be done by identifying changes in transmitter distribution following surgical or electrolytic lesion of the pathway (e.g. Cuello *et al.*, 1981; see Chapter 19) or by combining immunocytochemistry with a retrograde tract tracing procedure (e.g. Hökfelt *et al.*, 1979; Sofroniew and Schrell, 1981; Priestley *et al.*, 1981). Extension of such techniques to the EM level allows the ultrastructural description of transmitter-characterized identified projection neurons and also of nerve terminals synapsing with such neurons (Ruda, 1982). Immunocytochemistry has already been applied in combination with anterograde degeneration techniques (e.g. Hunt *et al.*, 1980; Barber *et al.*, 1978, 1979) and this gives information on the localization of transmitters interacting with the terminals of an identified neuronal pathway. Figure 19 shows an example of this approach used to examine the relationship between enkephalin and primary afferent terminals in the substantia gelatinosa. Also of interest are mapping techniques based on the uptake of specific antibodies following their *in vivo* administration. Thus, Jacobowitz and colleagues (1975) demonstrated that antibodies to the membrane-bound vesicular enzyme dopamine-β-hydroxylase (DBH) are taken up by noradrenergic fibres following its *in vivo* administration and are subsequently transported retrog-

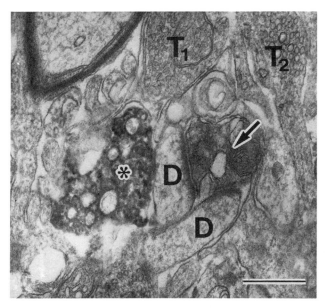

Figure 19   Combination of anterograde degeneration with immunocytochemistry. Substantia gelatinosa of the spinal trigeminal nucleus. A degenerating primary afferent terminal (arrow) makes synaptic contact with two dendrites (D). Close by is an enkephalin immunostained terminal (asterisk). Various unstained terminals are also visible, containing either ellipsoid (T_1) or spherical (T_2) synaptic vesicles. (Bar = 0.5 μm)

radely to their cell bodies (Ziegler *et al.*, 1976; see also Chapter 6 for protocol). More recently this procedure has been used at light microscopic level to study noradrenergic projections in the brain (e.g. Pasquier *et al.*, 1980), and at EM level to examine peripheral noradrenergic terminals (Llewellyn-Smith *et al.*, 1981). It has now been reported that similar uptake and retrograde transport occurs for antibodies directed against the neuropeptide substance P (Chan-Palay, 1979a) and the cytoplasmic enzyme L-glutamate decarboxylase (Chan-Palay *et al.*, 1979), and at light microscopic level this localization of substance P has been combined with transmitter autoradiography for 5-HT (Chan-Palay, 1979b; see also Chapter 17). If such uptake and retrograde transport of antibodies directed against transmitter-related antigens should prove to be a general phenomenon it will undoubtedly be a powerful tool for identifying transmitters involved in neuronal circuits.

A final area of potential future development involves the wider application of monoclonal antibodies to ultrastructural immunocytochemistry. The advantages of using monoclonal antibodies as pure reagents for PAP immunocytochemistry have already been mentioned (Section III.3). However, this approach can also be used for the production of highly specific antibodies directed against different components of an impure immunogen. Thus, various groups have obtained monoclonal antibodies against a range of neural antigens including various neuron-specific cell surface markers, synaptic membrane markers, and synaptic vesicles (McKay *et al.*, 1981). Most of the work done so far has been at light microscopic level, but many interesting questions concerning neuronal development and control of cell–cell interactions will ultimately only be solved as the distribution of these various membrane markers is explored at the ultrastructural level.

There are many questions of brain structure, neurochemistry, development, and function to which these techniques could make a vital contribution, and we hope that this chapter will prove useful to workers interested in exploring these problems applying EM immunocytochemistry.

APPENDIX 1 (see also Appendix 2 in Chapter 1)
PROTOCOL FOR PAP POST-EMBEDDING ULTRASTRUCTURAL IMMUNOCYTOCHEMISTRY

The following outline protocol is not intended to be a detailed experimental procedure and is given merely as a guide to the post-embedding staining approach. For more information the reader should consult Sternberger, 1979; Van Leeuwen *et al.*, 1976; Moriarty and Halmi, 1972; and Moriarty, 1976.

For post-embedding staining several authors recommend the use of buffered picric acid paraformaldehyde fixative (Zamboni and de Martino, 1967).

Tissue is perfusion fixed, dehydrated through graded ethanols, and embedded in Araldite. Light gold EM sections are cut and mounted on nickel grids. Sections are then stained using the following incubations:

—5 min in 5% aqueous H_2O_2
—washed by being dipped several times in distilled water, and blotted 'edgewise' on filter paper
—5 min in normal serum of link antibody
—blotted but not washed
—12 h in primary antiserum
—washed and blotted
—5 min in normal link serum followed by blotting
—5 min in link antibody (1/10 dilution)
—washed and blotted
—5 min in normal link serum followed by blotting
—5 min in PAP (1/50 dilution)
—washed but not blotted.

Sections are then dipped briefly (3 min) into a solution of 0.0125% DAB containing 0.0025% H_2O_2 in 0.05 M Tris pH 7.6. Grids are washed, blotted, and then treated with 4% OsO_4 for 20 min followed by washing and blotting. Staining is carried out by floating sections in drops of solutions in a paraffin wax layered Petri dish, and Sternberger (1979) recommends 0.05 M Tris saline pH 7.6 for making up all antiserum dilutions. During staining, grids should never be allowed to dry out completely.

APPENDIX 2
PREPARATION OF REAGENTS

(1) Fixative:
    4% paraformaldehyde 0.1% glutaraldehyde in 0.1 M phosphate buffer, pH 7.4.
    Prepare 8% paraformaldehyde stock solution as follows:
      Add 40 g paraformaldehyde (BDH) to 500 ml distilled water
      Heat to 58–60 °C
      Add 1 N NaOH dropwise until clear. Leave to cool, then filter.
    Prepare 0.2 M phosphate buffer (pH 7.4) stock solution as follows:
    (A) 0.2 M monobasic sodium phosphate
            (31.2 g $NaH_2PO_4 \cdot 2H_2O$ in 1000 ml H_2O)
    (B) 0.2 M dibasic sodium phosphate
            (71.7 g $Na_2HPO_4 \cdot 12H_2O$ in 1000 ml H_2)
    Add x ml A to B until required pH is reached (approx. 19 ml A to 81 ml B).
    For 250 ml fixative mix 125 ml paraformaldehyde stock, 125 ml buffer stock, and 1 ml 25% glutaraldehyde (EMscope).
(2) Phosphate buffer saline (PBS):
    For 2 litres mix: 100 ml 0.2 M buffer stock (see above)
                      17.52 g NaCl
                      400 mg KCl
                      1900 ml H_2O.
(3) Stain for semi-thin plastic-embedded sections: (courtesy J. Somogyi)
    (a) 0.5 g Azur II in 50 ml H_2O
    (b) 0.5 g toluidine blue + 0.5 g sodium tetraborate in 50 ml H_2O.
    Mix (a) and (b) and add 6 g sucrose. Warm gently to dissolve sucrose. Filter.

SUPPLIERS OF IMMUNOCHEMICALS

(1) Cappel Laboratories Inc., Cochranville, PA 19330, USA; *or*
    Dynatech Labs Ltd, Daux Road, Billingshurst, Sussex, England.

(2) Miles-Yeda Ltd, PO Box 1122, Kiryat Weizmann, Rehovet, Israel; *or*
    Miles Laboratories Inc., Research Products, Elkhart, Indiana 46514, USA; *or*

Miles Laboratories Ltd, Stoke Court, Stoke Poges, Slough, Bucks, England.

(3) Polysciences Inc., Paul Valley Industrial Park, Warrington, Pennsylvania 18976, USA; *or*
International Enzymes Ltd, Hanover Way, Vale Road, Windsor, Berks, England.

ACKNOWLEDGEMENTS

The development of the PAP pre-embedding protocol described in this chapter was carried out in collaboration with Dr Péter Somogyi, and the authors gratefully acknowledge his participation in the preparation of some of the material presented here.

This work was supported by grants to A.C.C. from The Wellcome Trust, The Royal Society, and E. P. Abraham Cephalosporin Trust. J.V.P. is a Beit Memorial Research Fellow and acknowledges support from the Medical Research Council (UK) and the British Council.

We would like to thank Drs V. Pickel, F. van Leeuwen, G. Childs, J. Kraehenbuhl, C. Ribak, and E. De Robertis for generously providing illustrative material. Thanks are also due to Klara Szigeti for expert technical assistance. Finally, thanks to Tonly Barclay, Brian Archer, and Terry Richards for preparing illustrations; Lorenza Eder for critically reading the manuscript, and Ella Iles for typing it.

BIBLIOGRAPHY

In the text reference is made both to original papers and to review articles. The reader may find it helpful to consult some of these reviews and so they are listed separately below under general subject classifications. The full reference for each review can be found in the references at the end of this chapter.

EM enzyme-labelled procedures:
Avrameas, 1970
Kuhlmann, 1977
Nakane, 1971.

Peroxidase–antiperoxidase procedure (PAP):
Sternberger, 1979.

PAP post-embedding procedure:
Moriarty, 1976
Van Leeuwen *et al.*, 1976
Williams, 1977.

PAP pre-embedding procedure:
Pickel, 1981
Ribak *et al.*, 1981
Vaughn *et al.*, 1981.

Comparison of pre- and post-embedding procedures:
Kraehenbuhl and Jamieson, 1974
Van Leeuwen, 1980b.

Criteria for specificity:
Vandesande, 1979.

Staining of surface markers:
De Petris, 1978.

REFERENCES

Avrameas, S. (1970). 'Enzymes as markers for the localisation of antigens and antibodies.' *Int. Rev. Cytol.*, **27**, 349–385.

Avrameas, S. and Ternynck, T. (1971). 'Peroxidase labelled antibody and Fab conjugates with enhanced intracellular penetration.' *Immunochemistry*, **8**, 1175–1179.

Avrameas, S. and Uriel, J. (1966). 'Méthode de marquage d'antigènes et d'anticorps avec des enzymes et son application en immunodiffusion.' *C.R. Acad. Sci. Paris*, **262**, 2543–2544.

Barber, R. P., Vaughn, J. E., Randall Slemmon, J., Salvaterra, P. M., Roberts, E., and Leeman, S. E. (1979). 'The origin, distribution and synaptic relationships of substance P axons in rat spinal cord.' *J. Comp. Neurol.*, **184**, 331–352.

Barber, R., Vaughn, J. E., Saito, K., McLaughlin, B. J., and Roberts, E. (1978). 'GABAergic terminals are presynaptic to primary afferent terminals in the substantia gelatinosa of the rat spinal cord.' *Brain Res.*, **141**, 35–55.

Beaudet, A., Pickel, V. M., Joh, T. H., Miller, R. J., and Cuénod, M. (1980). 'Simultaneous detection of serotonin and tyrosine hydroxylase or enkephalin containing neurons by combined radioautography and immunocytochemistry in the central nervous system of the rat.' *Soc. for Neuroscience Abstracts*, **6**, 353.

Beauvillain, J. C. and Tramu, G. (1980). 'Immunocytochemical demonstration of LH-RH, somatostatin, and ACTH-like peptide in osmium-postfixed resin-embedded medium eminence.' *J. Histochem. Cytochem.*, **28**, 1014–1017.

Beauvillain, J. C., Tramu, G., and Croix, D. (1980). 'Electron microscopic localisation of enkephalin in the medium eminence and the adenohypophysis of the guinea-pig.' *Neuroscience*, **5**, 1705–1716.

Berod, A., Hartman, B. K., and Pujol, J. F. (1981). 'Importance of fixation in immunohistochemistry: use of formaldehyde solutions at variable pH for the localisation of tyrosine hydroxylase.' *J. Histochem. Cytochem.*, **29**, 844–850.

Bigbee, J. W., Kosek, J. C., and Eng, L. F. (1977). 'Effects of primary antiserum dilution of staining of "antigen-rich" tissues with the peroxidase antiperoxidase technique.' *J. Histochem. Cytochem.*, **25**, 443–447.

Bugnon, C., Bloch, B., Lenys, D., and Fellman, D. (1977). 'Ultrastructural study of the LH-RH containing neurons in the human fetus.' *Brain Res.*, **137**, 175–180.

Buijs, R. M. and Swaab, D. F. (1979). 'Immunoelectronmicroscopical demonstration of vasopressin and oxytocin synapses in the limbic system of the rat.' *Cell Tiss. Res.*, **204**, 355–365.

Chan-Palay, V. (1979a). 'Immunocytochemical detection of substance P neurons, their processes and connections by *in vivo* microinjections of monoclonal antibodies: light and electron microscopy.' *Anat. Embryol. (Berl).*, **156**, 225–240.

Chan-Palay, V. (1979b). 'Combined immunocytochemistry and autoradiography after *in vivo* injections of monoclonal antibody to substance P and ^{3}H-serotonin: coexistence of two putative transmitters in single raphe cells and fiber plexuses.' *Anat. Embryol (Berl).*, **156**, 241–254.

Chan-Palay, V. and Palay, S. L. (1977). 'Ultrastructural identification of substance P and their processes in rat sensory ganglia and their terminal in the spinal cord by immunocytochemistry.' *Proc. Natl. Acad. Sci. USA*, **74**, 4050–4054.

Chan-Palay, V., Palay, S. L., and Wu, J. Y. (1979). 'Gamma-aminobutyric acid pathways in the cerebellum studied by retrograde and anterograde transport of glutamic acid decarboxylase antibody after *in vivo* injections.' *Anat. Embryol. (Berl).*, *157*, 1–14.

Consolazione, A., Milstein, C., Wright, B., and Cuello, A. C. (1981). 'The immunohistochemical detection of serotonin with monoclonal antibodies.' *J. Histochem. Cytochem.*, **29**, 1425–1430.

Coulter, H. D. and Terracio, L. (1977). 'Preparation of biological tissues for electron microscopy by freeze-drying.' *Anat. Rec.*, **187**, 477–493.

Cuello, A. C. and Milstein, C. (1981). 'Use of internally labelled monoclonal antibodies. In Bizollon, Ch. A. (ed.), *Physiological Peptides and New Trends in Radioimmunology*, pp. 293–305. Elsevier North Holland.

Cuello, A. C., Del Fiacco, M., Paxinos, G., Somogyi, P., and Priestley, J. V. (1981). 'Neuropeptides in striato-nigral pathways.' *J. Neural. Trans.*, **51**, 83–96.

Cuello, A. C., Galfre, G., and Milstein, C. (1979). 'Detection of substance P in the central nervous system by a monoclonal antibody.' *Proc. Natl. Acad. Sci. USA*, **76**, 3532–3536.

Cuello, A. C., Jessell, T., Kanazawa, I., and Iversen, L. L. (1977). 'Substance P: localisation in synaptic vesicles in rat central nervous system.' *J. Neurochem.*, **29**, 747–751.

Cuello, A. C., Milstein, C., and Priestley, J. V. (1980). 'Use of monoclonal antibodies in immunocytochemistry with special reference to the central nervous system.' *Brain Res. Bull.*, **5**, 575–587.

Cuello, A. C., Priestley, J. V., and Milstein, C. (1982). 'Immunocytochemistry with internally labelled monoclonal antibodies.' *Proc. Natl. Acad. Sci. USA*, **79**, 665–669.

De Petris, S. (1978). 'Immunoelectron microscopy and immunofluorescence in membrane biology.' In Korn, E. D. (ed.), *Methods in Membrane Biology*, vol. 9, pp. 1–201. Plenum Press, New York.

Dray, A. (1979). 'The striatum and substantia nigra: a commentary on their relationships.' *Neuroscience*, **4**, 1407–1439.

Dutton, A. H., Tokuyasu, K. T., and Singer, S. J. (1979). 'Iron–dextran antibody conjugate: general method for simultaneous staining of two components in high resolution immunoelectron microscopy.' *Proc. Natl. Acad. Sci. USA*, **76**, 3392–3396.

Falck, B. (1962). 'Observations on the possibilities of the cellular localisation of monoamines by a fluorescence method.' *Acta Physiol. Scand.*, **56**, Suppl. 197, pp. 1–25.

Geuze, J. J. and Slot, J. W. (1980). 'Double-labelling and quantitative immunoelectron microscopy on ultrathin frozen sections.' In *EMBO Practical Course Immunocytochemistry*, Abstracts, pp. 91, 92.

Goldsmith, P. C. and Ganong, W. F. (1975). 'Ultrastructural localisation of luteinizing hormone-releasing hormone in the median eminence of the rat.' *Brain Res.*, **97**, 181–193.

Gonatas, N. K., Stieber, A., Gonatas, J., Gambetti, P., Antoine, J. C., and Avrameas, S. (1974). 'Ultrastructural autoradiographic detection of intracellular immunoglobulins with iodinated Fab fragments of antibody. The combined use of ultrastructural autoradiography and peroxidase cytochemistry for the detection of two antigens (double labelling).' *J. Histochem. Cytochem.*, **22**, 999–1009.

Gonzalez Aguilar, F. and De Robertis, E. (1963). 'A formalin–perfusion fixation method for histophysiological study of the central nervous system with the electron microscope.' *Neurology*, **13**, 758–771.

Graham, R. C. and Karnovsky, M. J. (1966). 'The early stages of absorption of injected horseradish peroxidase in the proximal tubules of mouse kidney: ultrastructural cytochemistry by a new technique.' *J. Histochem. Cytochem.*, **14**, 291–302.

Halasz, N., Ljungdahl, A., Hökfelt, T., Johansson, O., Goldstein, M., Park, D., and Biberfield, P. (1977). 'Transmitter histochemistry of the rat olfractory bulb. I. Immunohistochemical localisation of monoamine synthesising enzymes. Support for intrabulbar peri-glomerular dopamine neurones.' *Brain Res.*, **126**, 455–474.

Hanker, J. S. (1979). 'Osmiophilic reagents in electronmicroscopic histochemistry.' *Prog. Histochem. Cytochem.*, **12** (1), 1–85.

Hanker, J. S., Yates, P. E., Metz, C. B., and Rustioni, A. (1977). 'A new specific sensitive and non-carcinogenic reagent for the demonstration of horseradish peroxidase.' *Histochem. J.*, **9**, 789–792.

Hartman, B. K. (1973). 'Immunofluorescence of dopamine-β-hydroxylase. Application of improved methodology to the localisation of peripheral and central noradrenergic nervous system.' *J. Histochem. Cytochem.*, **21**, 312–332.

Hayat, M. A. (1973). 'Specimen preparation.' In Hayat, M. A. (ed.), *Electron Microscopy of Enzymes: Principles and Methods*, vol. 1, pp. 10–35. Van Nostrand Reinhold Co., New York.

Hökfelt, T. and Ljungdahl, A. (1972). 'Modification of the Falck–Hillarp formaldehyde fluorescence method using the Vibratome: simple, rapid and sensitive localisation of catecholamines in sections of unfixed or formalin fixed brain tissue.' *Histochemie*, **29**, 324–339.

Hökfelt, T., Ljungdahl, A., Steinbusch, H., Verhofstad, A., Nilsson, G., Brodin, E., Pernow, B., and Goldstein, M. (1978). 'Immunohistochemical evidence of substance P-like immunoreactivity in some 5-hydroxytryptamine-containing neurons in the rat central nervous system.' *Neuroscience*, **3**, 517–538.

Hökfelt, T., Philipson, O., Kuypers, H. G. J. M., Bentivoglio, M., Catsman-Berrevoets, C. E., and Dann, O. (1979). 'Tracing of transmitter histochemically identified neuron projections: immunohistochemistry combined with fluorescent retrograde labelling.' *Neurosci. Lett.*, Suppl. 3, S.342.

Horisberger, M. and Rosset, J. (1977). 'Colloidal gold, a useful marker for transmission and scanning electron microscopy.' *J. Histochem. Cytochem.*, **25**, 295–305.

Hsu, S-M., Raine, L., and Fanger, H. (1981). 'Use of avidin–biotin–peroxidase complex (ABC) in immunoperoxidase techniques: a comparison between ABC and unlabelled antibody (PAP) procedures.' *J. Histochem. Cytochem.*, **29**, 577–580.

Hunt, S. P., Kelly, J. S., and Emson, P. C. (1980). 'The electron microscopic localisation of methionine-enkephalin within the superficial layers (I and II) of the spinal cord.' *Neuroscience*, **5**, 1871–1890.

Jacobowitz, D. M., Ziegler, M. G., and Thomas, J. A. (1975). '*In vivo* uptake of antibody to dopamine-β-hydroxylase into sympathetic elements.' *Brain Res.*, **91**, 165–170.

Johansson, O., Hökfelt, T., Jeffcoate, N., White, N., and Sternberger, L. A. (1980). 'Ultrastructural localisation of TRH-like immunoreactivity.' *Exp. Brain Res.*, **38**, 1–10.

Johnson, R. P., Sar, M., and Stumpf, W. E. (1980). 'A topographic localisation of enkephalin on the dopamine neurons of the rat substantia nigra and ventral tegmental area demonstrated by combined histofluorescence immunocyto-chemistry.' *Brain Res.*, **194**, 566–571.

Jones, E. G. and Hartman, B. K. (1978). 'Recent advances in neuroanatomical methodology.' *Ann. Rev. Neurosci.*, **1**, 215–296.

Kawari, Y. and Nakane, P. K. (1970). 'Localisation of tissue antigens on the ultrathin sections with peroxidase-labelled antibody method.' *J. Histochem. Cytochem.*, **18**, 161–166.

Köhler, G. and Milstein, C. (1975). 'Continuous cultures of fused cells secreting antibody of predefined specificity.' *Nature*, **256**, 495–497.

Kraehenbuhl, J. P. and Jamieson, J. D. (1973). 'Localisation of intracellular antigens using immunoelectron microscopy.' In Wisse, E. *et al.* (eds), *Electron-Microscopy and Cytochemistry*, pp. 181–192. North-Holland, Amsterdam.

Kraehenbuhl, J. P. and Jamieson, J. D. (1974). 'Localisation of intracellular antigens by immunoelectron microscopy.' *Int. Rev. Exp. Pathol.*, **13**, 1–53.

Kuhlmann, W. D. (1977). 'Ulastructural immunoperoxidase cytochemistry.' *Progress in Histochem. Cytochem.*, vol. **10** (1), pp. 1–57.

Larsson, L-I., Childers, S., and Snyder, S. H. (1979). 'Met- and Leu-enkephalin immunoreactivity in separate neurons.' *Nature*, **282**, 407–410.

La Vail, J. H. (1978). 'A review of the retrograde transport technique.' In Robertson, R. T. (ed.), *Neuroanatomical Research Techniques*, pp. 355–384. Academic Press, New York.

La Vail, J. H. and La Vail, M. M. (1974). The retrograde intra-axonal transport of horseradish peroxidase in the chick visual system: a light and electron microscopic study. *J. Comp. Neurol.*, **157**, 303–358.

Lidov, H. G. W., Grzanna, R., and Molliver, M. E. (1980). 'The serotonin innervation of the cerebral cortex in the rat: an immunohistochemical analysis.' *Neuroscience*, **5**, 207–227.

Lillie, R. D. and Pizzolato, P. (1972). 'Histochemical use of borohydrides as aldehyde blocking reagents.' *Stain Technol.*, **47**, 13–16.

Llewellyn-Smith, I. J., Wilson, A. J., Furness, J. B., Costa, M., and Rush, R. A. (1981). 'Ultrastructural identification of noradrenergic axons and their distribution within the enteric plexuses of the guinea-pig small intestine.' *J. Neurocytol.*, **10**, 331–352.

Marucci, A. A., DiStefano, H. S., and Dougherty, R. M. (1974). 'Preparation and use of soluble ferritin–antiferritin complexes as a specific marker for immunoelectron microscopy.' *J. Histochem. Cytochem.*, **22**, 35–39.

Mason, D. Y. and Sammons, R. (1978). 'Alkaline phosphatase and peroxidase for double immunoenzymatic labelling of cellular constituents.' *J. Clin. Pathol.*, **31**, 454–460.

Mason, T. E., Phifer, R. F., Spicer, S. S., Swallow, R. S., and Dreskin, R. D. (1969). 'New immunochemical techniques for localising intracellular tissue antigen.' *J. Histochem. Cytochem.*, **17**, 190–191.

Mazurkiewicz, J. E. and Nakane, P. K. (1972). 'Light and electron microscopic localisation of antigens in tissues embedded in polyethylene glycol with a peroxi-dase-labelled antibody method.' *J. Histochem. Cytochem.*, **20**, 969–974.

McKay, R., Raff, M. and Reichardt, L. (eds) (1981). *Cold Spring Harbor, Symposium on Monoclonal Antibodies against Neural Antigens.* Cold Spring Harbor, New York.

McLean, I. W. and Nakane, P. K. (1974). 'Periodate–lysine–paraformaldehyde fixative. A new fixative for immuno-electron microscopy.' *J. Histochem. Cyto-chem.*, **22**, 1077–1083.

Melamed, M. D. and Green, N. M. (1963). 'Avidin. 2. Purification and composition.' *Biochem. J.*, **89**, 591–599.

Moriarty, G. C. (1973). 'Adenohypophysis: ultrastructural cytochemistry. A review.' *J. Histochem. Cytochem.*, **21**, 855–894.

Moriarty, G. C. (1976). 'Immunocytochemistry of the pituitary glycoprotein hormones.' *J. Histochem. Cytochem.*, **24**, 846–863.

Moriarty, G. C. and Halmi, N. S. (1972). 'Electron microscopic study of the adrenocorticotropin-producing cell with the use of unlabelled antibody and the soluble peroxidase–antiperoxidase complex.' *J. Histochem. Cytochem.*, **20**, 590–603.

Nakane, P. K. (1968). 'Simultaneous localisation of multiple tissue antigens using the peroxidase-labelled antibody method: a study on pituitary glands of the rat.' *J. Histochem. Cytochem.*, **16**, 557–560.

Nakane, P. K. (1971). 'Application of peroxidase-labelled antibodies to the intracellular localisation of hormones.' *Acta Endocrinol.* (Suppl.). (KbH), **153**, 190–204.

Nakane, P. K. (1973). 'Ultrastructural localisation of tissue antigens with the peroxidase-labelled antibody method.' In Wisse, E. *et al.* (eds), *Electron Microscopy and Cytochemistry*, pp. 129–143. North-Holland, Amsterdam.

Nakane, P. K. and Kawaoi, A. (1974). 'Peroxidase-labelled antibody. A new method of conjugation.' *J. Histochem. Cytochem.*, **22**, 1084–1091.

Nakane, P. K. and Pierce, G. B. (1966). 'Enzyme-labelled antibodies: preparation and application for the localisation of antigens.' *J. Histochem. Cytochem.*, **14**, 929–931.

Notani, G. W., Parsons, J. A., and Erlandsen, S. L. (1979). 'Versatility of *Staphylococcus aureus* Protein A in immunocytochemistry.' *J. Histochem. Cytochem.*, **27**, 1438–1444.

Novikoff, A. B. (1980). 'DAB cytochemistry: artefact problems in its current uses.' *J. Histochem. Cytochem.*, **28**, 1036–1038.

Novikoff, A. B., Novikoff, P. M., Quintana, N., and Davis, C. (1972). 'Diffusion artefacts in 3,3'-diaminobenzidine cytochemistry.' *J. Histochem. Cytochem.*, **20**, 745–749.

Pasquier, D. A., Gold, M. A., and Jacobowitz, D. M. (1980). 'Noradrenergic perikarya (A5–A7, subcoeruleus) projections to the rat cerebellum.' *Brain Res.*, **196**, 270–275.

Pearse, A. G. E. (1968). *Histochemistry*, vol. 1. (3rd edn). Churchill-Livingstone, Edinburgh.

Pelletier, G., Leclerc, R., and Dube, D. (1976). 'Immunohistochemical localisation of hypothalamic hormones.' *J. Histochem. Cytochem.*, **24**, 864–871.

Pelletier, G. and Leclerc, R. (1979). 'Localisation of Leu-enkephalin in dense core vesicles of axon terminals.' *Neurosci. Lett.*, **12**, 159–163.

Pelletier, G., Puviani, R., Bosler, O., and Descarries, L. (1981). 'Immunocytochemical detection of peptides in osmicated and plastic-embedded tissue. An electron microscopic study.' *J. Histochem. Cytochem.*, **29**, 759–764.

Pickel, V. M. (1981). 'Immunocytochemical methods.' In Heimer, L. and Robards, M. J. (eds), *Neuroanatomical Tract Tracing Methods*, pp. 483–509. Plenum Press, New York.

Pickel, V. M., Joh, T. H., and Reis, D. J. (1975). 'Ultrastructural localisation of tyrosine hydroxylase in noradrenergic neurons of brain.' *Proc. Natl. Acad. Sci. USA*, **72**, 659–663.

Pickel, V. M., Joh, J. T., and Reis, D. J. (1976). 'Monoamine-synthesising enzymes in central dopaminergic, noradrenergic and serotonergic neurons. Immunocytochemical localisation by light and electron microscopy.' *J. Histochem. Cytochem.*, **24**, 792–806.

Pickel, V. M., Reis, D. J., and Leeman, S. E. (1977a). 'Ultrastructural localisation of substance P in neurons of rat spinal cord.' *Brain Res.*, **122**, 534–540.

Pickel, V. M., Joh, T. H., and Reis, D. J. (1977b). 'A serotonergic innervation of noradrenergic neurons in nucleus locus coeruleus: demonstration by immunocyto-chemical localisation of the transmitter specific enzymes tyrosine and tryptophan hydroxylase.' *Brain Res.*, **131**, 197–214.

Pickel, V. M., Joh, T. H., Reis, D. J., Leeman, S. E., and Miller, R. J. (1979). 'Electron microscopic localisation of substance P and enkephalin in axon terminals related to dendrites of catecholaminergic neurons.' *Brain Res.*, **160**, 387–400.

Pickel, V. M., Sumal, K. K., Beckley, S. C., Miller, R. J., and Reis, D. J. (1980). 'Immunocytochemical localisation of enkephalin in the neo-striatum of rat brain: a light and electron microscopic study.' *J. Comp. Neurol.*, **189**, 721–740.

Priestley, J. V. (1981). 'Ultrastructural localisation of substance P and enkephalin in the substantia gelatinosa of the spinal trigeminal nucleus.' *Br. J. Pharmacol.*, **74**, 893P.

Priestley, J. V., Somogyi, P., and Cuello, A. C. (1981). 'Neurotransmitter specific projection neurons revealed by combining PAP immunohistochemistry with retro-grade transport of HRP.' *Brain Res.*, **220**, 231–240.

Priestley, J. V., Somogyi, P., and Cuello, A. C. (1982). 'Immunocytochemical localisation of substance P in the spinal trigeminal nucleus of the rat: a light and electron microscopic study.' *J. Comp. Neurol.* **211**, 31–49.

Reid, N. (1975). 'Ultramicrotomy.' In Glauert, A. M. (ed.), *Practical Methods in Electron Microscopy*, vol. 3 (II), pp. 288–320. North-Holland, Amsterdam.

Ribak, C. E., Vaughn, J. E., and Barber, R. P. (1981). 'Immunocytochemical localisation of GABAergic neurons at the electron microscopic level.' *Histochem. J.*, **13**, 555–582.

Ribak, C. E., Vaughn, J. E., and Roberts, E. (1979). 'The GABA neurons and their axon terminals in rat corpus striatum as demonstrated by GAD immunocyto-chemistry.' *J. Comp. Neurol.*, **187**, 261–283.

Ribak, C. E., Vaughn, J. E., Saito, K., Barber, R., and Roberts, E. (1976). 'Immunocytochemical localisation of glutamate decarboxylase in rat substantia nigra.' *Brain Res.*, **116**, 287–298.

Ribak, C. E., Vaughn, J. E., Saito, K., Barber, R., and Roberts, E. (1977). 'Glutamate decarboxylase in neurons of the olfactory bulb.' *Brain Res.*, **126**, 1–18.

Robertson, R. T. (1978). *Neuroanatomical Research Techniques. Methods in Physio-logical Psychology*, vol. II. Academic Press, New York.

Rodning, C. B., Erlandsen, S. L., Coulter, H. D., and Wilson, I. D. (1978). 'Localisation of immunoglobulin antigens (IgA) on epoxy embedded tissue.' *J. Histochem. Cytochem.*, **26**, 223.

Roth, J., Bendayan, M., and Orci, L. (1980). FITC–protein A–gold complex for light and electron microscopic immunocytochemistry. *J. Histochem. Cytochem.*, **28**, 55–57.

Ruda, M. A. (1982). 'Opiates and pain pathways: Demonstration of enkephalin synapses on dorsal horn projection neurons.' *Science*, **215**, 1523–1525.

Sar, M. and Stumpf, W. E. (1979). 'Simultaneous localisation of steroid and peptide hormones in rat pituitary by combined thaw-mount autoradiography and immuno-histochemistry: localisation of dihydrotestosterone in gonadotopes, thyrotropes and pituicytes.' *Cell Tissue Res.*, **203**, 1–7.

Shahrabadi, M. S. and Yamamoto, T. (1971). 'A method for staining intracellular antigens in thin sections with ferritin-labelled antibody.' *J. Cell Biol.*, **50**, 246–250.

Silverman, A. J. (1976). 'Ultrastructural studies on the localisation of neurohypo-physial hormones and their carrier proteins.' *J. Histochem. Cytochem.*, **24**, 816–827.

Silverman, A. J. and Zimmerman, E. A. (1975). 'Ultrastructural immunocyto-chemical localisation of neurophysin and vasopressin in the medium eminence and posterior pituitary of the guinea-pig.' *Cell Tissue Res.*, **159**, 291–301.

Singer, S. J. (1959). 'Preparation of an electron-dense antibody conjugate.' *Nature*, **183**, 1523–1524.

Singer, S. J., Painter, R. G., and Tokuyasu, K. T. (1973). 'Ferritin–antibody staining of ultrathin frozen sections. In Wisse, W. *et al.* (eds), *Electron Microscopy and Cytochemistry*, pp. 171–180. North-Holland, Amsterdam.

Sladek, J. R. and McNeill, T. H. (1980). 'Simultaneous monoamine histofluorescence and neuropeptide immunocytochemistry. IV. Verification of catecholamine–neuro-physin interactions through single-section analysis.' *Cell Tissue Res.*, **210**, 181–189.

Slot, J. W. (1980). 'Light and electronmicroscopical immunolocalisation of amylase on pancreas tissue using cryokit sections (with special reference to the colloidal gold/protein-A method.' In: *EMBO Practical Course Immunocytochemistry*, Abstracts, pp. 237–242.

Smith, R. E. (1970). 'Comparative evaluation of two instruments and procedures to cut non-frozen sections.' *J. Histochem. Cytochem.*, **18**, 590–591.

Sofroniew, M. V. and Schrell, U. (1981). 'Evidence for a direct projection from oxytocin and vasopressin neurons in the hypothalamic paraventricular nucleus to the medulla oblongata: immunohistochemical visualisation of both the horseradish peroxidase transported and the peptide produced by the same neurons.' *Neurosci. Lett.*, **22**, 211–217.

Sofroniew, M. V., Weindl, A., Schinko, I., and Wetzstein, R. (1979). 'The distribu-tion of vasopressin-, oxytocin-, and neurophysin-producing neurons in the guinea-pig brain. I. The classical hypothalamo–neurohypophyseal system.' *Cell Tissue Res.*, **196**, 367–384.

Somogyi, P. (1978). 'The study of Golgi stained cells and of experimental degenera-tion under the electron microscope: a direct method for the identification in the visual cortex of three successive links in a neural chain.' *Neuroscience*, **3**, 167–180.

Somogyi, P., Hodgson, A. J., and Smith, A. D. (1979). 'An approach to tracing neuron networks in the cerebral cortex and basal ganglia. Combination of Golgi staining, retrograde transport of horseradish peroxidase and anterograde degenera-tion of synaptic boutons in the same material.' *Neuroscience*,**4**, 1805–1852.

Somogyi, P., Priestley, J. V., Cuello, A. C., Smith, A. D., and Bolam, J. P. (1982). 'Synaptic connections of substance P immunoreactive nerve terminals in the substantia nigra of the rat: a correlated light and electron microscopic study.' *Cell Tissue Res.*, **223**, 469–486.

Steinbusch, H. W. N., Verhofstad, A. A. J., and Joosten, H. W. J. (1978). 'Localisation of serotonin in the central nervous system by immunohistochemistry: description of a specific and sensitive technique and some applications.' *Neuro-science*, **3**, 811–819.

Stell, W. K. (1965). 'Correlation of retinal cytoarchitecture and ultrastructure in Golgi preparations.' *Anat. Rec.*, **153**, 389–398.

Sternberger, L. A. (1967). 'Electron microscopic immunocytochemistry: a review.' *J. Histochem. Cytochem.*, **15**, 139–159.

Sternberger, L. A. (1979). *Immunocytochemistry* (2nd edn). John Wiley, New York.

Sternberger, L. A. and Cuculis, J. J. (1969). 'Method for enzymatic intensification of the immunocytochemical reaction without use of labelled antibodies.' *J. Histochem. Cytochem.*, **17**, 190.

Sternberger, L. A., Donati, E. J., Cuculis, J. J., and Petrali, J. P. (1965). 'Indirect immuno-uranium technique for staining of embedded antigen in electron microscopy.' *Exp. Mol. Pathol.*, **4**, 112–125.

Sternberger, L. A., Hardy, P. H., Cuculis, J. J., and Meyer, H. G. (1970). 'The unlabelled antibody-enzyme method of immunohistochemistry. Preparation and properties of soluble antigen–antibody complex (horseradish peroxidase–antihorseradish peroxidase) and its use in identification of spirochetes.' *J. Histochem. Cytochem.*, **18**, 315–333.

Straus, W. (1971). 'Inhibition of peroxidase by methanol–nitroferricyanide for use in immunoperoxidase procedures.' *J. Histochem. Cytochem.*, **19**, 682–688.

Striker, G. E., Donati, E. J., Petrali, J. P., and Sternberger, L. A. (1966). 'Post-embedding staining for electron microscopy with ferritin-antibody conjugates.' *Exp. Mol. Pathol.*, Suppl. 3, pp. 52–58.

Swaab, D. F., Pool, C. W., and Van Leeuwen, F. W. (1977). 'Can specificity ever be proved in immunocytochemical staining?' *J. Histochem. Cytochem.*, **25**, 388–391.

Tokuyasu, K. T. (1978). 'A study of positive staining of ultrathin sections.' *J. Ultrastruct. Res.*, **63**, 287–307.

Tokuyasu, K. T. and Singer, S. J. (1976). 'Improved procedures for immunoferritin labelling of ultrathin frozen sections.' *J. Cell Biol.*, **71**, 894–906.

Tougard, C., Tixier-Vidal, A., and Avrameas, S. (1979). 'Comparison between peroxidase conjugated antigen or antibody and peroxidase–anti-peroxidase complex in a post-embedding procedure.' *J. Histochem. Cytochem.*, **27**, 1630–1633.

Vacca, L. L., Abrahams, S. J., and Naftchi, N. E. (1980). 'A modified peroxidase–antiperoxidase procedure for improved localisation of tissue antigens: localisation of substance P in rat spinal cord.' *J. Histochem. Cytochem.*, **28**, 287–307.

Vandesande, F. (1979). 'A critical review of immunocytochemical methods for light microscopy.' *J. Neurosci. Methods*, **1**, 3–23.

Van Leeuwen, F. W. (1977). 'Immunoelectron microscopic visualisation of neurohypophyseal hormones: evaluation of some tissue preparations and staining procedures.' *J. Histochem. Cytochem.*, **25**, 1213–1221.

Van Leeuwen, F. (1980a). 'Immunocytochemical specificity for peptides with special reference to arginine–vasopressin and oxytocin.' *J. Histochem. Cytochem.*, **28**, 479–482.

Van Leeuwen, F. W. (1980b). 'An introduction to the immunocytochemical localisation of neuropeptides and neurotransmitters.' *Acta Histochemica*, Suppl. Bd. XXIV, pp. 1–52.

Van Leeuwen, F. W. and Swaab, D. F. (1977). 'Specific immunoelectron-microscopic localisation of vasopressin and oxytocin in the neurohypophysis of the rat.' *Cell Tiss. Res.*, **177**, 493–501.

Van Leeuwen, F. W., Swaab, D. F., and Romijn, H. J. (1976). 'Light and electron microscopic immunolocalisation of oxytocin and vasopressin in rats.' In Feldmann, G. *et al.* (eds), *First International Symposium on Immunoenzymatic Techniques* (INSERM Symposium No. 2), pp. 345–353. North-Holland, Amsterdam.

Vaughn, J. E., Barber, R. P., Ribak, C. E., and Houser, C. R. (1981). 'Methods for the immunocytochemical localisation of proteins and peptides involved in neurotransmission.' In Johnson, J. E. (ed.), *Current Trends in Morphological Techniques*, vol. III. CRC Press, Florida. (In press.)

Verhofstad, A. A. J., Steinbusch, H. W. M., Penke, B., Varga, J., and Joosten, H. W. J. (1980). 'Use of antibodies to norepinephrine and epinephrine in immunohistochemistry.' In Eränkö, O. *et al.* (eds), *Histochemistry and Cell Biology* of Autonomic Neurons, SIF Cells and Paraneurons. *Advances in Biochemical Psychopharmacology*, vol. 25, pp. 185–193. Raven Press.

Weber, E., Voigt, K. H., and Martin, R. (1978). 'Concomitant storage of ACTH- and endorphin-like immunoreactivity in the secretory granules of anterior pituitary corticotrophs.' *Brain Res.*, **157**, 385–390.

Weir, D. M. (ed.) (1978). *Handbook of Experimental Immunology*, vol. 1, pp. 7.1–10.6. Blackwell Scientific Publications, Oxford.

Weir, E. E., Pretlow, Th. G., Pitts, A., and Williams, E. E. (1974). 'A more sensitive and specific histochemical peroxidase stain for the localisation of cellular antigen by the enzyme-antibody conjugate method.' *J. Histochem. Cytochem.*, **22**, 1135–1140.

Wendelschafer-Crabb, G., Erlandsen, S. L., and Walker, D. H. (1976). 'Ultrastructural localisation of viral antigens using the unlabelled antibody-enzyme method.' *J. Histochem. Cytochem.*, **24**, 517–526.

Williams, M. A. (1977). 'Autoradiography and immunocytochemistry.' In Glauert, A. M. (ed.), *Practical Methods in Electron Microscopy*, vol. 6.1. North-Holland, Amsterdam.

Wood, J. G., McLaughlin, B. J., and Vaughn, J. E. (1976). 'Immunocytochemical localisation of GAD in electron microscopic preparations of rodent CNS. In Roberts, E. *et al.* (eds), *GABA in Nervous System Function*, pp. 133–148. Raven Press, New York.

Zamboni, L. and deMartino, C. (1967). 'Buffered picric-acid formaldehyde: a new rapid fixation for electron microscopy.' *J. Cell Biol.*, **35**, 148A.

Ziegler, M. G., Thomas, J. A., and Jacobowitz, D. M. (1976). 'Retrograde axonal transport of antibody to dopamine-β-hydroxylase.' *Brain Res.*, **104**, 390–395.

Immunohistochemistry
Edited by A. C. Cuello
© 1983 IBRO

CHAPTER 12

The use of Protein A–Colloidal Gold (PAG) Complexes as Immunolabels in Ultra-thin Frozen Sections

JAN W. SLOT and HANS J. GEUZE

Centre for Electron Microscopy, Medical School, State University of Utrecht, Utrecht, The Netherlands

I INTRODUCTION

The various immunocytochemical techniques currently in use for the localization of intracellulair antigens by electron microscope can be classified according to the following three main aspects.

(a) *The accessibility of the antigens.* In *pre-embedding techniques*, the cellular membranes are made penetrable by chemical or mechanical treatment (see Chapters 1 and 11). In *post-embedding* techniques the immunoreaction is done on the surface of ultra-thin sections from tissue already embedded in materials like Epon, methacrylate, or glutaraldehyde cross-linked albumin. By *ultracryotomy* ultra-thin frozen sections are prepared from non-embedded tissue. After immunolabelling, such sections are embedded in order to protect the structures against shrinkage during drying.

(b) *The marker used to visualize the immunoreaction* (see Chapters 3, 9, and 11).

(c) *The binding of the marker to the antibody* (see also Chapters 3 and 11, Section II). In *direct techniques* the marker is conjugated to the primary antibody. The immunoreaction is a one-step procedure. In *indirect techniques* the marker is attached to the primary antibody via secondary carrier molecules. The carrier is often an antibody directed against the primary one, but it can also be staphylococcal protein A, or the biotin-avidin combination. Except for colloidal gold particles, which adsorb the carrier molecules to their surface by complicated physicochemical interaction (Geoghegan and Ackerman, 1977), in direct and indirect techniques the markers are covalently bound to the carriers. This is avoided in the *unlabelled antibody techniques* (see chapter 4).

In our laboratory we explored (Geuze *et al.*, 1981b; Slot and Geuze, 1981) the combination of ultracryotomy according to Tokuyasu (1978, 1980a,b) and indirect immunostaining with colloidal gold particles (Faulk and Taylor, 1971) and protein A as the marker–carrier (Romano and Romano, 1977). Here we give a detailed methodical description of this technique and demonstrate its applicability to different tissues. Special attention is paid to nervous tissue, since no work on this tissue with this technical approach has been reported so far. Finally, we summarize the reasons why we think that this technique is advantageous, especially when it comes to high-resolution immunocytochemistry.

II TECHNICAL REQUIREMENTS

II.1 Tissue Fixation

Fixation must be adjusted to the particular tissue and antigens studied. In the case of nervous tissue, working with several antigens, we achieve good results with perfusion fixation via the heart with mixtures of 2% paraformaldehyde and varying concentrations of (0.1–1%) glutaraldehyde in 0.1 M phosphate buffer, pH 7.4 (PB). These fixatives are also used for rat pancreas and liver. In the pancreas the fixative is injected into the interstitium and the liver is fixed by perfusion via portal vein. In each case, the *in situ* application of the fixative is followed by immersion fixation with the same fixative for 1 h. The tissue can be stored in the buffer for a couple of days. For longer periods Tokuyasu (1978) prescribes the addition of low concentrations (~0.3%) of paraformaldehyde. We store up to 1 month in 1 M sucrose + 2% paraformaldehyde in PB in the refrigerator.

II.2 Cryosectioning

Ultra-thin frozen sections are prepared by the technique developed by Tokuyasu (1976), and discussed by him recently (1980b). Small blocks of fixed tissue are immersed in 2.3 M sucrose for 30 min at room temperature. The blocks should be trimmed so that the cutting surface comprises a square of ~ 0.25 mm^2 or less. The base of the block has to be flat enough to ensure a stable fitting to the specimen holder of the microtome. Trimming facilities in the available ultracryotomes are poor. Therefore it is important to adjust the blocks as much as possible before freezing. A tissue block is placed in the proper position on the specimen holder to which it sticks by adhering sucrose. Then it is frozen rapidly by plunging in liquid nitrogen, and transferred to the cold chamber of the ultracryotome, set at -90 to -100 °C. We use the Porter Blum MT2B or LKB3 ultramicrotomes with cryo-attachment. Sections between 50 and 100 nm are cut with a dry glass knife. Section thickness can be judged by interference colours, as for plastic sections. This became easier after we replaced the microtome lamp by a fibre-optic light source, which produces a concentrated, bright bundle of cold light. Irregularities in thickness are common. First of all there are temperature instabilities of the microtome, especially during the first period of cooling. Variation in thickness within a ribbon of sections is probably not due to temperature instability. In such cases one has to ascertain that the knife is clean and sharp, that the knife angle is close to 45° (Tokuyasu, 1980b), and that the shape of the specimen is correct. Small rectangular sections give the best results. Some variation in thickness is advantageous and should not be avoided. Strong cell structures can be studied in very thin sections (~ 50 nm), but fragile structures are sensitive to surface tensions (see below) in too thin sections and can better be observed in thicker sections (~ 100 nm).

The sections are picked up from the knife by touching them with a small drop of 2.3 M sucrose in PB in a wire loop (loop diameter ~ 2 mm). A good way is to remove ribbons of about five sections from the knife edge and to 'park' them in a convenient position somewhere on the knife, so that they can be picked up later on without the risk of damage to the knife edge, or spilling sucrose on to it. During cutting, the sections sometimes tend to curl backwards to the knife edge. To avoid this the operator will be assisted by the use of an eyelash mounted on the tip of a 15 cm stick. This tool can also be used to collect sections from the knife edge. The sections have to be picked up very quickly since the sucrose solution in the loop freezes within a few seconds upon entering the cryochambre. Outside the cryochambre the sections stretch on the surface of the thawing sucrose drop. Stretching takes no more than 10 s and can be promoted by warm breath.

During cutting the section is often compressed and wrinkled parallel to the knife edge. Apparently this process is reversible, since the stretched

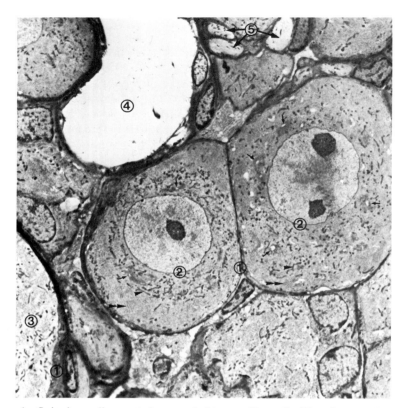

Figure 1   Spinal ganglion, rat. Surrounded by satellite cells (1), a few small ganglion cells (2) are shown and a large one (3) which is recognizable by its 'light' cytoplasm. The capillary lumen (4) is distended and empty as result of the perfusion fixation. Some nerve processes (5) are also visible. Even at this low magnification, Nissl substance (double arrowheads), mitochondria (arrowheads) and Golgi complexes (arrows) can be recognized. Damage, especially to the latter structures (see also Figure 5), in the cell to the right demonstrates its vulnerability to forces like surface tension and drying. The fact that the cell in the middle (close to the blood vessel) is much less damaged, supports our impression that proper and rapid fixation is very important for optimal preservation of the structure (×1260)

parts of the sections on the grids look flat and show no signs of compression (Figure 1). To minimize compression it is important to use clean and sharp knives and properly shaped tissue blocks. Compression can also be counteracted by lowering the temperature. When the temperature is too low sections become crumbly. Tokuyasu (1980b) suggests also that the sucrose concentration, in which the tissue is immersed, can be varied for finding the conditions for optimal flat sections. We have, however, experienced best results with the very high sucrose concentrations.

The sucrose drops with sections are put on carbon-coated formvar grids, with the sections downwards, so that these are pressed against the grids and covered by a layer of sucrose. The grids are then placed on a wet gel with the sections downwards, so that the sucrose can diffuse away. We use ~ 3 mm thick layers of 2% gelatin in PB, poured into small (3 m diameter) Petri dishes, which are kept in a larger pair of dishes, with moistened filter paper. The dishes are placed on ice so that the gelatin solidifies. When cutting is finished the dishes with the grids are placed at room temperature. The grids are left on the plates for ~ 15 min after liquefaction of the gel so that they are coated with gelatin. This prevents non-specific adherence of immuno-reagents.

II.3   Protein A–Gold (PAG) Complex

Spherical gold particles can easily be prepared in colloidal state by reducing chloroauric acid ($HAuCl_4$) in aqueous solution. The size of the particles depends partly on the reducing agent used, and partly on the intrinsic heterogeneity of each particular sol. To prepare PAG with a particular size, one first makes the appropriate crude sol by choice of a reducing agent. This crude preparation is then complexed with protein A (PA). Next, homogeneous fractions can be purified from the crude preparation by gradient centrifugation (see below). Recently we described this method (Slot and Geuze, 1981) for sols prepared by white phosphorus (Au_{phos}) (Faulk and Taylor, 1971) and sodium ascorbate (Au_{asc}) (Stathis and Fabrikanos, 1958). The average diameters of the particles in these crude sols were 5–6 and 11–12 nm respectively, and by gradient centrifugation homogeneous fractions could be prepared in the size ranges of 4.5–6.5 nm and of 8–13 nm respectively. In addition, by reducing $HAuCl_4$ with sodium citrate (Au_{citr}) (Frens, 1973), particles larger than 15 nm (up to 150 nm) can be prepared. The amount of citrate added determines the size of the particles. We used the finest gold sol after Frens, in which the average particle size was 15.5 nm. This sol was much more homogeneous than Au_{phos} and Au_{asc}, so that further sizing by gradient centrifugation was not necessary. Larger Au_{citr} particles have only limited value for high-resolution cytochemistry. To complete the list of gold sols used in immunocytochemistry, a new sol has to be mentioned, prepared by ethyl alcohol reduction (Au_{ea}) (Baigent and Müller, 1980). Although we have no experience with Au_{ea}, we included the preparation procedure in the list below. It works well as an immuno-marker when complexed with protein A (Müller and Baigent, 1980). The size range (6–10 nm) seems appropriate for bridging the small gap between Au_{phos} and Au_{asc}, but the particles appear rather variable. This shortcoming can presumably be obviated by gradient centrifugation.

III PROTOCOLS TO PREPARE GOLD SOLS

—*Au$_{phos}$*. Mix 1.5 ml of a 1% HAuCl$_4$ (Drijfhout & Zn's, Amsterdam or BDH, Poole, England) solution and 1.4 ml of 0.1 M K$_2$CO$_3$ in 120 ml distilled water. Add 1 ml of a solution of white phosphorus (Merck, Darmstadt) in diethylether and mix well. The phosphorus solution is made up by adding 4 parts of ether to 1 part of ether saturated with white phosphorus. Leave the solution for 15 min at room temperature. Boil under reflux until the colour turns from brownish to red ($\sim$ 5 min).

—*Au$_{asc}$*. Mix 1 ml of 1% HAuCl$_4$ and 1 ml of 0.1 M K$_2$CO$_3$ in $\sim$ 25 ml distilled water. While stirring, add quickly 1 ml of a 0.7% solution of sodium ascorbate (BDH, Poole, England). This reaction is done on ice. Higher temperature tends to increase the particle size. After adding the ascorbate the colour becomes immediately purple–red. Adjust the volume to 100 ml with distilled water and heat the solution until boiling so that the colour becomes red.

—*Au$_{citr}$*. Add 1 ml of 1% HAuCl$_4$ to 100 ml distilled water, followed by 2 ml 1% tri-sodium citrate · 2H$_2$O (Merck, Darmstadt). Boil the mixture under reflux for 15–30 min, on, until the colour becomes red. Cool and add 0.5 ml 0.1 M K$_2$CO$_3$.

—*Au$_{ea}$*. Add 0.6 ml of 1% HAuCl$_4$ to 50 ml distilled water. Neutralize the solution with 0.2 M K$_2$CO$_3$. Cool to 4 °C and add 1 ml ethyl alcohol. Subject this solution to ultrasonics by immersion of a flat-ended probe at 20 kHz and 125 W. Within 5 min a grey–blue colour appears which turns to deep burgundy–red after a while (Müller and Baigent, 1980).

All gold sols are to be made up in clean glass vials and can be stored for weeks. Optimal conditions for a protein to be adsorbed to gold particles (see below) are found at a pH range around and just above its isoelectric point (Geoghegan and Ackerman, 1977). The isoelectric point of PA is 5.1. Therefore, the amount of K$_2$CO$_3$ used in the recipes above is calculated so that the pH is a little below 6 (check by pH paper since the unstabilized colloid is harmful to the electrode of a pH meter).

IV PROTEIN GOLD COMPLEXES

IV.1 Complexing of Protein to Gold Particles

Gold sols are negatively charged hydrophobic sols. Such sols are unstable and precipitate upon the addition of electrolytes. When mixed with hydrophylic substances, such as proteins, these are adsorbed to the surface of the gold particles, resulting in a hydrophylic protein–gold sol which is stable when electrolytes are added. The stabilization occurs very rapidly after addition of a certain amount of protein. This amount can be determined easily (Horisberger and Rosset, 1977). Add to a series of 2 ml glass tubes increasing amounts of protein (for protein A in the range of 0–3 µg per tube). Then add 250 µl of the gold sol per tube mix, wait 5 min, and add 250 µl of a 10% NaCl solution. As long as the red colour turns to blue, not enough protein is added to stabilize the sol. We usually find 8, 6, and 5 µg PA necessary to stabilize 1 ml of Au_{phos}, Au_{asc}, and Au_{citr}, respectively. The minimal amount of PA required to stabilize a gold sol, is enough to saturate the surface of the particles completely. Excess PA is not adsorbed and remains in the supernatant when the particles are pelleted.

To prepare PAG, take 30 ml gold sol and add an amount of PA which exceeds the saturation point by 10%. Wait 5 min and add polyethylene glycol (PEG) (20,000 daltons) to a final concentration of 0.05% to be sure that the gold particles are stabilized maximally (Horisberger and Rosset, 1977). Then the complexes are pelleted by centrifugation: Au_{phos}, 45 min at $125,000\,g_{av}$; Au_{asc}, 45 min at $50,000\,g_{av}$, and Au_{citr}, 45 min at $15,000\,g_{av}$. This yields a pellet with a major loose part and a small, tightly packed part, which is not used. The supernatant is carefully removed. The loose part of the pellet is resuspended in PBS (0.15 M NaCl, 2.5 mM KCl, 0.01 M phosphate, pH 7.2) and centrifuged as described above. Again the supernatant is removed without disturbing the pellet. The loose part of this second pellet, which is called *crude preparation*, is resuspended in the remainder of the supernatant (the small part that cannot be removed without taking some of the pellet) and stored in siliconized caps.

IV.2 Sizing of PAG by Gradient Centrifugation

To make uniform subfractions, crude preparations of PAG from Au_{phos} and Au_{asc} are prepared as described above, except that the second centrifugation can be omitted. The loose part of the first pellet is resuspended in the remainder of its supernatant (~ 0.5 ml) and layered over a 10–30% continuous sucrose or glycerol gradient in PBS. The gradients are centrifuged in a SW41 rotor (Beckman) for 45 min at 41,000 r.p.m. in the case of Au_{phos} and for 30 min at 20,000 r.p.m. in the case of Au_{asc}. After centrifugation a column of ~ 7 cm, from ~ 1 cm under the top, down to the bottom of the gradient, is stained red by the PAG complex. We usually collect five successive fractions of ~ 1 ml from the upper half of the red zone, dialyse these against PBS in 50% glycerol and store at $-18\,°C$. The fractions thus achieved differ gradually in average particle size, and they are much more homogeneous than the crude preparation (Slot and Geuze, 1981).

V IMMUNOLABELLING

Grids with sections are picked up from the liquefied 2% gelatine and washed for a few minutes on drops of PBS containing 0.02 M glycine to quench reactive glutaraldehyde remnants in the tissue. This and all subsequent steps of the procedure are done at room temperature.

Next, the grids are placed for 20–30 min on 5–10 µl drops containing the antibody. A concentration of 10 µg/ml of specific antibody is sufficient. The antibody preparations here illustrated are: rabbit anti-rat pancreas amylase; and affinity-purified IgG fraction; a purified IgG fraction from a rabbit antiserum against a major pancreatic membrane glycoprotein, GP 2 (Geuze *et al.*, 1981b); rabbit anti-tubulin, an affinity-purified IgG fraction (from Dr S. J. Singer, San Diego); rabbit anti-clathrin, an affinity-purified IgG fraction (from Dr D. Louvard, Heidelberg); a rabbit antiserum with reactivity against neurofilaments (from Dr F. W. van Leeuwen, Amsterdam); rabbit anti-rat serum albumin, an affinity:purified IgG preparation. The technique requires the application of complete immunoglobulins. Active fragments, such as Fab or F(ab')$_2$ (bivalent antigen binding fragments) can not be used, since PA binds to the Fc (constant fragments) part of the molecules. PA binds to most mammalian IgG's, but not to those of goat and sheep. If such a non-PA reactive antibody has to be used, an intermediate PA reactive antibody, directed against the first, can be applied. After the incubation, excess antibody is washed away by passing the grids over several drops of PBS.

Subsequently the grids are placed, for 20–30 min, on 5–10 µl drops with the PAG complex. PAG is used in a concentration equivalent to a 5–10 times dilution of the original crude complex before centrifugation. This means for PA a concentration of 0.5–1 µg/ml. Before use some protein such as 1% BSA or diluted serum can be added to prevent non-specific adherence. We use goat serum from which IgG is removed by precipitation with 50% ammonium sulphate. After the incubation with PAG the grids are washed thoroughly. They are passed over four successive drops of PBS on each of which they are left for at least 5 min.

VI DOUBLE-LABELLING

Multiple antigens can be localized in a tissue section by a simple extension of the immunolabelling procedure (Geuze *et al.*, 1981b). After the last washing, the protocol above is repeated for another antibody. The PAG complex by which this second antibody is labelled should be distinguishable from the one used to visualize the first antibody reaction by the size of the gold particles. It is advisable to incubate the section during ~5 min with a free PA solution (0·1 mg/ml) immediately following the staining with the first gold marker. This is to be sure that all IgG molecules of the first antibody are occupied by PA, so that the second marker can only bind to the second antibody, which is brought on the sections subsequently.—

VII PROCESSING OF THE SECTIONS FOR EM OBSERVATION

When frozen sections are dried without any further treatment, except a few seconds wash on distilled water to remove the saline, the delineation of cell structures is poor (Figure 2). Tokuyasu developed several methods for

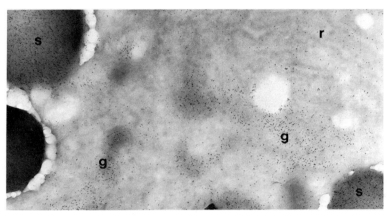

Figure 2 Exocrine pancreas, rat. Immunolabelling with anti-amylase, marked with 4.5 nm PAG. The section is not stained with uranyl and not embedded in MC–PEG. Therefore delineation of structures, RER (r) and Golgi complex (g), is very poor. The absence of embedding material also caused damage during drying, for example around the secretory granules (s) (×28 000)

negative or positive staining of frozen sections and for their embedding in supporting material to prevent drying artefacts. His procedures for positive staining with uranyl (Tokuyasu, 1978) or uranyl adsorption staining (Tokuyasu, 1980a) with embedding in a mixture of methyl cellulose (MC) and polyethylene glycol (PEG) (Tokuyasu, 1980a) will be dealt with briefly.

For positive staining, the grids are washed in water and placed on a drop of a neutral uranyl solution. This is prepared by mixing equal volumes of 4% uranyl acetate and 0.3 M potassium oxalate. Adjust the pH to 7–8 with KOH. After 10 min and two quick passages over water, the grids are put on drops of an aqueous solution of 0.1–2% uranyl acetate for 5–10 min. Rinse for a few seconds and place them on a mixture of 0.4% MC (400 centipoise) and 1.6% PEG (MW 1540) in water for a few minutes. The grids are then picked up in a wire loop with an inner diameter just exceeding that of the grids. Excess solution is then sucked off by filter paper from the edge of the loop so that a film of uniform and minimal thickness is left on the grid.

Another, so-called adsorption staining method, proposed by Tokuyasu, differs from the procedure above in omitting the aqueous uranyl staining. Instead, a very low concentration of uranyl acetate (0.01–0.02%) is added to the MC–PEG embedding mixture. The idea is that most of the uranyl is adsorbed to the tissue, so that excess need not to be washed away.

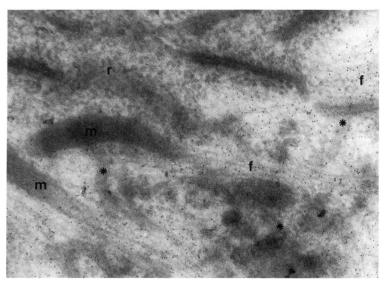

Figure 3 Spinal ganglion, rat. Immunolabelling with an antiserum reacting with neurofilaments, marked with 4.5 nm PAG. Perikaryon with free ribosomes and RER (r), smooth ER (asterisks), and bundles of neurofilaments (f); m = mitochondria (×39,900)

All figures, except 2 and 14, show sections stained by the adsorption method. Positive staining prior to embedment can give a very good contrast (Figure 14), but this is less reproducible, possibly because the uranyl is easily extracted from the sections.[1]

VIII   IMMUNOFLUORESCENCE STAINING

An important feature of the EM immuno-technique we described above is that the observations can be extended very easily towards light microscope level by immunofluorescence staining of cryosections. The technique has to be modified in the following respects.

1 Recently we modified the uranyl-methylcellulose treatment upon a suggestion from Dr G. W. Griffiths (Griffiths *et al.*, 1982) as follows: (a) 5 min staining in 2% neutral uranyl solution. (b) wash over three drops of distilled water. (c) 5 min staining in 2–4% uranyl-acetate. (d) transfer grids, without washing, from the uranyl over three drops of 1.5% methylcellulose (Tylose MH 300, Fluka). After 30 seconds pick the grids up in 3 mm wireloop, remove excess methylcellulose solution. This modification improved the contrast and was very advantageous for further reduction of drying artefacts.

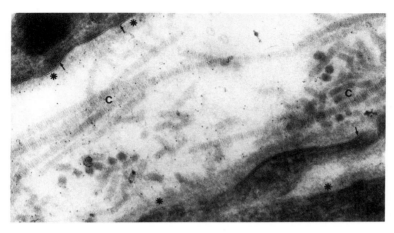

Figure 4   Same section as in Figure 3. Interstitium with collagen fibrils (c) and basal lamina (asterisks). The bilaminar structure of the plasma membranes of satellite cells (arrows) is clearly visible. Immunolabelling of the interstitium is due to an impurity which often occurs in rabbit antisera and which can be removed by adsorption to rat erythrocytes (×39,900)

We usually cut thicker sections (~250 nm) for immunofluorescence, at higher cutting temperature (−60 to −70 °C). This allows larger section surface (up to 1 mm²).

The sections, picked up with sucrose, are placed on microscope slides, coated with 1% gelatin in 0.1% KCr (SO₄). Carefully degreased slides may also be used. The sucrose is allowed to diffuse away in drops of phosphate buffered (0.1 M; pH 7.4) 2% gelatin.

In the immunolabelling procedure PAG is replaced by a carrier, bearing a fluorescing probe. We use a secondary antibody tagged with fluorescein or rhodamin.

Finally the section is embedded in 60% glycerol and covered by glass. The edges of the coverglasses can be fixed by some kit (i.e. nail polish). The specimens can be stored for weeks in the refrigerator.

IX   GENERAL PROPERTIES OF CRYOSECTIONS AND PAG IMMUNOLABELLING

IX.1   Frozen Sections

In some respects ultracryotomy does not work as smoothly as conventional plastic ultramicrotomy. In the first place, section thickness is difficult to control and the sections are not always spread out over the grid perfectly. We have earlier mentioned some hints to avoid this (see also Tokuyasu, 1980b),

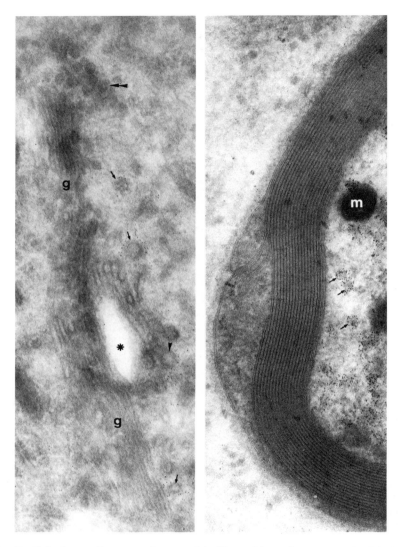

Figure 5 Spinal ganglion, rat. Immunolabelling with anti-coat protein (clathrin), marked with 4.5 nm PAG. Clathrin is demonstrated on the cytoplasmic face of vesicles in the environment of (arrows) or attached to (arrowhead) the trans-side Golgi cisternae. No significant labelling occurs in the remaining part of the cisternae (g) or in the vesicles at the margins of the Golgi stacks (double arrowhead). Damage in the stack of cisternae is indicated with an asterisk (×36,400)

Figure 6 Spinal ganglion, rat. Immunolabelling with anti-tubulin, marked with 4.5 nm PAG. Part of a myelinated nerve process. Label is mainly located at the outer faces of the cross-sectioned neurotubules (arrows); m = mitochondria (×39,200)

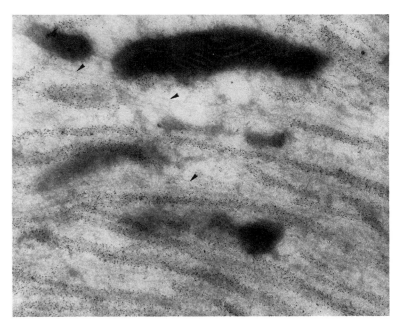

Figure 7   Same section as Figure 6. Longitudinal section of an unmyelinated nerve process. Between the labelled neurotubules, some non-labelled filaments are visible (arrowheads) (×25,200)

but with the equipment and knowledge now available, frozen sections remain inferior to plastic ones in this respects. Nevertheless, with some patience, grids with sections in the right range of thickness and with stretched parts can always be collected. An experienced operator can cut 10–20 reasonable ribbons from one or two tissue blocks within about 2 h.

Secondly, the sections are subjected to damaging forces at a few stages of the procedure. (a) Freezing may cause ice-crystal damage. This is largely prevented by infusion of the specimen block with 2.3 M sucrose. This simple measure means that more complicated freezing methods such as in slush-nitrogen or nitrogen-cooled freon need not to be considered. (b) Tearing of cell structures by surface tension on the sucrose drop. Some protein (e.g. 0.75% gelatin, Tokuyasu, 1980b) may be added to the sucrose to lower the surface tension; on the other hand this also counteracts stretching of the sections. We had some success by embedding fragile tissues, after fixation, in 10% gelatin. The gelatin was then fixed with 0.2% glutaraldehyde prior to sucrose infusion and freezing. The gelatin gives, in the sections, some support against surface tension (Geuze *et al.*, 1979). (c) Damage by surface tension at the moment of drying (Figure 2). This problem has been obviated largely by

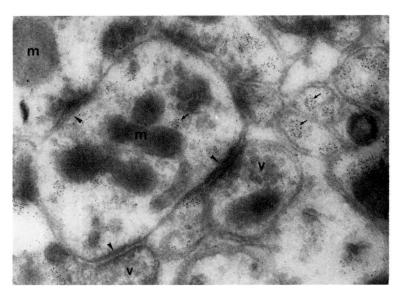

Figure 8 Cerebellum, synaptic structures in the molecular layer of the cortex, rat. Immunolabelling with anti-tubulin, marked with 4.5 nm PAG. Dense labelling occurs over cross-profiles of neurotubules (arrows). Labelling of the cytoplasmic matrix seems more significant here than in other parts parts of the nerve processes, indicating the presence of higher concentrations of free tubulin. Arrows = synapses; v = pre-synaptic vesicles; M = mitochondria (×32,900)

the embedment of the sections in a hydrophylic MC–CW matrix prior to drying, (see footnote on page 332). Yet some damage usually remains in certain vulnerable structures like the Golgi complex (Figure 5), the rims of secretory granules (Figure 2), and myelin sheaths. Sometimes it seems as if clefts occur in or between membranes (Figure 5). Possibly low concentrations of proteins at these sites result in discontinuities of the three-dimensional meshwork of glutaraldehyde cross-linked protein, which are vulnerable to tearing in thin sections. Also, local differences in fixation are likely to attribute to heterogeneity in the tissue (e.g. differences between the neurons in Figure 1). These observations demonstrate the importance of a proper fixation.

IX.2   The Quality of Ultrastructure in Frozen Sections

The ultrastructure in frozen sections is generally consistent with that in plastic ones. At low magnification substructures appear less sharply deline-ated than in plastic sections. Nevertheless, most tissue components are recognizable in survey pictures, as is shown for the spinal root ganglion in Figure 1. At high magnification the marked contours of cellular membranes

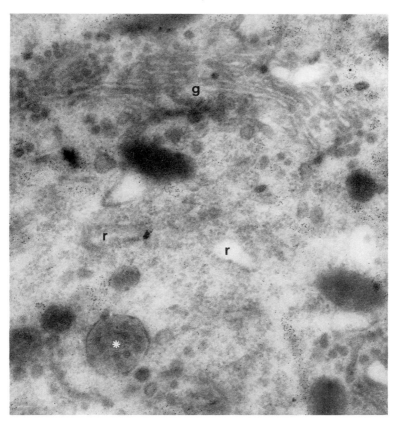

Figure 9   Same section as in Figure 8. Detail of perikaryon of a Purkinje cell. As in Figure 8 most of the label is concentrated over neurotubules but some occurs in the cytoplasmic matrix. Golgi cisternae (g), RER (r), and multi-vesicular body (asterisk), are not labelled (×30,100)

come through, as is shown for smooth and rough endoplasmic reticulum (Figure 3), the Golgi complex (Figures 5 and 9), multi-vesicular bodies (Figure 9), and cell membrane (Figure 4). Also cell membrane specializations like junctions, synapse (Figure 8) and myelin sheaths (Figure 6) can easily be discerned. The same holds for non-membranous structures, such as nuclei and ribosomes (Figure 3), filamentous structures in muscle cells (Tokuyasu, 1980b; Griffiths and Jockusch, 1980) and neurons (Figures 3 and 7), and collagen fibrils (Figure 4). On the other hand, coated vesicles (Figure 6) and neurotubules (Figure 6–9) are difficult to identify.

In conclusion, the Tokuyasu technique for the preparation of ultra-thin frozen sections appears very suitable for immunocytochemistry. The sections

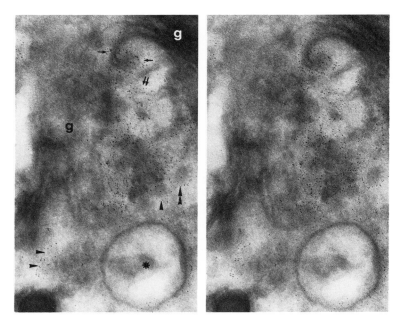

Figure 10 Spinal ganglion, rat. Immunolabelling with anti-coat protein (clathrin), marked with 4.5 nm PAG. The stereo image provided by this pair of micrographs shows that the label is penetrated all through the section, probably because the antigen was accessible via the loose cytoplasmic matrix. Most of the label occurs in the central part of the Golgi complex, between two stacks of cisternae (g), the lower of which is sectioned obliquely. Clathrin is detectable on a part of the inner Golgi cisternae with an attached vesicle (arrows), on a vesicle attached to GERL-like membranes (double arrow), on one side of an mvb-like structure (asterisk) and on free vesicles (arrowheads) some of which are labelled on one side (double arrowhead). Tilting angle was
± 6° (×34,300)

can be prepared without too much difficulty, and offer a structural quality that can largely meet the 'plastic' standard.

IX.3   Immunolabelling with PAG

PAG complexes are reactive immunoreagents. This has been shown with the post-embedding technique (Bendayan *et al.*, 1980) as well as with ultra-thin frozen sections (Geuze *et al.*, 1981a,b; Slot and Geuze, 1981). In pre-embedding techniques PAG is only used for labelling of surface antigens (Romano and Romano, 1977; Müller and Baigent, 1980).

Here we demonstrate the suitability of ultra-thin frozen sections with the immunolabelling of three structural components of nerve cells: neurofilaments (Figure 3), coated membranes (Figures 5 and 10), and neurotubules

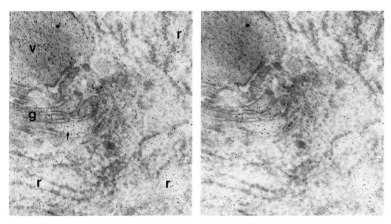

Figure 11   Exocrine pancreas, rat. Immunolabelling with anti-amylase, marked with 4.5 nm PAG. This stereo-view of various cell structures shows that the label penetrates completely into the RER cisternae (r) and partly into the cis-Golgi cisternae (arrow). (Sometimes we observed complete penetration into these cisternae.) In the trans-side cisternae (g) and condensing vacuoles (v) label is restricted to the section surface. Tilting angle was ± 6° (×28,000)

(Figures 6–9). Theoretically, the resolution of the PAG technique is determined by (1) the distance between the antigen binding site and the C-terminal end of the IgG molecule (~ 10 nm); (2) the size of the PA molecule (to be approximated to maximally 55 nm); and (3) the diameter of the gold particle used. The distance between gold particles and antigenic sites can thus be estimated at ~ 15 nm, which is about three times the diameter of the small gold marker. This cannot directly be demonstrated in the sections since the antigenic sites themselves remain obscure. However, the alignment of gold particles along neurotubules, neurofilaments, and coated membranes, and the distance between the particles and the pancreas membranes (Figure 15), indicate that this calculation is fairly realistic.

Non-specific adherence of antibody and PAG to the sections can be judged in sections stained with non-reactive IgG prior to the PAG complex, and in cell structures in specifically stained sections that are not supposed to be labelled. Usually the non-specific labelling is very low with the exception of nuclei and mitochondria which sometimes show some background.

The sensitivity of immunocytochemical techniques is predominantly determined by the accessibility of the antigenic sites to the immunoreagents. Accessibility of immunoreactive sites is influenced by both the location of the antigen and the penetrability of the tissue. If, for example, antigens are enclosed in vacuoles, the vacuole membrane hinders passage of immunoreagents to the interior of the vacuole (Figure 13). In the case where thick

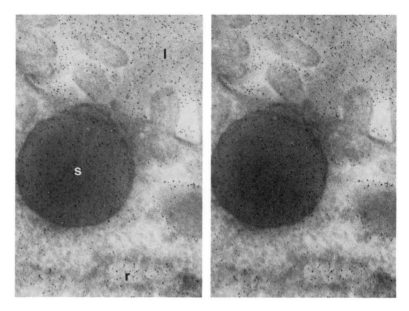

Figure 12   As Figure 11. Detail of the cell apex. This stereo pair shows that the label in the secretory granule (s) is mainly located at the upper surface of the section, as is the case for the label over the secretory material in the lumen (l). RER (r) contents is labelled all through the section. Some label occurs in the cytoplasmic matrix. This may be due to grazing sections through RER but also to amylase leaked from the secretory compartments, which happens very easily when fixation is not perfect (×48,300)

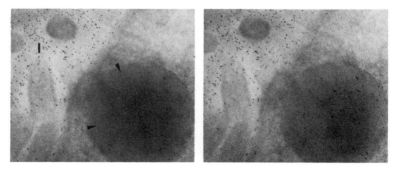

Figure 13   As Figure 12. In this case the immunoreagents apparently could penetrate into the secreted material in the lumen (l). The secretory granule is cut in such a way that only a small profile is present at the upper face of the section where the antibody is applied, whereas a large profile faces the formvar film on the grid. The stereo-view demonstrates that only the small profile is labelled. The sloping edge of the granule inside the section is not labelled (arrowheads). This indicates that the granule membrane is an impermeable barrier for the immunoreagents (×48,300)

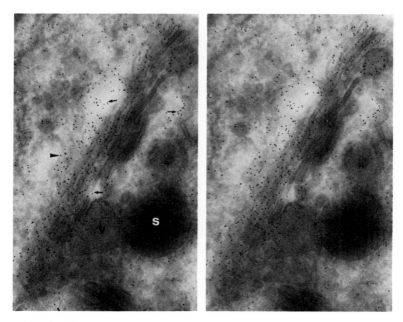

Figure 14 As Figure 11, but marked with 8 nm PAG. This stereo pair of a Golgi complex shows that the marker occurs only on the section surface, except for some artificial pits where the label seems to penetrate deeper (arrows). At some sites the under-surface of the section is also labelled (arrowheads). The upper surface of the section does not contain a profile of the secretory granule (s), so that it remained unlabelled. The condensing vacuole (v), close to it, is only partly exposed to the upper surface, which explains its partial labelling (×28,700)

sections or even tissue slices are immunolabelled, incomplete penetration may seriously interfere with the resulting labelling pattern. This difficulty is largely overcome by working with ultra-thin sections in which most of the membrane-bound intracellular structures are cut so that their contents and the inner face of their membranes are exposed.

As compared to plastic sections, frozen sections allow the immunoreagents to penetrate deeper. Penetration depth depends on the molecular density of the substructure under study, as well as on the effective size of the immunorea-gents. For instance, the loosely packed cytoplasmic matrix can be permeated easier than the compact contents of secretory granules. Likewise, small PAG particles penetrate deeper into frozen sections than larger ones. We used stereo-pictures to observe the depth of immunostaining. It appeared that the 4–5 nm PAG particles labelled the clathrin coating at the cytoplasmic side of membranes all through the section thickness (Figure 10). On the other hand, penetration varied in the secretory compartments of pancreatic cells. Staining

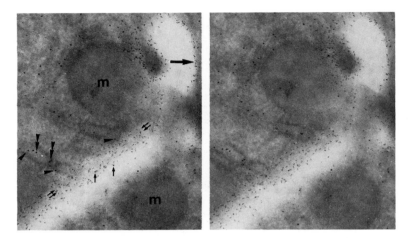

Figure 15   Stereo micrographs of the border between two exocrine pancreatic cells. Double-labelling. Immunolabelling sequence: (1) antiserum against the major glyco-protein (GP-2) in pancreatic membranes; (2) 4.5 nm PAG; (3) anti-amylase; (4) 8 nm PAG. GP-2 is labelled along the entire slope of the obliquely cut plasma membrane (between pairs of arrows). In cross-section the close approximation of the marker and the membrane can be observed (large arrow). The larger marker for amylase labels the RER on the upper (double arrowheads) and under (arrowheads) surface of the section. Only a few 8 nm particles (small arrows) contaminate the reaction with the 4.5 nm particles. Tilting angle ± 6° (×28,700)

for amylase occurred throughout the section thickness in the case of wide RER-cisternae near the Golgi complex (Figures 11 and 12), but reaction depth was variable in the cis-Golgi cisternae (Figure 11) and the secreted material in the lumen (Figures 12 and 13). The labelling in trans-Golgi cisternae (Figure 11), condensing vacuoles (Figure 11), and secretory granules (Figures 12 and 13) was always restricted to the surface of the sections.

These observations prove that the target antigens within the sections become rapidly inaccessible with increasing density of the surrounding material. If we used 8 nm PAG, penetration was considerably less (Figures 14 and 15). This is in line with the tendency of lower yield of label when larger gold particles were used (Slot and Geuze, 1981). So, the combination of ultra-thin frozen sections and the 5 nm PAG marker offers optimal conditions for a sensitive immunoreaction. At some places the sections were labelled at both sides (Figures 14 and 15). Apparently in these cases the immunoreagents could penetrate between the section and the formvar film.

The differential accessibility of antigens can easily lead to misinterpretation of the labelling patterns. For instance in a two-dimensional image, the density of anti-amylase labelling is about the same in the RER and secretory granules

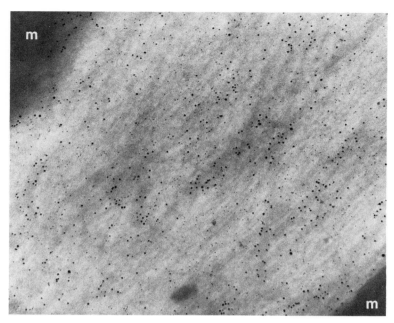

Figure 16 Spinal ganglion, rat. Detail of a nerve process. Double-labelling. Immuno-labelling sequence: (1) antiserum reactive with neurofilaments; (2) 4.5 nm PAG; (3) anti-tubulin, (4) 10 nm PAG. Close observation shows that the 4.5 nm particles are associated with the neurofilaments whereas the 10 nm particles accompany the course of the neurotubules. m = mitochondrion (×40,600)

(Figures 11 and 12). This gives the misleading impression of equal concentrations of amylase in these compartments.

Particular markers, such as ferritin and colloidal gold, make quantitation of immunoreactions possible (Kraehenbuhl *et al.*, 1980; Bendayan *et al.*, 1980). However, varying depths of the immunoreaction into ultrathin frozen sections make direct conclusions on the concentration of the antigens in the various cell compartments impossible. To get around this problem, one can exclude penetration completely by using a post-embedding technique with plastic sections (Bendayan *et al.*,1 1980). However, an important part of the immunoreaction is then lost. At the moment, quantitative work with particulate labels on frozen sections is only possible when penetration depth can be ignored, as in the case of measurements within one homogeneous compartment, or when the distribution of two antigens relative to each other is studied in the same compartments.

Double-labelling with gold particles of different sizes has for the first time been described for lectin–gold complexes (Horisberger, 1979; Roth and Binder, 1979). Recently we reported a simple procedure for double-labelling

Immunohistochemistry

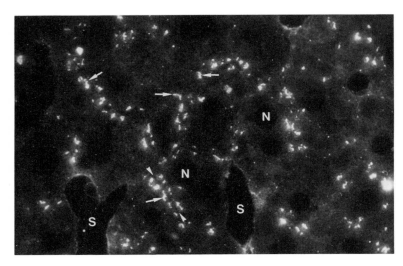

Figure 17 Immunofluorescence in a 250 nm section of rat liver, immunolabelled with rabbit-anti-albumin, stained with rhodamin–goat–anti-rabbit IgG. A weak reaction occurs in the cytoplasm, which can be attributed to the endoplasmic reticulum (Geuze *et al.*, 1981a). The Golgi complexes (arrows), located along the bile canaliculi (arrowheads) fluoresce very brightly. Nuclei (N) are negative, as are the sinusoids (S) from which the serum albumin was removed during perfusion (×700)

with two sizes of PAG complexes (Geuze *et al.*, 1981b). The method is based on the monovalency of IgG molecules for PA so that contamination of the first immunoreaction with the second gold probe is low. Sites where only the first labelled antigen occurs, offer the best opportunity to check this; e.g. the exterior of the plasma membrane for the pancreatic membrane protein in Figure 15. Since distinct size classes of PAG can be obtained by gradient centrifugation, double-labelling with two particles of less than 10 nm is now possible (Figures 15 and 16) (Slot and Geuze, 1981).

The availability of an extensive assortment of gold probes makes the PAG technique very flexible. For instance, it is convenient to mark an antigen in separate grids with different sizes of PAG particles, so that the reaction can be observed at different levels of magnification. In addition, the technique is extended very easily towards light microscope level (Figure 17). Prior to, or after, cutting cryosections for EM, with some minor modifications, sections from the same tissue block can be prepared for immunofluorescence studies (Geuze and Slot, 1980). It is even possible to stain a grid simultaneously for fluorescence and EM observation of an immunoreaction (Tokuyasy *et al.*, 1978). Immunofluorescence on thin cryosections is a powerful technique. Its resolution is optimal for light microscopy allowing accurate observations on intracellular distribution of antigens. On the other hand it gives a good impression of the overall distribution in a tissue, as in the liver (Figure 17), where albumin was found evenly distributed in all hepatocytes (Geuze *et al.*, 1981a).

X CONCLUDING REMARKS

The combination of ultra-thin frozen sections prepared according to Tokuyasu and PAG probes is, in our judgement, one of the most powerful immunocytochemical techniques presently available. The technique is especially suitable for high-resolution electron microscope studies on intracellular antigens, and can in the same run be extended to fluorescence microscopy with some simple adaptations. At the ultrastructural level, accurate determination of labelled sites is possible thanks to the particular image of the label and its small size. PAG probes made of Au_{phos} are to our knowledge the smallest known immunolabels and allow a resolution of less than 20 nm.

PAG probes of various sizes can easily be obtained by gradient centrifugation. This opens the field of multiple labelling in one section with particles of less than 10 nm. In addition PAG labelling allows quantification of the immunoreaction. However, comparison of data from different structures is hampered by the phenomenon of different penetration depths of the immunoreaction in loose and compact structures. Finally, the technique is highly sensitive because of a maximal accessibility of the antigens in the ultra-thin sections of non-embedded specimens.

REFERENCES

Baigent, C. L. and Müller, G. (1980). 'A colloidal gold prepared with ultrasonics.' *Experienta*, **36**, 472–473.

Bendayan, M., Roth, J., Perrelet, A., and Orci, L. (1980). 'Quantitative immunocytochemical localization of pancreatic secretory proteins in subcellular compartments of the rat acinar cell.' *J. Histochem. Cytochem.*, **28**, 149–160.

Faulk, W. P. and Taylor, G. M. (1971). 'An immunocolloid for the electron microscope.' *Immunochemistry*, **8**, 1081–1083.

Frens, G. (1973). 'Controlled nucleation for the regulation of the particle size in monodisperse gold suspensions.' *Nature Phys. Sci.*, **241**, 20–22.

Geoghegan, W. D. and Ackerman, G. A. (1977). 'Adsorption of horseradish peroxidase ovomucoid and anti-immunoglobulin to colloidal gold for the indirect detection of concanavalin A, wheat germ agglutinin and goat anti-human immunoglobulin G on cell surfaces at the electron microscope level: a new theory and application.' *J. Histochem. Cytochem.*, **25**, 1187–1200.

Geuze, H. J. and Slot, J. W. (1980). 'Disproportional immuno-staining patterns of two secretory proteins in guinea pig and rat exocrine pancreatic cells. An immunoferritin and fluorescence study.' *Eur. J. Cell Biol.*, **21**, 93–100.

Geuze, H. J., Slot, J. W., and Brands, R. (1981a). 'The occurrence of albumin in the rat liver. A light and electron microscope immunocytochemical study.' *Cell Biol. Int. Reports.* **5**, p. 463.

Geuze, H. J., Slot, J. W., van der Ley, P. A., and Scheffer, R. C. T. (1981b). 'The use of colloidal gold particles in double-labelling immunoelectronmicroscopy of ultrathin frozen tissue sections. Observations on a major glycoprotein in zymogen granules of the rat pancreas.' *J. Cell Biol.* **89**, 653–655.

Geuze, H. J., Slot, J. W., and Tokuyasu, K. T. (1979). 'Immunocytochemical localization of amylase and chymotrypsinogen in the exocrine pancreatic cell with special attention to the Golgi complex.' *J. Cell Biol.*, **82**, 697–707.

Griffiths, G. W. and Jockush, B. M. (1980). 'Antibody labelling of thin sections of skeletal muscle with specific antibodies: a comparison of bovine serum albumin (BSA) embedding and ultracryotomy.' *J. Histochem. Cytochem.*, **28**, 969–978.

Griffiths, G., Brands, R., Burke, B., Louvard, D and Warren, G. (1982). 'Viral membrane proteins acquire galactose in Trans Golgi cisternae during intracellular transport.' *J. Cell Biol:* **95**, 781–792.

Horisberger, M. (1979). 'Evaluation of colloidal gold as a cytochemical marker for transmission and scanning electronmicroscopy.' *Biol. Cellulaire*, **36**, 253–258.

Horisberger, M. and Rosset, J. (1977). 'Colloidal gold, a useful marker for transmission and scanning electronmicroscopy.' *J. Histochem. Cytochem.*, **25**, 295–305.

Kraehenbuhl, J. P., Racine, L., and Griffiths, G. W. (1980). 'Attempts to quantitate immunocytochemistry at the electron microscope level.' *Histochem. J.*, **12**, 317–332.

Müller, G. and Baigent, C. L. (1980). 'Antigen controlled immunodiagnosis—"ACID test".' *J. Immunol. Methods*, **37**, 185–190.

Romano, E. L. and Romano, M. (1977). 'Staphylococcal protein A bound to colloidal gold: a useful reagent to label antigen-antibody sites in electron microscopy.' *Immunochemistry*, **14**, 711–715.

Roth, J. and Binder, M. (1978). 'Colloidal gold, ferritin and peroxidase as markers for electron microscopic double labelling lectin technique.' *J. Histochem. Cytochem.*, **26**, 163–169.

Slot, J. W. and Geuze, H. J. (1981). 'Sizing of protein A–colloidal gold probes for immunocytochemistry.' *J. Cell Biol.* **90**, 533–536.

Stathis, E. C. and Fabrikanos, A. (1958). 'Preparation of colloidal gold.' *Chem. Ind.*, **27**, 860–861.

Tokuyasu, K. T. (1978). 'A study of positive staining of ultrathin frozen sections.' *J. Ultrastruct. Res.*, **63**, 287–307.

Tokuyasu, K. T. (1980a). 'Adsorption staining method for ultrathin frozen sections.' *38th Ann. Proc. Electro. Microsc. Soc. Amer.*, San Francisco, Calif., pp. 760–763.

Tokuyasu, K. T. (1980b). 'Immunochemistry on ultrathin frozen sections.' *Histochem. J.*, **12**, 381–403.

Tokuyasu, K. T., Slot, J. W., and Singer, S. J. (1978). 'Simultaneous observations of immunolabeled frozen sections in LM and EM.' *9th Int. Congr. Elect. Microsc. Toronto*, **2**, 164–165.

Immunohistochemistry
Edited by A. C. Cuello
© 1983 IBRO

CHAPTER 13

The Preparation of Immunoglobulin Gold Conjugates (IGS Reagents) and their use as Markers for Light and Electron Microscopic Immunocytochemistry

JAN R. DE MEY

Laboratory of Oncology, Janssen Pharmaceutica, Research Laboratories, B-2340 Beerse, Belgium

I INTRODUCTION

Since the introduction of the fluorescent antibody technique (Coons *et al.*, 1955) the use of antibodies as specific probes for detection of antigens has greatly expanded. Soon afterwards, with the introduction of ferritin and enzyme immunocytochemistry, localization studies at the ultrastructural level became possible (for review, see Sternberger, 1979; Singer and Schick, 1961; Nakane and Pierce, 1966). Of these, the peroxidase–antiperoxidase (PAP) technique (see Chapter 4) has been particularly widely used in neuro-immunocytochemistry (Sternberger *et al.*, 1970). Enzyme immunohisto-chemistry yields stable preparations that can be observed in a normal microscope. Fluorescence microscopy, however, is also very attractive. The method is extremely simple and emitted light is easily percepted by the human eye. A recent improvement, eliminating the problem of bleaching, will certainly reinitiate interest in using the immunofluorescence technique (Johnson *et al.*, 1981). The use of enzymes as tracer molecules above all allows the combination of light and electron microscopy of the same sample under study. The pre-embedding approach, involving the peroxidase staining of thick unembedded histological sections, followed by plastic embedding and thin sectioning of selected areas (Pickel *et al.*, 1975) is a good example that has been used with success for localizing specific antigens in the nervous system. The pre-embedding approach can also be used for immunoelectron microscopy of whole tissue culture cells (De Brabander *et al.*, 1977).

The immunoenzyme cytochemical methods have also been proven very helpful for post-embedding localization work, especially the labelling of thin sections of plastic-embedded tissue (Hardy *et al.*, 1970). The major problem of enzyme immunocytochemistry in general is, however, that the reaction product is not always clearly localized and/or distinguishable. In cells or tissues, labelled with the pre-embedding approach, the peroxidase reaction tends to damage the fine structure. On thin sections the reaction product masks the fine structural detail of the labelled areas. This is often a serious problem, because the purpose of the labelling is indeed in many cases to determine the ultrastructural characteristics of the labelled structures (e.g. form and size of secretory granules).

To overcome this drawback the serial thin/thin (Dacheux *et al.*, 1976) or semi-thin/thin section methods (Baetens *et al.*, 1977) can be used. These procedures, however, are tedious and time-consuming.

Many of the inherent disadvantages of enzyme immunoelectron micro-scopy could in principle be overcome by using a particulate label. For many years ferritin (Singer and Schick, 1961) has been the only one available. The production of well-defined ferritin–antibody conjugates is, however, compli-cated and the yield is rather low. In addition, ferritin has a relatively low electron-density. The recently introduced ferritin-bridge technique (Willingham, 1980) is relatively unknown in the field of neurobiology and deserves more attention. For example, by fluoresceinating the ferritin molecules, one could probably use this method in the pre-embedding approach for tissues. The principle of this technique offers the same advantages of specificity and sensitivity as the PAP technique and increases both resolving power and tissue preservation, relative to the PAP procedure (De Brabander *et al.*, 1981). A minor drawback is that it requires four incubations, and the ferritin label is not always localized within the shortest possible distance of the antigen. Iron–dextran particles have recently been introduced, mainly for surface antigen labelling, but most interestingly, also for labelling of ultra-thin frozen sections. One of these, Imposil (Dutton *et al.*, 1979), has proved to be useful in combination with ferritin.

All of the above tracing systems can be used, in combination with antibodies. In recent years, however, other detection principles, such as protein A (Biberfeld *et al.*, 1974), or the biotin–avidin system (Heitzmann and Richard, 1974; Guesdon *et al.*, 1979; Hsu *et al.*, 1981) have been introduced. They offer additional possibilities for double or multiple labelling experiments. This holds true especially when a third marker system is considered: the colloidal gold system. Colloidal gold can be prepared in various sizes as monodisperse particles. It is a negatively charged hydrophobic sol. Under appropriate conditions it will bind macromolecules by non-covalent electrostatic adsorption. This adsorption often results in little or no change in the bioactivity of the bound macromolecule.

Initially, colloidal gold has been used as tracer for TEM (transmission electron microscopy) (Feldherr and Marshall, 1962). The high electron opacity of gold particles makes them indeed a very distinct marker, even in their smallest available size (about 3 nm). The first application, 10 years ago, of colloidal gold in immunocytochemistry involved adsorption of whole serum (Faulk and Taylor, 1971). Soon afterwards, purified antibodies proved to be superior (Romano *et al.*, 1974; Horisberger and Vonlanthen, 1977), but problems were reported in making sufficiently stable conjugates (Romano *et al.*, 1974). The introduction of protein A–gold conjugates (Romano and Romano, 1977) and their use for labelling thin sections (Roth *et al.*, 1978) has strongly increased the interest in the colloidal gold system. The demonstration that protein A–gold can be used for double labelling studies on ultra-thin frozen sections (Geuze *et al.*, 1981) indicates that this approach has great potential for localizing antigens in nervous tissue. Antibody–gold conjugates, can also be used for labelling of thin sections (Horisberger and Vonlanthen, 1977; Probert *et al.*, 1981). Recently, the basic methodology for adsorbing proteins to colloidal gold has been established (Geoghegan and Ackerman, 1977; Geoghegan *et al.*, 1980; Horisberger, 1979; Horisberger and Vonlanthen, 1979), resulting in improved success of labelling antibodies with gold. Recently, however, it has been reported that considerable amounts of antibodies (and in general of other proteins) will be released from gold particles with time and under the influence of competing proteins (Goodman *et al.*, 1981). This may be one of the reasons why, until now, antibody–gold complexes have not been widely used. Other possible reasons will be discussed below.

Interestingly, it was shown that colloidal gold can be used as a marker for light microscopy (Geoghegan *et al.*, 1978). This observation has recently been extended by results involving labelling of surface differentiation antigens on leucocytes (De Waele *et al.*, 1981; De Mey *et al.*, 1982), microtubules in cultured cells (De Mey *et al.*, 1981) and tissue antigens in histological sections (Gu *et al.*, 1981). Colloidal gold can be used subsequent to peroxidase immunocytochemistry for double labelling experiments (De Mey *et al.*, 1980a; Gu *et al.*, 1981). It produces an intense red colour when large numbers of gold particles accumulate over antigen-containing structures.

These results are based on the production of highly effective and stable antibody–gold conjugates with minimal amounts of antibodies free in solution (De Mey *et al.*, 1981; Moeremans and De Mey, in preparation). Such conjugates, made with very small-sized gold can be used for the intracellular labelling of antigens in tissue cultures, with preservation of an acceptable fine structure, adding another field of application for the colloidal gold system (De Mey *et al.*, 1981).

In this chapter we give a detailed description of the production of antibody–colloidal gold complexes. Emphasis is given to specific problems inherent to the use of antibodies for coupling. At the same time the simplicity of the procedure will become very clear. In view of the wide range of applications of colloidal gold-labelled antibodies in both light and electron microscopy, we have called the technique, using such conjugates, the immunogold staining method or IGS method. The immune reagents are called IGS reagents.

One of the most important new developments in recent years has been the introduction of the hybridoma technology for the production of monoclonal antibodies (Köhler and Milstein, 1975). More and more monoclonal antibodies are becoming available. Those made against neuropeptides and neurotransmitter molecules are of particular interest for neurobiologists (Cuello *et al.*, 1979; Consolazione *et al.*, 1981). The fact that they can be metabolically labelled with isotopes has given rise to a new technique: radioimmunocytochemistry (Cuello *et al.*, 1980). The fact that isolated monoclonal antibodies are homogeneous with respect to their isoelectric point makes them a material of choice for conjugating to colloidal gold. This has recently been demonstrated (De Mey *et al.*, 1982). Here we include the modification needed for successfully conjugating monoclonals to various sizes of colloidal gold.

II ANTIBODY GOLD CONJUGATES

II.1 General Remarks

Colloidal gold can be made in various useful sizes: 3–5 nm is about the smallest particle size that is still easily visible in the electron microscope at the usual magnifications and that will still efficiently bind antibodies; 20 nm is the size that will produce enough colour to be seen in a bright-field light microscope. For a limited number of applications larger particles (e.g. 40 nm) may give optimal results. The overview of the procedure for making conjugates is: (1) prepare a purified antibody; (2) make gold particles of the right size; (3) conjugate them with the purified antibody; and (4) wash the conjugate to obtain a clear, stable reagent. It is obvious that the final reagent will be no better than the antibody. Since preservation of ultrastructure is a major concern in high-resolution immunocytochemistry (Novikoff, 1980), it is of particular interest to know whether the antibody to be conjugated will react with antigen after glutaraldehyde or mixed aldehyde fixations. It is also highly recommended to use affinity-purified antibodies for conjugation to colloidal gold. For serum antibodies (e.g. secondary antibodies), this can be achieved by antigen affinity chromatography. For monoclonal antibodies or serum immunoglobulin, protein-A affinity chromatography is often used. Otherwise, a 50% ammonium sulphate fraction followed by DEAE ion exchange chromatography can be used.

II.2 Affinity-purification of Serum Antibodies

Antigen affinity chromatography is relatively simple to perform. Because of its importance for producing highly specific and effective IGS reagents, a general one-step procedure from serum is described here. It yields monospecific antibodies with 95% immunoglobulin content as judged by analytical SDS–PAGE.

The antigen is coupled to Sepharose-4B-CNBr (Pharmacia) according to the instructions of the manufacturer. Other carriers may be used. Usually, 5–10 mg of the antigen is coupled per gram dry gel to give a total gel volume of 3.5 ml. This amount of gel is added to ± 15 ml antiserum and incubated for 2–3 h at room temperature with gentle shaking or rolling. The serum/gel mixture is poured into a column and washed with 10 mM Tris buffered saline (TBS) at pH 7.6 until the OD of the effluent is equal to zero.

Then the gel is washed with TBS + 1 M NaCl to elute a small peak of non-specifically absorbed material. The salt is removed from the gel by washing with TBS. To elute the specifically bound antibody the column is washed with 0.1 M glycine–HCl buffer, pH 2.8, until the base-line is almost reached. The trailing peak is collected entirely since the antibodies that are released more slowly are those with the highest affinity. The acid eluant is neutralized with ± 10% of 1 M Tris/HCl buffer pH 8.5. This is done during the elution step. Aliquots are stored at −20 or −70 °C without further treatment. The gel is removed from the column, washed with 10^{-2} M HCl (pH 2) on a scintered glass filter and re-equilibrated with TBS + 2.10^{-2} M NaN_3 for storage at 4 °C.

II.3   Making the Gold Particles

II.3.1   *General points*

Three major methods are found in the literature for the making of monodisperse colloidal gold sols. The methods are all based on the controlled reduction of an aqueous solution of chloroauric acid using as reducing agents either phosphorus-saturated ether (Weiser, 1933) and sodium ascorbate (Stathis and Fabrikanos, 1958; Horisberger, 1979) for small particles (5 and 12 nm), or sodium citrate (Frens, 1973) for larger particles (17–150 nm). The latter technique is the one providing gold particles appropriate for light microscopic use and SEM (scanning electron microscopy). Particles produced by the first two methods are excellent for TEM studies.

Very clean glassware is required. After usual good washing procedures, boil in double-distilled deionized water. Siliconized glassware is useful but not absolutely necessary. All solutions are microfiltered (0.22 μm). The mean size of the gold particles is measured by electron microscopy. Formvar-coated grids are contacted with a drop of colloidal gold. The grids are then air-dried and photographed in the EM.

II.3.2   *5 nm particles*

Make a saturated solution of white phosphorus (Merck) in 100% diethyl ether. The phosphorus reacts rapidly with air. Keep the sticks under water. Cut off a small piece while under water, then transfer it quickly to 10 ml of 100% ether. Close the vial and swirl for at least 2 h to insure saturation. Centrifuge down remaining solids in a glass centrifuge tube. Mix 1 part saturated solution with 4 parts 100% ether. Meanwhile, make a 1% solution of $HAuCl_4$ (Merck) in H_2O. Microfilter through a 0.22 μm millipore filter. Add 3 ml of 1% $HAuCl_4$ to 240 ml H_2O in an Erlenmeyer flask fitted with a water-cooled reflux tube. Add 5.4 ml of 0.2 M K_2CO_3 to increase the pH to ± 9. Add 2 ml of the diluted phosphorus ether to the $HAuCl_4$ solution, by pipetting it in below the surface to minimize contact with air. Mix this combination slowly at room temperature for 15 min. Then heat and reflux for 20–30 min to remove the ether and to drive the reaction. Cool to 4 °C. Use the colloidal gold solution within 14 days.

II.3.3   *12 nm particles* (after Horisberger, 1979)

A 0.07% sodium ascorbate solution (10 ml) is added at room temperature as fast as possible to a rapidly stirred solution consisting of 1% $HAuCl_4$ (1 ml), 0.2 N K_2CO_3 (1.5 ml), and water (25 ml). The volume is immediately adjusted to 100 ml with distilled water. All the solutions, except the sodium ascorbate, are microfiltered (0.22 μm).

II.3.4   *17–20 nm particles*

Make a 4% stock solution of $HAuCl_4$. Microfilter 0.22 μm. Add 0.5 ml 4% $HAuCl_4$ to 200 ml H_2O for a final concentration of 10^{-2}%. Boil and then add 6 ml 1% Na citrate under vigorous mixing. Reflux for 30 min. Cool to 4 °C. Use within 14 days.

II.3.5   *40 nm particles*

Identical. Use 3 ml 1% Na-citrate.

II.4   Adsorbing Antibodies to Colloidal Gold

II.4.1   *Terminology*

As mentioned above, we call immunoglobulin–gold conjugates 'IGS reagents'. IGS means immuno-gold staining, in analogy with immunofluorescence staining. The first symbols (e.g. GAR, GAM, R, M) designate the kind of immunoglobulin used. For example GAR is affinity-purified goat anti-rabbit IgG; R is protein-A Sepharose purified rabbit immunoglobulin G. G followed by a figure designates the size class of the colloidal gold. For example G5 means colloidal gold with a mean diameter of 5 nm.

II.4.2   *General background*

Successful attempts to label antibodies with colloidal gold particles are far less numerous than for other macromolecules. It has been reported (Romano *et al.*, 1974) that human and rabbit antibodies will not stabilize gold while horse antibodies will. For an excellent review on the colloidal gold system, I refer to Goodman and collaborators (1980). The adsorption of proteins to colloidal gold is influenced by parameters such as particle size, ionic concentration, pH, and protein concentration (Geoghegan and Ackerman, 1977; Geoghegan *et al.*, 1980; Goodman, *et al.*, 1981). Most of the applications using gold-labelled antibodies in the literature involve labelling of antigens in TEM and SEM, either at the surface of plasma membranes or of thin plastic sections (see Horisberger and collaborators 1975, 1977, 1979 and also Goodman *et al.*, 1980; Probert *et al.*, 1981). For applications involving surface labelling, the presence of antibodies, free in solution (Goodman *et al.*, 1981) could, at worst, reduce labelling efficiency by the introduction of competing antibodies in the solution. We have found that such competing antibodies will totally abolish efficient labelling in applications in which the gold-labelled antibodies have to penetrate into well-preserved cells. One of the major reasons for the reported problems with the production of stable immunoglobulin/gold conjugates (Romano *et al.*, 1974; Goodman, *et al.*, 1981) may be inherent to the nature of the antibodies themselves. Antibodies isolated from antisera, even by antigen affinity chromatography, are not very stable in low salt solutions at neutral pH, and consist of many different immunoglobulins displaying a wide range of isoelectric points. Monoclonal antibodies form an interesting exception here, because they show a very narrow range of isoelectric points. With the above in mind we have introduced a small number of modifications in the general methodology. The aim was to produce gold-labelled antibodies that are stable, and in which release of antibody in free solution is minimal.

This work and the evaluation of the results will be published elsewhere (Moeremans and De Mey, in preparation) and is summarized below:

(a) To overcome the instability of immunoglobulins in low salt solutions at neutral pH, we have used dialysis or gel filtration of the antibody solution against a 2 mM borax buffer, pH 9.

(b) It has been clearly demonstrated that the adsorption of protein to gold is pH-dependent (Geoghegan and Ackerman, 1977). Maximal binding takes place just at, or just on the basic side of, the isoelectric point. It has also been shown that immunoglobulins will stabilize gold sols over a pH range from 6.5 to 9 (Geoghegan and collaborators, 1977, 1978, 1980). We have found that for serum antibodies pH 9 is optimal in producing gold-labelled antibody reagents that will subsequently remain more stable than reagents coupled at neutral pH.

(c) Until now, PEG 20,000 (Carbowax 20 M) (Horisberger *et al.*, 1975) has been most often used as a 'quenching' or 'stabilizing' agent. The purpose is to stop further adsorption of protein to gold and to block free binding sites still present at the gold surface. It is said that this also minimizes possible aggregation and enhances probe stability. Other reagents such as polyvinyl pyrollidone (PVP) (Geoghegan and collaborators, 1977, 1978) or BSA (Romano *et al.*, 1974) have occasionally been used. Our studies have further evaluated BSA in this respect. It was found that, when used under proper conditions, BSA is as effective as PEG. In addition BSA containing IGS reagents proved to perform better in applications involving penetration of the probe. Therefore, we now routinely use BSA as stabilizing reagent.

(d) Removal of unstabilized marker and free or loosely bound antibodies is performed by washing the IGS reagent. This is done by centrifugation. The mobile pool has to be resuspended in an isosmotic buffered salt solution. We use 20 mM Tris buffered saline, pH 8.2 supplemented with 10 mg/ml BSA (Sigma, Type V). Using ^{125}I-labelled antibodies, we found that washing of the IGS reagent is essential for the production of stable and efficient probes. Several washings were initially included in the protocol of Faulk and Taylor (1971), but this has subsequently been omitted in many cases. After the coupling at least three washes, spaced in time, are necessary. The yield in gold may vary between 50 and 90%. Slot and Geuze (1981) have recently introduced a sizing method for producing gold–protein-A probes that are very homogeneous in size. This step will also eliminate most of the free proteins. We feel nevertheless that washing colloidol gold reagents at least three times should be encouraged. There are indeed many indications that there exists a population of protein molecules that are not very tightly bound. These are slowly released when the saline buffer is added, thus yielding colloidal gold particles that will not afterwards be optimally stabilized. Washing steps eliminate these less well-stabilized particles. Sizing of gold after three washing steps, then, is a very elegant way of producing high-quality and highly stable reagents.

In conclusion, the method described below for the preparation of gold-labelled immunoglobulin yields IGS reagents that are stable for several months at 4 °C and that can be used in a wide variety of applications, including high-resolution labelling of intracellular antigens.

II.4.3   *Preparation of the antibody for adsorption*

The protein concentration is adjusted to about 1 mg/ml. Protein is then dialysed *versus* 2 mM borax buffer at pH 9.0. Alternatively, gel chromatography may be used to exchange the buffer. It is recommended to keep the antibodies only for short periods in this low salt buffer. Immediately before use the protein solution is centrifuged at 100,000 g for 1 h at 0 °C to clarify.

II.4.4   *Determination of the optimally stabilizing protein concentration*

This is done by constructing a concentration variable adsorption isotherm (Geoghegan and collaborators, 1977, 1978, 1980). For serum antibodies the pH of the gold sol is adjusted to 9 with 0.2 M K_2CO_3. Just before use the pH of the gold sol is measured with a gel-filled combination electrode (e.g. Orion). This type of electrode has the advantage of having a low electrolyte flow rate. Other types of electrodes tend to be quickly plugged by flocculating gold at the electrode/solution interphase. The contact between electrode and gold sol is kept as short as possible.

The test involves (a) making a dilution series with small volumes of antibody; (b) adding a standard amount of gold colloid; (c) letting them react; (d) then adding a standard amount of salt to try to destabilize the colloid, and finding the amount of protein that is just enough to protect the colloid against salt destabilization. This destabilization is visualized by a colour change towards the blue that can be quantitated by an increase in absorbance at 580 nm.

For example, to work with 20 nm particles, start with a $1:3–1:5$ dilution of the centrifuged, dialysed antibody in 2 mM borax buffer pH 9.0. Make a linear dilution series.

⎰ Amount AB solution	100 µl	90 µl	. . . 10 µl	—
⎱ Amount borax buffer	—	10 µl	. . . 90 µl	100 µl

Centrifuge pH adjusted gold sol to remove any aggregates: $3000\,g$ for 15 min for 5 and 12 nm; $500\,g$ for 15 min for 20 and 40 nm. Add 1 ml of centrifuged gold to each tube in dilution series. Vortex, let stand 2 min, then add 100 µl of 10% (w/v) NaCl in H_2O. Measure $OD_{580\,nm}$ after 5 min. A typical example with affinity-purified GAR/Ig and 20 nm gold is shown in Figure 1. The optimal amount of antibody is determined by the point where the curve appears asymptotic with the X-axis.

For 5 and 12 nm gold a $1:2$ dilution of the dialysed antibody will be more appropriate, since this gold requires more protein to stabilize the colloid. This is because of the greater surface-to-volume ratio of the smaller particles. We have found that pH 9 is compatible with all kinds of serum immunoglobulins (e.g. mouse, goat, rat, human).

For monoclonal antibodies it is necessary to determine the optimal pH for protein adsorption. This is best done by isoelectric focussing in polyacrylamide or agarose gels, under native conditions. The monoclonal antibody is also dialysed *versus* 2 mM borax buffer, pH 9. The pH of the gold sol, however, is adjusted to the pI of the monoclonal antibody. Mixture of protein and gold sol will only result in a slight shift of pH, that will not influence the adsorption efficiency. Using these conditions a concentration-variable adsorption isotherm is constructed in the same way as for serum antibodies. It is not necessary to construct a pH-variable adsorption isotherm (Geoghegan and Ackerman, 1977), when the pI has been determined with isoelectric focussing.

II.4.5 *Preparation of an IGS reagent*

Once the optimal amount of antibody has been determined, the amount is increased by 10%, and any desired volume of pH-adjusted gold sol is mixed

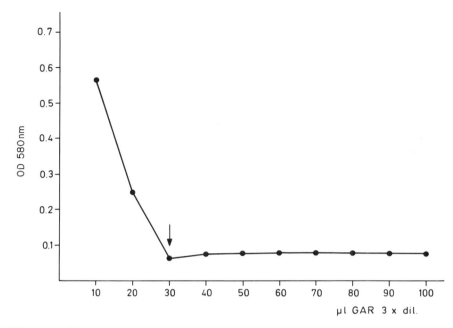

Figure 1 Concentration variable isotherm for 20 nm gold and GAR/Ig, diluted 1:3. The arrow indicates the amount of GAR/Ig that stabilizes the 20 nm gold sol against flocculation by 1% NaCl

with the appropriate volume of antibody solution (now undiluted). After 2 min of reaction, add a 10% BSA (Sigma, type V) solution to make a final concentration of 1% BSA. The 10% BSA solution is prepared in distilled water. The pH of the BSA solution is adjusted to 9 with NaOH. The solution is microfiltered (0.22 μm).

II.4.6 *Washing the conjugate*

Make up 1% BSA in 20 mM Tris buffered saline, pH 8.2 (1% BSA buffer). Microfilter (0.22 μm).

Spin down the gold particles with conjugated Ab. Use 60,000 g for 1 h at 4 °C to pellet 5 and 12 nm; 14,000 g for 1 h at 4 °C for 20 and 40 nm. These are g max values in the tube. As a result, a mobile pool of material, at the bottom, not a hard pellet, should be obtained. Most of the supernatant is carefully aspirated and the pool resuspended in the small remaining volume. Normally, nearly 100% of the gold sol is easily resuspended at this step. Then the tube is filled to the original volume with 1% BSA buffer.

After 15–30 min equilibration (overnight is even better), the centrifugation step is repeated. The supernatant is again aspirated and this washing step is repeated once. Then the gold is spun down a final time and resuspended in 1% BSA buffer containing 2×10^{-2} M azide to a volume such that, when diluted 1/20 in 1% BSA buffer, the OD at 520 nm will be 0.35 for 40 nm gold, 0.5 for 20 nm and 0.25 for 5 nm. 1% BSA buffer is used as the blank. Of course these values are arbitrary and serve only for standardization of different batches. If there were visible aggregates in the liquid at any time during washing, use a low-speed spin before the high-speed spin and discard the pellet. For 5 and 12 nm use $4800\,g$ for 20 min; for 20 and 40 nm use $250\,g$ for 20 min. The final product may be sterile filtered through 0.22 μm and stored under sterile conditions, if azide is not desired.

Using iodinated antibodies, it was determined that only minimal amounts (1–4%) of radioactivity were released from the gold reagents over a period of several months (unpublished observation). These preparations, when stored at 4 °C, maintained unchanged labelling activities for at least 3 months. During the first washing step in 1% BSA buffer, sometimes more then 50% of the gold particles may become aggregated irreversibly. The amount lost decreases sharply with subsequent washing steps. This suggests that the washing steps eliminate a fraction of the particles that became destabilized by addition of the physiological salt buffer. In the majority of the cases, however, a yield of 70–80% has been obtained.

II.4.7   *Sizing IGS reagents*

For double-labelling experiments, sizing of the gold particles, as previously introduced for protein A–gold, may be desirable (Slot and Geuze, 1981). Sizing may also be useful for selecting the smallest unaggregated particles out of the crude 5 nm IGS reagent. These can be used for high-resolution labelling. To this end, the final pool of the last washing step (in 1 ml) is layered on a 10–30% sucrose gradient in 1% BSA buffer that was formed in a centrifuge tube. For 5 nm gold, $150,000\,g$ for 1 h will produce an even distribution of the gold particles over the gradient. Fractionation yields particles with diameter from 3 to 8 nm. The smaller particles are more appropriate for applications involving penetration of the label. We have not yet attempted to size gold sols of other dimensions. Two different monoclonals, each adsorbed to different sized gold particles respectively, (e.g. 4 and 8 nm) will provide a very powerful tool for direct double high-resolution labelling experiments.

III   FIELDS OF APPLICATION

III.1   General Remarks

The use of colloidal gold-labelled antibodies in neuroimmunocytochemistry is still limited to a few examples (Gu *et al.*, 1981; Wharton *et al.*, 1981; Probert *et al.*, 1981). Much more work has to be done to evaluate its potential. Both light and electron microscopic applications in fields other than neurobiology are already described.

Light microscopic applications include:

(1) detection of surface differentiation antigens with both monoclonal and serum antibodies on cell suspensions or cell monolayers (Geoghegan *et al.*, 1978; De Waele *et al.*, 1981; De Mey *et al.*, 1982);
(2) the localization of certain intracellular antigens in cultured monolayers (De Mey *et al.*, 1980a, 1981);
(3) detection of antigens in histological and semi-thin sections (Gu *et al.*, 1981).

At the light microscopic level, the IGS method can so far best be seen as a complementary method that could be useful when other markers present problems such as background or endogenous enzyme activity. The sensitivity of the method is in many cases satisfactory but it has not yet systematically been studied whether it reaches the sensitivity offered by immunoenzyme histochemical methods. The major drawback of IGS reagents used for LM is the need for using relatively concentrated preparations. The amount of stain is indeed proportional to the number of gold particles accumulating at the antigen consuming site. By applying two layers of gold-labelled immunoglobulins—the first containing a secondary antibody and the second a pre-immune immunoglobulin recognized by the secondary antibody—very intense staining could be obtained (Gu *et al.*, 1981). The red colour is very useful subsequent to an enzyme histochemical method in double-labelling experiments. Further advantages of the LM IGS methods are the simplicity, through the direct production of stain, and the absence of background formation.

IGS reagents could become increasingly successful markers for immunoelectron-microscopy. With the increasing number of available monoclonal antibodies, direct high-resolution labelling could soon become common practice. For medium high-resolution work indirect labelling techniques may also be used for convenience. Sandwich IGS techniques do not seem to be specifically advantageous for EM, because with colloidal gold there is no need for amplifying the signal, and use of affinity-purified antibodies eliminates specificity problems. As has been outlined (Slot and Geuze, 1981; see also Chapter 12), double-labelling experiments can best be done by using two relatively small sizes of gold particles, because the use of larger particles decreases the labelling density.

EM applications of IGS reagents include detection of:

(1) surface antigens on cell suspensions and cell monolayers (Horisberger

and collaborators, 1975, 1979; Geoghegan and Ackerman, 1977; Yeger and Kalnins, 1978; Trejdosiewicz *et al.*, 1981; De Mey *et al.*, 1982);
(2) intracellular antigens in cultured monolayers (De Mey *et al.*, 1981);
(3) tissue antigens (Wharton *et al.*, 1981; Probert *et al.*, 1981).

For labelling surface antigens on cell monolayers, it may be interesting to use the approach of whole-cell mounts (Wolosewick and Porter, 1976; De Mey *et al.*, 1981). This methodology permits observation of large numbers of whole cells with high-resolution TEM. It consists in growing cells on formvar-coated grids, doing the labelling experiment, and critical-point drying the specimen. This can then be observed in the transmission electron microscope. By using stereovisualization techniques, information about the structures underlying the labelled areas can be obtained. One limitation of this approach is that it works only with well-spread cells. This methodology can also be used for the localization of intracellular antigens (De Mey *et al.*, 1981). When the antigen is associated with fibrillar structures such as microtubules or microfilaments, it enables unequivocal determination as to whether the label is really associated with the structures or is free in the cytoplasm. A detailed description of this relatively unknown approach is given below.

For the localization of tissue antigens, with the pre-embedding approach, the colloidal gold method does not seem to be very useful. This is due to penetration problems, also encountered with, for example, the PAP method. In addition, the pre-embedding approach is much dependent on the previous light microscopic visualization and subsequent selection of the area to be studied by EM. This is not possible with the smaller-sized gold, unless using fluorescently labelled antibodies for conjugation to the gold particles.

IGS reagents are very powerful, on the contrary, for labelling of thin sections of plastic-embedded tissue (Wharton *et al.*, 1981; Probert *et al.*, 1981) and potentially also to thin frozen sections as previously shown for protein A–gold (Geuze *et al.*, 1981). The plastic sections have the disadvantage that only their surfaces can be labelled. The high electron-density of the gold particles facilitates contrast of the sections with the usual uranyl and lead stains, and makes it possible to obtain full information on the fine structure of labelled areas. The problem of penetration is partly solved when frozen sections are used, and recent improvements have considerably increased imaging of ultrastructural detail (Tokuyasu, 1978; see also Chapter 12).

III.2   General Procedures

IGS reagents are used in exactly the same way as other reagents for immunocytochemistry. As outlined in Figure 2, four procedures are in principle possible: the direct, indirect, bridge, and combined indirect and bridge procedures. The two latter procedures give stronger staining for light microscopic applications because they increase the number of gold particles

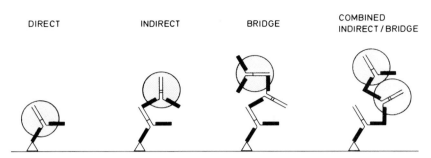

DIRECT   INDIRECT   BRIDGE   COMBINED
                                            INDIRECT / BRIDGE

Figure 2 Different ways of using colloidal gold-labelled antibodies (IGS reagents). The direct and indirect method are most useful for EM studies. The bridge and combined indirect/bridge techniques give enhanced staining at the light microscopic level. For simplicity, only one antibody molecule/gold granule has been drawn. This is the case for 5nm gold. With 20 nm gold, 20–30 antibody molecules are adsorbed/gold granule. It has, however, often been noticed that 5 nm gold gives a denser labelling than the 20 nm particles (Slot and Geuze, 1981; De Mey *et al.*, 1981). Steric hindrance between molecules could explain this phenomenon

accumulating near the antigen-containing sites. The bridge procedure also allows one to use pre-immune immunoglobulins of the same species as the primary antibody, coupled to gold particles, instead of the more precious secondary antibodies. In general, signal amplification is not needed for EM, and is even undesired when the work involves quantitation or when high resolution is needed.

A general indirect procedure for fixed preparations (cells or sections) is described below. For the bridge procedure, the primary antibody is followed by an unlabelled secondary antiserum, and then, the procedure is continued from step (c) on. For labelling of living cells, isosmotic phosphate buffers can be used instead of the Tris buffer recommended below.

(a) Preparation of samples will differ from application to application. The most suitable method will not differ very much from standard methods that give satisfactory results with other labelling methods. We refer to different chapters of this book for specific examples of tissue preparation.

(b) Incubate the preparation with 5% normal serum (same species as secondary antibody) made up in 0.1% BSA buffer (20 mM Tris, 150 mM NaCl, 1 mg/ml BSA, pH 8.2).

(c) Remove excess normal serum and replace by appropriate dilution of primary antibody made up in 0.1% BSA buffer supplemented with 1% normal serum. When the optimal dilution is unknown, it should be determined by making up a series of serial dilutions. Incubate for times ranging from a couple of hours to overnight, at room temperature in a moist atmosphere.

(d) Wash the preparations with 0.1% BSA buffer. Use three changes of ±10 min each.
(e) Incubate with the IGS reagent diluted in 1% BSA buffer. The optimal dilution and incubation time should be determined. Centrifuge the diluted reagent for 10 min at low speed to remove small aggregates of denatured reagent ($250g$ for G20 and G40, $4800g$ for G5 and G12). In most light microscopic applications the development of stain can be followed under the microscope.
(f) Wash the preparations with 0.1% BSA buffer as in (d).
(g) Fix with 1% glutaraldehyde in fixing buffer.
(h) Process the preparations according to standard procedures for light microscopy (dehydration and permanent mounting) or for electron microscopy.

III.3   Special Application 1: Labelling Cultured Cells, Grown on Formvar-coated Grids for TEM

III.3.1   *Growing cells on formvar-coated grids*

Golden grids, 200 mesh, are rinsed with acetone and ether and dried. Formvar (0.7% in chloroform) films (±60 × 25 min) are made on microscopy slides and are floated on clean deionized water. Two groups of four grids, each group fitting in a square of 18 × 18 mm, are put on the formvar film, coarse side down. Two clean coverslips (18 × 18 mm) are positioned over the grids and attached to the formvar film. The total assembly is covered with a sheet of paper, 80 × 40 mm, taken from a parafilm roll. The paper is lifted and the whole is put, formvar film up, in a Petri dish, on filter paper.

After air-drying (drops of water are carefully sucked off with pieces of filter paper), coverslips are sterilized under UV light at both sides. Dissociated cell suspensions in a suitable growth medium are seeded in Petri dishes (30 mm) containing one grids/coverslip assembly, in the usual way and cultivated to the desired density in an incubator with water-saturated air and 5% CO_2 at 37°C.

III.3.2   *Preparations for immunocytochemistry*

Depending on the kind of labelling (intracellular or extracellular) and type of antigen, fixation conditions will differ.

When ultrastructural preservation of the total cell is important, fixation should also be checked by thin sectioning work after plastic embedding. Glutaraldehyde (double-distilled, high purity grade), 0.25–1% or mixed aldehyde: 2–4% paraformaldehyde/0.1–0.2% glutaraldehyde for 10 min are the minimal conditions that give acceptable preservation. Formaldehyde alone does not usually give satisfaction for EM. We have obtained good results with the following buffer, which is called buffer [I] (Small and Celis, 1978).

—Make a stock solution of double Hanks salt solution per litre:

KCl	0.8 g
NaCl	16 g
KH_2PO_4	0.12 g
Na_2NPO_4	0.095 g
$NaHCO_3$	0.7 g

—The buffer [I] is made as follows, for 1 litre:
   —double Hanks, 500 ml
   —PIPES (Sigma) 100 mм, 50 ml   5 mм final concentration
   —EGTA 500 mм, 4 ml (neutralized with KOH)   2 mм final concentration
   —$MgCl_2$ 1 м, 2 ml   2 mм final concentration

Add H_2O up to 1 litre, after adjusting pH to 6.0 with 1 N HCl. Other buffers, such as 0.1 м cacodylate, pH 7.2 will also be adequate in many cases. The following fixation protocol is also suitable for cells grown on cover-slips without grids or directly on plastic (for embedding and thin sectioning) and works well with the indirect fluorescence, PAP, or ferritin bridge procedures (De Mey *et al.*, 1980; De Brabander *et al.*, 1981).

Fixation is done by removing the culture medium and adding the fixative. Removal of medium and subsequent solutions is done with a Pasteur pipette, fixed in a stand and connected to a vacuum line and flask. After a short time the fixative is replaced by fresh one. After 10 min, fixative is aspirated and the grids/coverslip mount is washed with buffer [I]. For permeabilization (detection of intracellular antigens), 0.5% Triton X-100 in buffer [I] is used (30 min). Do not include this step when surface labelling is the purpose.

Now the cells have to be treated with $NaBH_4$ in order to reduce remaining free aldehyde groups.

To this end the grids must be carefully separated from the coverslips. With fine-pointed forceps, the formvar around the coverslip is disrupted, and the grid is lifted and transported into a special grid-holder (Polysciences catalogue no. 7332) placed in buffer [I] in a Petri dish. Each holder has a perforated bottom, and also the corresponding place in the cover is perforated. This allows for free passage of fluids. An identical grid-holder is used for washing the grids after each incubation.

The closed grid-holder, containing the grids, is placed in a freshly prepared 50% ethanol/50% buffer [I] mixture, containing 0.5 mg/ml $NaBH_4$, for 15 min. The $NaBH_4$ is extremely hydrophilic and should be stored in a dessicator.

For surface labelling, freshly prepared $NaBH_4$, 0.5 mg/ml in buffer [I] for 15 min should be used. To stop the reaction with $NaBH_4$, the grid-holder with grids is placed in a Petri dish containing 0.1% BSA buffer. From then on, the usual series of incubations (see general scheme above) is carried out.

For the incubation steps, the grids are immersed in small drops (20 μl) placed in the individual wells of microtest plates (Falcon or other supplier).

For washing, the grids are simply transferred from the wells into the special grid-holder, bathing in 0.1% BSA buffer in a Petri dish. The holder is closed and placed in a beaker (±250 ml) containing 0.1% BSA buffer. This is slowly stirred for 20 min. This simple procedure is very gentle and has the advantage of built-in order. Many different antibodies and different concentrations can be run in one experiment. After the final washing in 0.1% BSA buffer the grids with cells are briefly rinsed in buffer [I] and post-fixed with 1% glutaraldehyde in buffer [I] for 10 min. After rinsing in buffer [I] they are treated with 0.5% OsO_4 in 0.05 M veronal acetate buffer, pH 7.4 at 4 °C for 15 min. The veronal buffer is made as follows:

(a) veronal acetate buffer, stock:

sodium acetate, cryst	9.71 g
sodium barbiturate	14.71 g
distilled water	500 ml

(b) veronal acetate buffer 0.05 M, pH 7.4:

veronal acetate buffer, stock	2 parts
HCl 0.1 N	2 parts
distilled water	6 parts

Fixation and osmication can also be done in the wells of microtest plates.

After the osmication the grids are dipped in H_2O and transferred to the grid-holder, bathing in H_2O in a Petri dish. From there, they are mounted in a grid-holder for a critical-point drying apparatus and dehydrated through a series of ethanol or acetone. Extra contrast can be obtained by reacting the samples with 0.2% uranyl acetate in 15% acetone for 15 min. After critical-point drying, a layer of carbon is evaporated on the cells and these can then be viewed by normal or high-voltage EM.

Figures 3 and 4 show an example: PtK_2 rat kangaroo cells grown on formvar-coated grids and labelled as described above with rabbit antibodies to tubulin and GAR G5. They were viewed in a Philips 300 microscope at 100 kV. The microtubules are densely labelled. Label can also be found that is not associated with microtubules. Stereo imaging can be used to distinguish surface label from cytoplasmic label (not shown). The controls of specificity are identical to those used with other markers. Gold, like ferritin, presents the advantage that each granule can be detected. Its greater electron-density allows it to be seen against the high contrast of the critical-point dried cell.

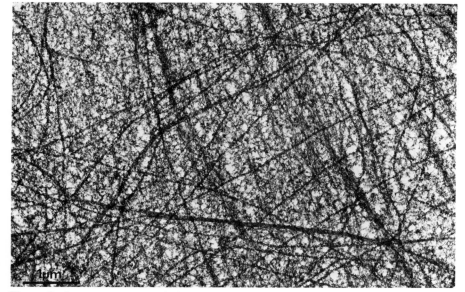

Figure 3 Low-power transmission EM view of a whole-cell mount of PtK$_2$ cells. The three-dimensional distribution of the densely labelled microtubules can be studied relative to unlabelled stress fibres and tonofilaments

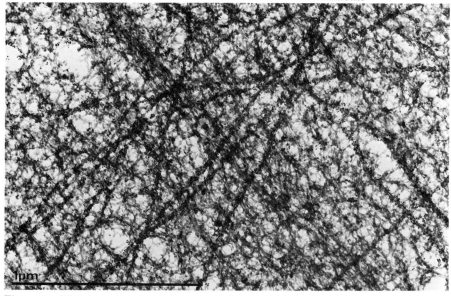

Figure 4 High-power view of the same cell as in Figure 3. Label, not associated with microtubules, can be clearly seen. Stereo-techniques could reveal its exact three-dimensional localization. The whole-cell mount approach is the only way of easily determining whether the label is associated with the microtubules, or is free in the cytoplasm

Preliminary results have shown that the label is also clearly visible in pictures of cells viewed with the high-voltage EM (1000 kV).

III.4   Special Application 2: Labelling of Antigens in Thin Plastic Sections

In principle, the method is very similar to immunostaining of ultra-thin sections, previously described (Roth *et al.*, 1978; Larsson, 1979; Batten and Hopkins, 1979) and identical to Probert *et al.* (1981).

The convenient way of handling EM grids described above can also be used for labelling thin sections. Normally, plastic sections are etched with 10% H_2O_2 for 15 min. This can be done in the wells of the microtest plates. Etching is necessary for tissues that have already been osmicated. A number of antigens seem to resist osmication. This results in excellent ultrastructural detail. The use of colloidal gold does not mask this detail to a great extent, as is often the case with reaction products of enzymes.

(a) Thin sections of plastic-embedded tissues are mounted on EM grids.
(b) They are etched with 10% H_2O_2 for 15 min. The drops (20 μl) of H_2O_2 are placed in wells of microtest plates (Falcon), and the grids simply immersed in the drops.
(c) The grids are rinsed by dipping them in a beaker with water and immersed in drops (20 μl) 5% NGS in 0.1% BSA buffer. For transfer of grids away from the microtest plates, two fine forceps are used. One (left) is used for tilting the grid, the other for holding the grid.
(d) The grids are transferred to drops (in wells) of diluted specific antibody in 1% NGS/0.1% BSA buffer and incubated for 2 h.
(e) For washing, the grids are transferred to a special grid-holder (Polysciences, Lot No. 7332) bathing in 0.1% BSA buffer in a Petri dish. The holder has a perforated bottom; the cover is also perforated over each place. This allows for free passage of fluids when the holder is closed. The closed grid-holder with grids is moved to a beaker with 150 ml 0.1% BSA buffer which is slowly stirred for 15 min. This washing procedure is efficient but very mild, and especially helpful when formvar-coated slot grids are used.
(f) The grid-holder is again moved to a Petri dish with 0.1% BSA buffer and opened. Care is taken to ensure that the grids are not damaged. These are then transferred to appropriately diluted IGS (immuno gold staining) reagent in 1% BSA buffer and (in wells) incubated for 1 h.
(g) Washing as in (e).
(h) The grids are post-fixed with glutaraldehyde and the sections contrasted with uranyl acetate and lead citrate, rinsed, and dried as usual.

Figure 5 shows a specific example obtained with antibodies against substance P.

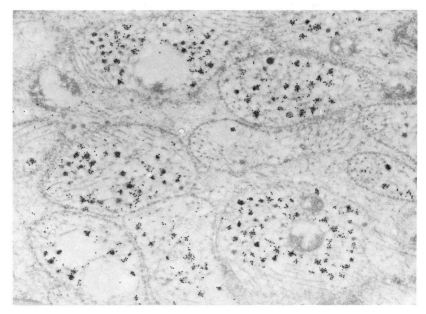

Figure 5 Substance P-like immunoreactivity in guinea-pig myenteric plexus, revealed with rabbit anti substance-P and GAR G20

IV CONCLUSIONS

The growing interest in the colloidal gold system as a versatile, extremely flexible marker for light and electron microscopic labelling studies seems fully justified. Conjugating all kinds of ligands to colloidal gold is extremely simple and does not need special skill.

This chapter has been devoted to the specific problems of conjugating antibodies to colloidal gold, and is intended to stimulate other workers to couple their own antibodies and evaluate their potential as probes for light and electron microscopic immunocytochemistry. Colloidal gold as a light microscopic marker will prove to be very useful in certain areas such as the labelling of cell subpopulations on the basis of specific cell surface antigens (De Waele *et al.*, 1981). It is not yet possible to claim whether this will also be the case in neuroimmunocytochemistry. There exist, indeed, excellent methods at present. However, the exploitation of certain characteristics of colloidal gold, such as its dichroism, or its potential of reflecting incident light, may open totally new vistas in the near future (Inoué *et al.*, 1981; De Mey, unpublished results).

The clear-cut potential of colloidal gold in neuro-immunocytochemistry lies in the use of colloidal gold as a marker for transmission electron microscopy. Larger particles are suitable for SEM.

Small-sized colloidal gold is now firmly established as a marker for high-resolution immuno-electron microscopy. When applied to thin plastic sections, it allows specific detection of antigens with optimal delineation of ultrastructural detail. It has also great potential for double or even multiple labelling experiments, responding, for example, to a growing need for understanding the anatomical relationship of different neurotransmitter (peptidergic and other) systems. In neurobiology too, there is growing interest in performing tissue culture experiments (see Chapter 15). The special procedure described in this chapter should allow visualization, for example, of specific receptors and allow study of their relationship with underlying structures (e.g. coated pits, microfilaments, etc.). There also, double labelling experiments could yield interesting data. Colloidal gold is the first-choice marker for use in the whole-cell mount approach (see Chapter 14).

Indirect techniques with IGS reagents or protein A–gold will always be convenient. The expected wave of available monoclonals, and the demonstration that they are first-choice material for conjugation to colloidal gold (De Mey *et al.*, 1982), lead me to speculate that, very soon, direct antibody labelling at the ultrastructural level will become common practice. This evolution will increase both specificity and resolving power of immunocytochemical techniques, as well as enhancing the possibilities of performing multiple labelling experiments.

Problems such as co-localization of different substances, and anatomical relationship between different systems, will then be easier to challenge. The procedures will also become much more simple and less time-consuming.

Much evaluating work remains to be done. It seems, however, justified to claim that IGS reagents will gain a firm position among the many other possible ligands and markers available today. A certain experience is needed to choose the right marker system suitable for a given problem. It should not be forgotten, however, that the localization method will not be better than the antibody used, and the tissue preservation achieved. It looks as though we are far from solving these major problems in the field of immunocytochemistry.

ACKNOWLEDGEMENTS

My colleagues of the laboratory of Oncology—M. De Brabander, M. Moeremens, G. Geuens, and R. Nuydens—are gratefully acknowledged for their participation in this work. Thanks are also expressed to the group of the Histochemistry Department of Hammersmith Hospital, London—especially J. Polak, L. Probert, F. Tapia, I. Varndell, and J. Gu—for the fruitful collaboration involving the use of IGS reagents on the neuroendocrine system, and for the photographs they kindly provided.

This work has been supported by a grant from the IWONL (Instituut ter bevordering van wetenschappelijk onderzoek in landbouw en nijverheid, Brussels).

REFERENCES

Baetens, D., De Mey, J., and Gepts, W. (1977). 'Immunohistochemical and ultra-structural identification of the pancreatic polypeptide-producing cell in the human pancreas.' *Cell Tissue Res.*, **185**, 239–246.

Batten, T. F. C. and Hopkins, C. R. (1979). 'Use of protein A-coated colloidal gold particles for immuno-electronmicroscopic localization of ACTH on ultrathin sections.' *Histochemistry*, **60**, 317–320.

Biberfeld, B., Ghetie, V., and Sjöquist, J. (1974). 'Demonstration and assaying IgG antibodies in tissues and on cells by labelled Staphylococcal protein A.' *J. Immunol. Methods*, **6**, 249–259.

Consolazione, A., Milstein, C., Wright, B., and Cuello, A. (1981). 'Immunocytochemical detection of serotonin with monoclonal antibodies.' *J. Histochem. Cytochem.*, **29**, 1425–1430.

Coons, A. M., Leduc, E. M., and Connolly, J. M. (1955). 'Studies on antibody production. I. A method for the histochemical demonstration of specific antibody and its application to a study of the hyperimmune rabbit.' *J. Exp. Med.*, **102**, 49–60.

Cuello, A. C., Galfré, G., and Milstein, C. (1979). 'Detection of substance P in the central nervous system by a monoclonal antibody.' *Proc. Natl. Acad. Sci. USA*, **76**, 3532.

Cuello, A. C., Milstein, C., and Priestley, J. V. (1980). 'Use of monoclonal antibodies in immunocytochemistry with special reference to the central nervous system.' *Brain Res. Bull.*, **5**, 575–587.

Dacheux, F., Dubois, M., and Hall, H. (1976). 'Electron-microscopical immunohistochemical study of the localization in the anterior pituitary of an antiserum against a low molecular weight adenohypophyseal constituent.' *J. Histochem. Cytochem.*, **24**, 1034.

De Brabander, M., De Mey, J., Joniau, M., and Geuens, G. (1977). 'Immunocytochemical visualization of microtubules and tubulin at the light- and electron microscopic level.' *J. Cell Sci.*, **28**, 283–301.

De Brabander, M., Bulinski, J., Geuens, G., De Mey, J., and Borisy, G. (1981). 'Immuno-electron microscopic localization of the 210,000 mol wt microtubule-associated protein in cultured cells of primates.' *J. Cell Biol.*, **91**, 438–445.

De Mey, J., Moeremans, M., Geuens, G., Nuydens, R., Van Belle, H., and De Brabander, M. (1980a). 'Light- and electron microscopic localization of calmodulin in mitotic cells.' *Eur. J. Cell Biol.*, **22**, 297a.

De Mey, J., Moeremans, M., Geuens, G., Nuydens, R., Van Belle, H., and De Brabander, M. (1980b). Immunocytochemical evidence for the association of calmodulin with microtubules of the mitotic apparatus.' In De Brabander, M., and De Mey, J. (eds), *Microtubules and Microtubule Inhibitors*, pp. 227–241. Elsevier/North-Holland, Amsterdam.

De Mey, J., Moeremans, M., Geuens, G., Nuydens, R., and De Brabander, M. (1981). 'High resolution light and electron microscopic localization of tubulin with the IGS (immuno gold staining) method.' *Cell Biol. Int. Rep.*, **5**, 889–899.

De Mey, J., Moeremans, M., De Waele, M., Geuens, G., and De Brabander, M. (1982). 'The IGS (immuno gold staining) method used with monoclonal antibodies.' In Peeters, H. (ed.), *Prot. Biol. Fluids*, Vol. 29, pp 943–947. Pergamon Press, Oxford.

De Waele, M., De Mey, J., Moeremans, M., and Van Camp, B. K. G. (1981). 'The immuno gold staining method: an immunocytochemical procedure for leukocyte characterization by monoclonal antibodies.' In Knapp, W. (ed.), *Leukemia Markers*, pp. 173–176. Academic Press, London.

Dutton, A., Tokuyasu, K. T., and Singer, S. J. (1979). 'Iron-dextran antibody conjugates: general method for simultaneous staining of two components in high-resolution immuno-electron microscopy.' *Proc. Natl. Acad. Sci. USA*, **76**, 3392–3396.

Faulk, W. P. and Taylor, G. M. (1971). 'An immunocolloid method for the electron microscope.' *Immunochemistry*, **8**, 1081–1083.

Feldherr, C. M. and Marshall, J. M. (1962). 'The use of colloidal gold for studies of intracellular exchange in amoeba *Chaos chaos*.' *J. Cell Biol.*, **12**, 640–645.

Frens, G. (1973). 'Controlled nucleation for the regulation of particle size in monodisperse gold suspensions.' *Nature Phys. Sci.*, **241**, 20–22.

Geoghegan, W. D. and Ackerman, G. A. (1977). 'Adsorption of horseradish peroxidase, ovomucoid and anti-immuno-globulin to colloidal gold for the indirect detection of concanavalin A, wheat germ agglutinin and goat anti-human immuno-globulin G on cell surfaces at the electron microscopic level: a new method, theory and application.' *J. Histochem. Cytochem.*, **25**, 1187–1200.

Geoghegan, W. D., Scillian, J. J., and Ackerman, G. A. (1978). 'The detection of human B lymphocytes by both light- and electron microscopy utilizing colloidal gold labelled anti-immuno-globulin.' *Immunol. Commun.*, **7**, 1–12.

Geoghegan, W. D., Ambegaonkar, S., and Calvanico, N. (1980). 'Passive gold agglutination. An alternative to passive hemagglutination.' *J. Immunol. Methods*, **34**, 11–21.

Geuze, H., Slot, J., Van der Ley, P., Schuffer, R., and Griffith, J. (1981). 'Use of colloidal gold particles in double-labelling immuno-electron microscopy of ultrathin frozen tissue sections.' *J. Cell Biol.*, **89**, 653–665.

Goodman, S. L., Hodges, G. M., and Livingston, D. C. (1980). 'A review of the colloidal gold marker system.' In Johari, O. (ed.), *Scanning Electron Microscopy*, vol. II, pp. 133–145. SEM Inc., Chicago, Ill., USA.

Goodman, S. L., Hodges, G. M., Trejdosiewicz, L., and Livingston, D. C. (1981). 'Colloidal gold markers and probes for routine application in microscopy.' *J. Microscopy*, **123**, 201–213.

Gu, J., De Mey, J., Moeremans, M., and Polak, J. (1981). 'Sequential use of the PAP and immuno gold staining methods for the light microscopical double staining of tissue antigens. Its application to the study of regulatory peptides in the gut.' *Regulat. Pept.*, **1**, 365–374.

Guesdon, J. L., Ternynck, T., and Avrameas, S. (1979). 'The use of avidin-biotin interaction in immunoenzymatic techniques.' *J. Histochem. Cytochem.*, **27**, 1131–1139.

Hardy, P. H., Meyer, H. G., Cuculis, J. J., Petrali, J. P., and Sternberger, L. A. (1970). 'Postembedding staining for electron microscopy by the unlabelled antibody peroxidase method.' *J. Histochem. Cytochem.*, **18**, 684.

Heitzmann, H. and Richards, F. M. (1974). 'Use of the avidin–biotin complex for specific staining of biological membranes in electron microscopy.' *Proc. Natl. Acad. Sci. USA*, **71**, 3537–3541.

Horisberger, M. (1979). 'Evaluation of colloidal gold as a cytochemical marker for transmission and scanning electron microscopy.' *Biol. Cellul.*, **36**, 253–258.

Horisberger, M., Rosset, J., and Bauer, H. (1975). 'Colloidal gold granules as markers for cell surface receptors in the scanning electron microscope.' *Experientia*, **31**, 1147–1149.

Horisberger, M. and Vonlanthen, M. (1977). 'Localization of mannan and chitin on thin sections of budding yeasts with gold markers.' *Arch. Microbiol.*, **115**, 1–7.

Hsu, S., Raine, L., and Fanger, H. (1981). 'Use of avidin–biotin–peroxidase complex (ABC) in immunoperoxidase techniques: a comparison between ABC and unlabelled antibody (PAP) procedures.' *J. Histochem. Cytochem.*, **29**, 577–580.

Inoué, S., Bajer, A., and Molè-Bajer, J. (1981). 'Dichroism of mitotic microtubules displayed by gold-conjugated anti-tubulin.' *J. Cell Biol.*, **91**, 321a.

Johnson, G., Gloria, M., and Noghueira Araujo, C. (1981). 'A simple method of reducing the fading of immunofluorescence during microscopy.' *J. Immunol. Methods*, **43**, 349–350.

Köhler, G. and Milstein, C. (1975). 'Continuous cultures of fused cells secreting antibody of predefined specificity.' *Nature*, **265**, 495.

Larsson, L.-I. (1979). 'Simultaneous ultrastructural demonstration of multiple peptides in endocrine cells by a novel immunocytochemical method.' *Nature*, **282**, 743–746.

Nakane, P. K., and Pierce, G. B. Jr (1966). 'Enzyme-labelled antibodies: preparation and application for the localization of antigens.' *J. Histochem. Cytochem.*, **14**, 929.

Novikoff, A. (1980). 'DAB cytochemistry: artifact problems in its current uses.' *J. Histochem. Cytochem.*, **28**, 1036–1038.

Pickel, V. M., Joh, T. H., Field, P. M., Becker, C. G., and Reis, D. J. (1975). 'Cellular localization of tyrosine hydroxylase by immunohistochemistry.' *J. Histochem. Cytochem.*, **23**, 1–12.

Probert, L., De Mey, J., and Polak, J. (1981). 'Distinct subpopulations of enteric p-type neurones contain substance P and vasoactive intestinal polypeptide.' *Nature*, **294**, 470–471.

Romano, E. L., Stolinski, C., and Hughes-Jones, N. C. (1974). 'An antiglobulin reagent labelled with colloidal gold for use in electron microscopy.' *Immunochemistry*, **11**, 521–522.

Romano, E. L. and Romano, M. (1977). 'Staphylococcal protein A bound to colloidal gold: a useful reagent to label antigen-antibody sites in electron microscopy.' *Immunochemistry*, **14**, 711–715.

Roth, J., Bendayan, M., and Orci, L. (1978). 'Ultrastructural localization of intracellular antigens by the use of protein A-gold complex.' *J. Histochem. Cytochem.*, **26**, 1074–1081.

Singer, S. J. and Schick, A. F. (1961). 'The properties of specific stains for electron microscopy prepared by conjugation of antibody with ferritin.' *J. Biophys. Cytol.*, **9**, 519.

Slot, J. and Geuze, H. (1981). 'Sizing of protein A–colloidal gold probes for immuno-electron microscopy.' *J. Cell Biol.*, **90**, 533–536.

Small, J. V. and Celis, J. E. (1978). 'Filament arrangements in negatively stained cultured cells: the organization of actin.' *Cytobiologie*, **16**, 308–325.

Stathis, F. C. and Fabrikanos, A. (1958). 'Preparation of colloidal gold.' *Chem. Ind. (Lond.)*, **27**, 860–861.

Sternberger, L. A. (1979). *Immunocytochemistry*. Wiley, London.

Sternberger, L. A., Hardy, P. H., Cuculis, J. J., and Meyer, H. G. (1970). 'The unlabelled antibody enzyme method of immunohistochemistry. Preparation and properties of soluble antigen–antibody complex (horseradish-peroxidase–antihorseradish peroxidase) and its use in the identification of spirochetes.' *J. Histochem. Cytochem.*, **18**, 315–333.

Toduyasu, K. T. (1978).'A study of positive staining of ultrathin frozen sections.' *J. Ultrastruct. Res.*, **63**, 287–307.

Trejdosiewicz, L. K., Smolira, M. A., Hodges, G. M., Goodman, S. L., and Livingston, D. C. (1981). 'Cell surface distribution of fibronectin in cultures of fibroblasts and bladder derived epithelium: SEM-immunogold localization compared to immunoperoxidase and immunofluorescence.' *J. Microsc.*, **123**, 227–236.

Weiser, H. B. (1933). *Inorganic Colloid Chemistry*. Wiley, London.

Wharton, J., Polak, J., Probert, L., De Mey, J., McGregor, G., Brijant, M., and Bloom, S. (1981). 'Peptide containing nerves in the ureter of the guinea-pig and cat.' *Neuroscience*, **6**, 969–982.

Willingham, M. C. (1980). 'Electron microscopic immunocytochemical localization of intracellular antigens in cultured cells: the EGS and ferritin bridge procedures.' *Histochem. J.*, **12**, 419–434.

Wolosewick, J. J. and Porter, K. R. (1976). 'Stereo high-voltage electron microscopy of whole cells of human diploid line, WI-38.' *Am. J. Pathol.*, **147**, 303–324.

Yeger, H. and Kalnins, V. (1978). 'Immunocytochemical localization of Gp 70 over virus-related submembranous densities in its mutant Rauscher murine leukemia virus-infected cells at the nonpermissive temperature.' *Virology*, **91**, 489–492.

Immunohistochemistry
Edited by A. C. Cuello
© 1983 IBRO

CHAPTER 14

Immunohistochemistry on Whole Mount Preparations

M. COSTA and J. B. FURNESS

Centre for Neuroscience and Departments of Human Physiology and Morphology, School of Medicine, the Flinders University of South Australia

I INTRODUCTION

Whole mount preparations for the study of the arrangements of nerves in the periphery were widely used during the last century; whole mount and sections made with hand-held knives were the major methods of preparing tissue. From the middle of the nineteenth century, with the gradual introduction of microtomes capable of yielding thin and even tissue sections, the use of thin sections increased although whole mounts continued to be used by some investigators. Some tissues are sufficiently thin to be viewed directly but in other cases it is necessary to separate the tissues into layers. In some early studies this was done by maceration in acid; for example, Meissner (1857) first described the submucous plexus after scraping the macerated mucosa from the intestine. Subsequently, the staining techniques developed for nerves were applied to whole mount preparations. In particular, the use of methylene blue, introduced by Erlich (1886), soon became widespread; and since then there have been hundreds of papers using this technique in whole mount preparations. Worthy of mention is the pioneering work of Dogiel who used this technique to describe the nerve cell types in the intestine (1899a) and nerves in the heart (1899b).

In this century, some of the most comprehensive work on the arrangement of autonomic nerves in viscera has been performed in whole mounts. For example, the nerve plexuses in the intestine have been thoroughly studied in whole mount preparations with methylene blue, silver impregnation, and osmium impregnation (Hill, 1927; Schabadasch, 1930a,b; Rintoul, 1960; Taxi, 1965; Stach, 1971). Similarly, methylene blue staining in whole mount preparations has been used to investigate, amongst other things, the distribution of nerves to the heart and to the blood vessels (Huber, 1899; Busch, 1929; Mitchell, 1956; Hillarp, 1959), to the respiratory apparatus (Larsell, 1922), and to the cornea (Zander and Weddell, 1951). Precise information on the innervation of various organs has been achieved in more recent times with the development of histochemical techniques that demonstrate specific components in nerves. Thus, noradrenaline-containing nerves have been localized by histofluorescence techniques introduced by Falk (1962) and the method has been applied to whole mount preparations of a variety of organs including the iris (Malmfors, 1965), the heart and blood vessels (Falk, 1962; Furness and Malmfors, 1971; Furness, 1971; Sachs, 1970), autonomic ganglia (Costa and Furness, 1973b) and intestine (Costa and Gabella, 1971; Furness and Costa, 1975). Enzymes present in neurons have also been localized in whole mount preparations. The respiratory enzyme NADH: nitro-BT oxidoreductase (EC 1.6.9.3) has been demonstrated in enteric nerve cells in whole mount preparations of the intestinal wall (Gabella, 1969). A combined technique for the localization of noradrenergic nerves and of this enzyme in neuronal cell bodies in the intestine has been developed (Costa and Furness, 1973a). The presence of neurons capable of decarboxylating amino acid precursors into amines has been discovered in the enteric plexuses (Costa *et al.*, 1976; Furness and Costa, 1978) although these nerve cells do not contain any of the known amine transmitter substances (Furness *et al.*, 1980a). The enzymes acetylcholinesterase (EC 3.1.1.7) and monoamine oxidase (EC 1.4.3.4) have been localized in whole mount preparations (Filogamo, 1960; Ellison, 1971; Furness and Costa, 1972; Owman *et al.*, 1974; Stach and Hung, 1979).

With the discovery of small peptides in peripheral nerves (for review see Hökfelt *et al.*, 1980; Furness and Costa, 1980) it was natural to attempt to apply immunohistochemical techniques for the localization of neuropeptides to whole mount preparations also. The first reasonably successful attempts

(Costa *et al.*, 1977; Franco *et al.*, 1979) were followed by the development of a more effective and reliable procedure (Costa *et al.*, 1980a). The use of this technique has proved very useful in investigating the distribution and projections in the guinea-pig intestine of somatostatin-containing neurons (Costa *et al.*, 1980d), of substance P-containing neurons (Costa *et al.*, 1980b, 1981b) and of vasoactive intestinal polypeptide (VIP) containing neurons (Furness and Costa, 1979; Costa *et al.*, 1980c; Furness *et al.*, 1981a) and the distribution of substance P immunoreactive nerves to blood vessels (Furness *et al.*, 1981b), rat iris and cornea (Miller *et al.*, 1981). For a general interpretation of these findings in relation to intestinal function the reader is referred to review articles from this laboratory (Furness and Costa, 1980a,b, 1980b). In this chapter the procedure for immunohistochemical techniques applied to whole mounts, their advantages, their pitfalls, and some of the applications are discussed in detail.

II METHODOLOGY

The principles of immunohistochemistry applied to whole mount preparations do not differ substantially from those of the immunohistochemical techniques applied to tissue sections, and the reader is referred to other chapters in this book. With whole mount preparations additional problems of penetration of antibodies and non-specificity of staining of the background arise because of the thickness of the tissue. The basic steps include the preparation and fixation of the tissue, the incubation with primary and secondary labelled antibodies or other reagents, mounting and examination of the specimens, and photography.

II.1 Preparation of the Tissues

The main aim of this step is to ensure that the tissue is flattened and stretched so that the tissue becomes as thin as possible. The neuropeptides seem to be retained unaltered within the tissue of freshly killed animals allowing the necessary manipulations to occur before fixation without affecting immunohistochemical detection of the peptides. The tissues are placed for dissection in isotonic saline solution at neutral pH; a simple 0.9% NaCl solution at pH 7.3 buffered with 0.01 M sodium phosphate buffer was found to be suitable for dissection for all the neuropeptides investigated in this laboratory.

A sheet of balsa wood of about 3–5 mm thick provides a suitable flat surface onto which the tissue can be gently stretched and pinned flat, either by using normal sewing pins or, for thinner and more delicate tissues, using the different sizes of fine entomology pins. The pins are pushed through the balsa sheet and the emerging tip cut off with pliers. Thin sheets of tissue, such as

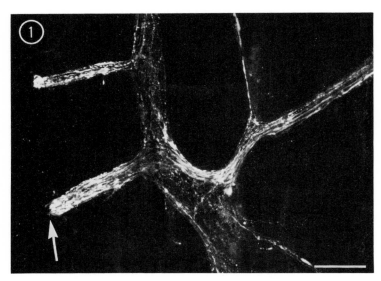

Figure 1 Accumulation of somatostatin-like immunoreactivity in nerves of the guinea-pig myenteric plexus following the crushing of the nerves *in vitro* (arrow). Whole mount preparation of the myenteric plexus attached to the longitudinal muscle. (Bar = 100 μm)

mesentery, pericardium, or iris, only need to be slightly distended flat on the balsa and pinned down, while hollow viscera such as large blood vessels, intestine, stomach, gall bladder, or bladder need first to be cut open and then pinned stretched on the balsa. The way in which the tissue is pinned, either facing up or down, does not appear to affect fixation or the immunohisto-chemical reaction, and tissues as thick as human intestine can be processed in this manner (Figure 2). In order to facilitate the subsequent steps of dis-section, the organs should be slit open at the entrance of their vascular supply,
i.e. for the intestine at the mesenteric border. In order to investigate the effect of drugs *in vitro* the tissue may require incubation in physiological solutions prior to fixation. For instance, incubation of tissues in a Kreb's solution containing colchicine (10^{-5} g/ml) for a few hours facilitates the visualization of neuropeptides in some nerve cell bodies (Costa *et al.*, 1980b). Incubation in Kreb's solution prior to fixation is also necessary when the accumulation of neuropeptides or other neuronal components following the interruption of axonal flow is to be investigated (Figure 1). Application of the procedure of interrupting neuronal pathways *in vitro* can be found in several papers from this laboratory (Costa *et al.*, 1980d; Furness and Costa, 1979, 1981; Furness *et al.*, 1980b; Costa *et al.*, 1981b) in which the direction within

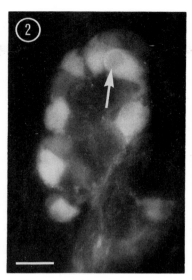

Figure 2 Ganglion in the submucosa of human duodenum showing nerve cell bodies with substance P-like immunoreactivity. The nucleus is visible in focus in one of the neurons (arrow). (Bar = 20 μm)

the intestinal wall of neuronal processes immunoreactive for substance P, VIP, somatostatin, enkephalins, and 5-hydroxytryptamine (5-HT) was established. For incubation before fixation it was found convenient to pin the tissue onto a balsa sheet of a size suitable to fit small pots. In this laboratory 20 mm diameter polyurethane vials, which hold about 20 ml, and are kept at 37 °C in a thermostatically controlled bath, proved adequate for most purposes. The balsa sheets are cut to fit into the vials snugly so that they do not float when placed vertically in the vial.

II.2   Fixation of the Tissues

All immunohistochemistry performed at present in this laboratory is on fixed tissues. The tissues are pinned on balsa sheets and floated face down on the fixative liquids in Petri dishes. After fixation the tissues are removed from the balsa.

Different fixative mixtures have been used in this laboratory: 4% formaldehyde in 0.1 M phosphate buffer pH 7.3; Bouin's fluid; a mixture of 4% formaldehyde and 0.5% glutaraldehyde in 0.1 M phosphate buffer, pH 7.0 (Faglu) (Furness *et al.*, 1977); a picric acid–formaldehyde mixture (Zamboni fixative; Stefanini *et al.*, 1967) and 0.5–2.5% glutaraldehyde in 0.1 M phosphate buffer (pH 7.3). The choice of the optimal fixative was found to depend on the ways in which the tissue was subsequently processed and on the type of substance to be localized. For all the neuropeptides investigated, the best fixative was found to be the formaldehyde–picric acid mixture (Costa *et al.*, 1980a). Formaldehyde alone also gave adequate fixation and retention of antigenicity. A weak neuropeptide immunoreactivity could be detected in tissues fixed with the Faglu mixture only with the best of the antibodies available to us. With Bouin's fluid and glutaraldehyde alone no neuropeptide immunoreactivity could be detected in the tissues studies. However, the formaldehyde–picric acid mixture, which was developed originally to improve the penetration of the fixative in the tissue (see Stefanini *et al.*, 1967), does not preserve the antigenicity of all neuronal substances equally well. Antigenicity of the enzyme DBH was found to be preserved better by formaldehyde than by the picric acid–formaldehyde mixture (unpublished results) and similar results were found for the 5-HT-like immunoreactivity in intestinal nerves (Costa *et al.*, 1982).

If the tissue was allowed to dry on a slide before being fixed, the immunorectivity of neuropeptides was found to be patchy and limited to the most superficial structures. However this procedure was found to be satisfactory for the localization of DBH (Costa *et al.*, 1976). The duration of fixation affects the various substances to be visualized differently. For the neuropeptides fixation in the picric acid–formaldehyde mixture for 18–24 h was found to be optimal, although good immunohistochemical staining can be obtained with as short a fixation time as 4 h. Prolonging the fixation to more than 24 h does not improve the staining. Indeed fixation longer than 24 h begins to impair the immunohistochemical detectability of neuropeptides. For the visualization of 5-HT immunoreactivity, fixation with 4% formaldehyde for 2–3 h was found to be optimal while longer periods impaired the staining (Costa *et al.*, 1981a). In most cases the fixation is carried out near 4°C, particularly with prolonged fixations.

In unfixed tissues processed for immunohistochemistry using the whole mount technique no neuropeptides could be detected. This may be attributed to loss of antigenicity, lack of penetration of the antibody, or excessive non-specific binding of the antibodies with a resulting too high background stain. On the other hand, the enzyme dopamine β-hydroxylase (DBH) could be visualized by immunohistochemistry in whole mount preparations of unfixed blood vessels, atria, intestine, etc. (Costa *et al.*, 1976). The tissues were prepared in thin laminae by opening them and dissecting their different layers apart (see below) and then stretching them on glass slides and allowing them to dry in the laboratory atmosphere (about 18°C and 45% humidity). The appearance of the immunohistochemical localization of the noradrenergic neurons containing DBH was found to be granular and the axons appeared slightly fragmented, probably due to artifacts occurring in the process of drying. It was subsequently found that DBH immunoreactivity in peripheral noradrenergic axons could be visualized better in tissues fixed with 4% formaldehyde.

No attempts have been made in this laboratory to fix the tissues by perfusing the animal and dissecting the tissues. Areas of tissue suitable for the preparation of flat laminae, which are necessary for this method, are rarely encountered in perfused animals. In some cases the tissues to be investigated are already flat *in situ*. The iris (Figure 3) and the cornea are examples, and suitable fixation can be achieved by immersing the whole eyeball into the fixative prior to dissection (Miller *et al.*, 1981).

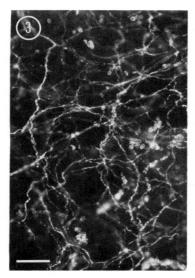

Figure 3   Dense network of substance P immunoreactive nerves in a whole mount of the dilator of the rat iris. (Bar = 50 μm)

II.3   Procedures for Rendering Tissues Permeable to Antibodies

The main difference between tissue sections and whole mount preparations from the immunohistochemistry point of view is that in tissue sections the cells are sectioned and usually frozen and thawed or treated with organic solvents so that their intracellular components are directly exposed to the antibodies. In whole mount preparations, however, most cells have intact membranes that represent barriers to the penetration of antibodies and these must be broken down before intracellular antigens can be visualized. The commonly used methods of permeabilization of membranes for immuno-histochemistry, i.e. freezing and thawing or treatment with detergents (Triton X-100) (see Hartman *et al.*, 1972; Schultzberg *et al.*, 1979) failed to improve the immunohistochemical reactions in whole mount preparations. In most cases the nerves showing neuropeptide immunoreactivity appeared disrupted and fragmented. Following fixation and washing with 0.01 M phosphate buffer solution (PBS) pH 7.3, incubation with antibodies without further processing of the tissue did not produce reliable and effective staining of neuropeptide-containing nerves, although the initial observations of somatostatin immunoreactivity in whole mount preparations of guinea-pig intestine were performed in tissues processed in this manner (Costa *et al.*, 1977).

the most effective way to allow the penetration of the antibodies to localize neuropeptides was found to be the treatment of the fixed tissue with ethanols. After fixation with the picric acid–formaldehyde mixture the tissues are cut free from the pins and the balsa sheet and are placed in 80% ethanol for 15–30 min or until the yellow colour of the picric acid has disappeared. The tissue are then dehydrated further in 95% and two changes of 100% ethanol and cleared in two changes of 100% xylol (15–30 min each change). The tissues are then rehydrated through a descending series of ethanol solutions (100%, 95%, 80%) with changes of 10–30 min, depending on the size and thickness of the tissue, and usually placed in PBS. Although complete dehydration, clearing, and rehydration were found to be optimal for neuropeptides, good results were also obtained with partial dehydration to 80% ethanol before storing in PBS for all neuropeptides studied. The incomplete dehydration procedure was found to be optimal for the immunohistochemical localization of 5-HT. In fact, the 80% ethanol washing is crucial for this substance and at least 10 changes of 10 min each were found necessary to visualize the 5-HT immunoreactivity. Dehydration in ethanol significantly reduces the immunoreactivity of DBH and should be avoided. After formaldehyde fixation and thorough washing in PBS antibodies can penetrate the tissue sufficiently to visualize this enzyme. After these procedures the tissues can be stored in PBS at 4 °C for several days with only a slow loss of immunoreactivity.

II.4   Separation of Tissue Layers (Laminae)

With the exception of thin tissue such as the iris, the pericardium, and the mesentery, most tissues are too thick to serve as single laminae for whole mount preparations without further dissection. Thus, in PBS after storage and before incubation with antisera the different layers of the organs need to be dissected. This procedure varies in difficulty with the nature of the layers and of the organs. Where the layers are well identified and separated by clear cleavage planes, they peel off very easily, as in the intestine. In organs with thick walls such as the heart the separation of thin layers of musculature is more difficult. After trimming the tissue with scissors the dissection is performed with watchmaker's forceps, and a scalpel of necessary, while the tissue is kept in PBS at room temperature. It is important to identify clearly the location and the origins and the orientation the small strips of tissue so prepared for the proper interpretation of the subsequent immunohisto-chemistry. The strips of tissue can be stored in separate containers in PBS until the dissection is completed.

The intestinal wall with its different layers lends itself to the separation of laminae (Furness and Costa, 1978). Following fixation this procedure is very easy but the fixed tissue is more brittle and less elastic than unfixed tissue. The following layers can be prepared from the intestine of the guinea-pig: the longitudinal muscle with the attached myenteric plexus, the circular muscle with the deep muscular plexus, the submucosa, the mucosal glands attached to the muscularis mucosae, and the villi. Because of the excellent penetration of antibodies and the low non-specific staining, laminae containing several layers can also be prepared for the visualization of neuropeptides and 5-HT (Figures 4 and 5). Thus, the circular muscle may be left attached to the longitudinal muscle so that the connections between the myenteric plexus and the muscular plexus could be visualized. The circular muscle can also be left attached to the submucosa and good visualization of some neuropeptides has been achieved in laminae of the longitudinal and circular muscle layers with

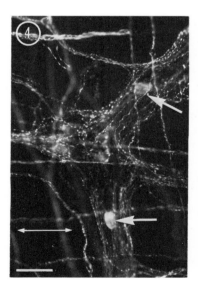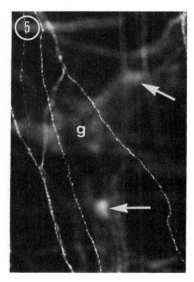

Figures 4 and 5 A thick lamina from the rabbit ileum shown at two levels of focus. The lamina includes the circular muscle (direction indicated by bipointed arrow), the myenteric ganglia (g) and the longitudinal muscle. Substance P Immunoreactive axons are present in all three layers and can be focussed in different planes. Substance P Immunoreactive nerve cell bodies are arrowed. (Bar = 50 μm).

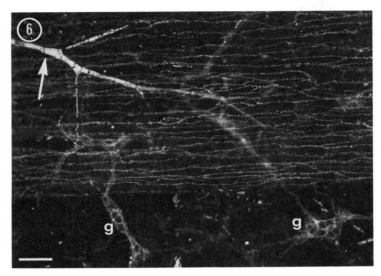

Figure 6 Whole mount preparation of the submucosa of the guinea-pig ileum showing the non-specific fluorescence of red blood cells filling submucous blood vessels (arrow), the ganglia (g) of the submucous plexus with substance P immunoreactive nerve fibres and the dense network of substance P axons in the deep part of the circular muscle attached to the submucosa (upper two-thirds of the preparation). (Bar = 100 μm)

the submucosa (Figure 6). In such preparations the two ganglionated plexuses, the myenteric and the submucous plexuses, can be observed in the same preparation. Similarly the bases of the glands can be left attached to the submucosa after removal of the villi, or the whole mucosa can be separated from the submucosa and these treated as single laminae.

Depending on the tissue, laminae of different sizes can be prepared. The whole width of several centimetres of intestine can be prepared as a lamina so that the projections of enteric neurons along the intestine can be investigated (see for example Furness *et al.*, 1980b).

III IMMUNOHISTOCHEMICAL PROCEDURES

III.1 Incubation with Primary Antisera

Incubation with antibodies is carried out on tissue laminae either in the small wells of disposable plastic serological trays for small 5–10 mm laminae or on glass slides for longer laminae. The laminae are incubated at room temperature in a humid chamber. Simple procedures that give optimal results are described below.

(a) Small laminae up to 1 cm² are dissected and placed on a large drop of PBS in the numbered cells of a disposable plastic serological tray. When all laminae have been placed in the wells, excess PBS is sucked off with thin strips of filter paper ensuring that the laminae do not dry. The plate containing the wells is then placed in a plastic container with a tightly fitting top (the plastic boxes for storage of food in freezers are adequate), and distilled water in the bottom. A support keeps the plates just above the water level. Diluted antiserum, 10–50 µl, is then pipetted over the laminae so that they are completely humid chamber is then sealed shut. The optimal time of incubation has been found to be 15–24 h, i.e. an overnight incubation, at room temperature. Short incubation of 1–3 h produces a much weaker reaction.

(b) If the laminae are several cm long they are placed after dissection onto a glass slide in a large drop of PBS. Before the antiserum is added, excess PBS is removed by filter paper. The slide around the tissue must be well dried so that the antiserum remains localized over the lamina and does not spread too thinly over the slide. The slides are then placed in the humid chamber in a perfectly horizontal position and incubated overnight in the sealed humid chamber.

For most of the antisera that we have used, dilutions from 1 : 150 to 1 : 3000 have been tried and optimal dilutions for most were found to be between 1 : 100 and 1 : 1000. After the incubation with the primary antisera the laminae are transferred to wells or small beakers containing PBS and washed in two or three changes of PBS for 5 min each. If the laminae contain much loose connective or elastic tissue, as do the adventitia of large blood vessels, the washing should be vigorous and more changes of PBS are needed.

III.2 Localization of the First Layer Antibody

III.2.1 *The indirect or sandwich immunofluorescence staining*

The site of binding of the primary antiserum to the substance to be localized can be demonstrated by incubating the tissue with antibodies against the γ-globulin of the species in which the first antiserum was raised according to the indirect immunofluorescence technique (Coons, 1954; Sternberger, 1974). The second layer antibodies are available commercially and are conjugated either with fluorescein isothiocyanate (FITC) which fluoresces green, or with rhodamine, which fluoresces red. Dilutions of the second layer antibodies of 1:40 or 1:80 have proved adequate for the visualization of neuropeptides, DBH and 5-HT. The procedure for incubation of the laminae is identical to that for the first layer antiserum. Incubation for 1 h is adequate for the visualization of the antigenic sites. The tissues are then washed thoroughly in several changes of PBS, the number of changes depending on the size of the tissue, and mounted in a mixture of PBS and glycerol (1 : 1 or 3 : 1) buffered at pH 8.6 (Sternberger, 1974).

Two antigens can be simultaneously localized in whole mount preparations as shown in Figures 18 and 19. The submucous neuron in Figure 18 shows immunoreactivity for somatostatin and is visualized with a second layer FITC labelled antibody, while Figure 19 shows another cell in the same ganglion with immunoreactivity for VIP and is visualized with a rhodamine-labelled second antibody.

III.2.2 *The peroxidase–antiperoxidase (PAP) technique*

Following incubation with the first antibody, the second layer antibody can be used as a bridge for the PAP staining technique (Sternberger, 1974). For this purpose the bridging antibody (which can still be labelled with FITC or rhodamine if desired) must be used at lower dilutions, i.e. at 1 : 4, 1 : 20, or 1 : 100. (If FITC or rhodamine-conjugated antibodies are used, the laminae can be temporarily mounted in buffered glycerol after this 1 h incubation to check with the fluorescence microscope whether the immunohistochemical reaction had occurred and unmounted again into PBS for subsequent processing.) The laminae are incubated for a further hour in a 1 : 40 dilution of PAP antiserum at room temperature, then washed in PBS three times for 5 min and transferred to 0.1 M Tris–HCl buffer, pH 7.2. The laminae are subsequently incubated with freshly prepared mixture of 4 chloro-1-naphthol- and H_2O_2 until the immunoreactive sites became visible (see Nakane, 1968). The preparations are then washed in distilled water several times (3×5 min at least) and mounted in pure glycerol (Figure 7).

III.3 Mounting the Tissue

The mounting of laminae preparations is a critical step since variations in thickness or folding of the laminae severely impair the microscopic observations and the photography. The laminae are placed on clean microscope slides in small drops of mounting medium and slightly stretched. A minimum amount of mounting medium should be used so that the capillary action of the medium between the slide and the coverslip flattens the laminae. Care should be taken to avoid the formation of air bubbles remaining trapped over or around the tissue.

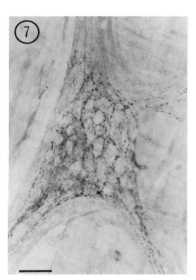

Figure 7 Somatostatin immunoreactivity in a myenteric ganglion of the guinea-pig colon demonstrated with the peroxidase–antiperoxidase technique. Varicose immunoreactive axons form pericellular endings around non-immunoreactive myenteric nerve cell bodies. (Bar = 50 μm)

III.4 Non-specific Staining

Non-specific binding represents a problem for immunohistochemical techniques in whole mount preparations even more than in tissue sections. In the laminae preparation it was found that with most antisera raised against neuropeptides the background was too high to be able to identify the specific antigenic sites unless the tissue had been fixed and treated with ethanol. The passage through various strengths of ethanols significantly reduces the non-specific staining. As yet, we have no explanation for this phenomenon.

The use of a primary antiserum raised in the same species as that under investigation poses problems of binding of the second layer antibodies to all γ-globulins of the tissue studied, not only to the γ-globulins which are bound specifically to the antigen under study. It is necessary therefore to absorb the second antiserum with a source of proteins that includes γ-globulins from the species studied. The commercially available liver powders are adequate in most circumstances. For example, in order to visualize substance P in rat by using anti-substance P antiserum raised in rats the laminae are first incubated with this antiserum and then with the second layer fluorescent labelled anti-rat γ-globulin which has been preincubated with rat liver powder. The final tests of specificity encompassed all the standard procedures including the absorption of the primary antiserum with the antigen and omission of the first layer antibody in the procedure or its replacement with pre-immune or non-immune serum (see Chapter 1 for specificity criteria).

IV   MICROSCOPY OF WHOLE MOUNT PREPARATIONS

Fluorescence or conventional white light microscopy are used for the observation and photography of immunoreactivity in whole mount preparations, depending on whether the indirect immunofluorescent or PAP technique are used. Most of the problems which are peculiar to whole mount preparations, either in the analysis or in the photography of the specimens, arise from the thickness of the tissue which contains several layers of intact cells. The immunoreactive nerve fibres are arranged in the three dimensions within the laminae and at high magnification many of them always appear out of focus (Figure 8). This difficulty can be ameliorated by using lower-power

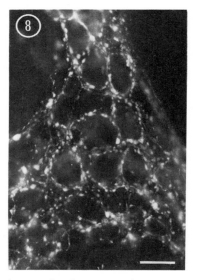

Figure 8   High-power micrograph of a myenteric ganglion of the guinea-pig colon showing a dense network of substance P immunoreactive varicose axons around non-immunoreactive ganglion cells. (Bar = 20 μm)

objectives with longer depth of focus. For example, most VIP immunoreactive axons in the preparation of longitudinal muscle–myenteric plexus shown in Figure 9 appear in focus in the low magnification photomicrograph, while at high magnification many axons are out of the plane of focus (Figure 10).

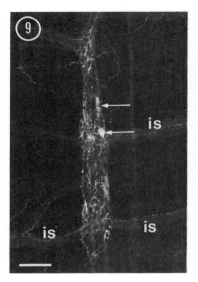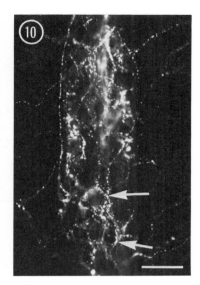

Figure 9 Low-power micrograph of a ganglion of the myenteric plexus of the guinea-pig ileum showing VIP immunoreactive nerves. Two VIP immunoreactive nerve cell bodies are visible (arrows). is: internodal strands. (Bar = 100 μm)

Figure 10 Higher magnification of a myenteric ganglion in the guinea-pig ileum showing VIP immunoreactive nerves which form a loose network within the ganglion with some varicose axons arranged as pericellular baskets (arrow). (Bar = 50 μm)

V   DISADVANTAGES OF IMMUNOHISTOCHEMISTRY ON WHOLE MOUNT PREPARATIONS

There are some disadvantages in the use of whole mount preparations and investigators must be fully aware of them to avoid misinterpreting the results. With the exception of those tissues that can be prepared as single-sheet laminae the separation of layers or strips from thicker tissues represents a disruption of the tissue, particularly at the interface between layers. Often these cleavage planes follow the connective tissue. Therefore, after stripping, the collagen and elastic fibres may remain loosely arranged at the surface of the lamina, they can easily trap labelled antibodies and can therefore be mistaken for fine nerve fibres.

It is difficult to predict how effectively antibodies will penetrate different tissues. Therefore, any unsuccessful staining with a particular antiserum in a tissue investigated for the first time cannot be regarded as conclusive evidence that the tissue antigen under investigation is not present in the tissue. Often the non-specific background staining in a thick tissue may mask very faint

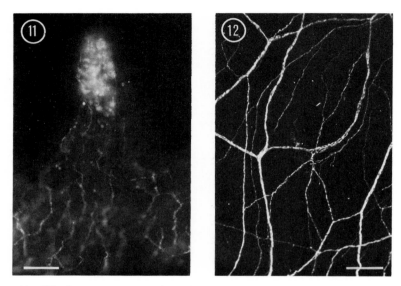

Figure 11   Whole mount preparation of a villus from the guinea-pig ileum showing a delicate subepithelial plexus of substance P, immunoreactive nerves. Non-specific fluorescence is present in cells at the apex of the villus. (Bar = 100 μm)

Figure 12   Substance P immunoreactive nerves running singly or in small bundles in the guinea-pig pericardium. (Bar = 200 μm)

immunoreactive staining. Since the laminae are several cell layers thick, there may be problems in identifying immunoreactive cells masked by overlying structures that are stained non-specifically or that possess autofluorescence. For instance, the delicate subepithelial network of substance P immunoreactive axons in the intestinal villi is partially masked by non-specific autofluorescent granules in the epithelium (Figure 11). Similar problems may arise in the identification of weakly immunoreactive nerve cell bodies embedded in the thickness of the laminae. Often the fluorescence of the cytoplasm may mask the non-immunoreactive nucleus. Many of these drawbacks can be overcome by fine focussing through the thickness of the preparation.

The major limitations of the use of whole mount preparations are the ones which led the histologists of last century to seek a method for cutting thin sections in different planes by using embedding techniques. The whole mount preparations are arranged in one plane only, and it is often difficult to achieve a full understanding of the three-dimensional arrangement of the cells in the tissue and particularly of nerve networks. The whole mount technique should therefore be used, whenever possible, in conjunction with immunohisto-chemistry in tissue sections.

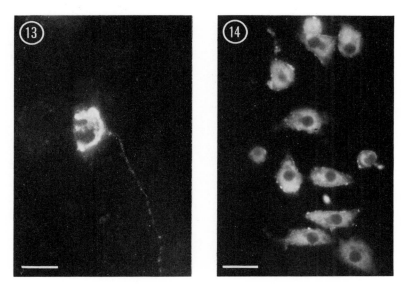

Figure 13 Single nerve cell body with single process immunoreactive for somatostatin in the myenteric plexus of the rat small intestine. Note that the immunoreactivity is concentrated in perinuclear clumps. (Bar = 20 μm)

Figure 14 Primary culture of bovine adrenal medulla cells stained with anti-leu enkephalin antiserum. (Bar = 20 μm)

VI ADVANTAGES AND APPLICATIONS OF IMMUNOHISTOCHEMISTRY ON WHOLE MOUNT PREPARATIONS

The extensive information that has been gained since last century in the study of both somatic and visceral nerves by using whole mount preparations is in itself the best indication of the usefulness of this method. It is therefore not surprising that immunohistochemical techniques applied to whole mount preparations are proving extremely useful in investigating the distribution in various organs of antigenic substances present in nerves. The main advantages can easily be identified:

(a) Large areas of tissue can be studied and the pattern of distribution of immunoreactive cells can be easily detected without the need for reconstructions from serial sections.

Thin tissues, such as the iris, the pericardium (Figure 12) and the mesentery lend themselves to this type of investigation. Immunohistochemistry on whole mount preparations has allowed the determination of the relative proportions of various classes of nerve cell bodies in the

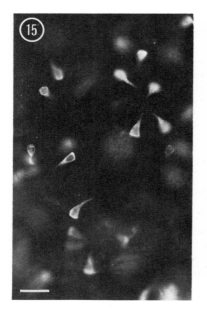 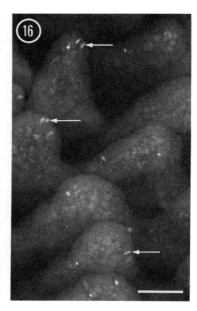

Figure 15 Enterochromaffin cells in the submucosa of the guinea-pig ileum, showing 5-HT immunoreactivity. Many cells are in different planes of focus. (Bar = 30 μm)

Figure 16 Whole mount preparation of the mucosa of the guinea-pig small intestine showing several somatostatin immunoreactive endocrine cells (arrows). (Bar = 200 μm)

enteric plexuses. Not only have the proportions of the total number of neurons containing each substance been investigated (substance P: Costa *et al.*, 1980b; somatostatin: Costa *et al.*, 1977; vasoactive intestinal polypeptide: Costa *et al.*, 1980c; enkephalin: Furness and Costa, 1980; and 5-HT-like indolamine: Costa *et al.*, 1981a), but from the morphology of the neurons and the distribution of their processes it was possible to conclude that they represent separate populations of enteric neurons. The ability to scan large areas of tissue provided by the whole mount technique has been essential for detecting the changes in the number and pattern of distribution of immunoreactive nerves following micro-operations. Thus it has been possible to establish the direction and the lengths of the processes of various classes of enteric neurons. Thus the projections of somatostatin, substance P, VIP, enkephalin, and 5-HT-like containing neurons could be determined in the guinea-pig intestine (Furness and Costa, 1979; Costa *et al.*, 1980d, 1981a,b; Furness *et al.*, 1980b, 1981a; Furness and Costa, 1981).

(b) Another advantage of whole mounts is that the immunoreactive struc-

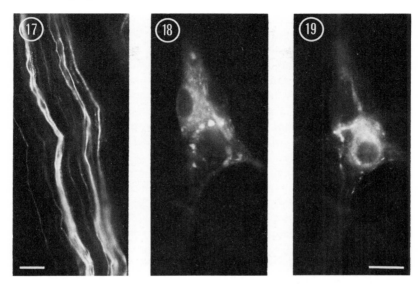

Figure 17 Small bundles of the vagus nerve showing substance P immunoreactive axons. (Bar = 20 μm)

Figures 18 and 19 Double staining of submucous neurons in the guinea-pig small intestine. Figure 18 shows a nerve cell body and varicose nerve fibre showing somatostatin immunoreactivity stained in green with FITC-labelled second antibody. Figure 19 shows the same ganglion as Figure 18, showing VIP immunoreactive nerve cell body and varicose nerve fibres stained in red with rhodamine-labelled second antibody. Note that the neuropeptides are localized in separate neurons. (Bar = 20 μm)

tures can be studied throughout the thickness of the tissue and even the three-dimensional arrangements of immunoreactive neurons can be established (see Figures 4, 5 , and 6), since the laminae are much thicker than routine histological sections and contain several cell layers or often several layers of tissue from an organ. Also since entire cells are embedded in the thickness of whole mount preparations their morphological appearance can be determined at a single glance and neuronal processes can be easily identified (Figure 13).

(c) Also worthy of mention is the advantage of the simplicity of procedure compared with that for routine histological or cryostat sections. As a result large numbers of observations or experimental tissues can be performed without lengthy and time-consuming preparative procedures.

The whole mount method is of course not restricted to the study of nerve tissue. In principle any tissue antigen could be investigated in whole mount preparations and there is no doubt that it will be used in the future for a variety of purposes. One of the potentially highly rewarding applications is the study of substances in endocrine cells, particularly those which are scattered in tissues, such as the endocrine cells in the intestinal mucosa. Figure 15 shows, for example, how the 5-HT-immunoreactive enterochromaffin cells in the intestinal mucosa appear in whole mount preparation of the base of the glands. Figure 16 shows even more dramatically th this immunohistochemical technique. The whole intestinal mucosa has been stained with antisomatostatin antiserum and prepared as whole mount with a good three-dimensional effect of the villi, with endocrine cells which contain somatostatin easily visible.

The application of these methods is not restricted to investigations on tissue laminae. The presence of specifically immunoreactive nerve fibres in nerve trunks can easily be demonstrated by teasing out small bundles and processing them in whole mounts (Figure 17).

The procedure for immunohistochemistry on whole mount preparations can be easily applied to tissue-cultured cells. Figure 14, for instance, shows bovine adrenal cells in culture stained with antiserum raised against enkephalin. Suitable modifications to the immunohistochemical procedure were adopted. The cells were cultured on coverslips which could be easily removed and processed. Fixation was briefer, 2–4 h instead of overnight. A brief wash in 80% ethanol (4 × 5 min) before returning to PBS avoided detachment of the cells from the slide and ensured adequate antibody penetration. The dilution of the antiserum may also need to be adjusted to the cultured preparation. In the case described the antiserum was diluted 5-fold more than that used for the staining of laminae of tissues.

Our experience has been that different antigens and different tissue preparations require different treatments for optimal immunohistochemical detection. It is therefore advised that the basic procedure be varied in any novel situation.

With a full awareness of its advantages and disadvantages, the marriage between immunohistochemistry and whole mount preparation is likely to provide invaluable information in many immunohistochemical problems. Appendix 1 summarizes some of the techniques for immunohistochemistry applied to whole mount preparations.

ACKNOWLEDGEMENTS

We would like to thank the following colleagues for the provision of antisera: A. Arimura, O. Crivelli, A. C. Cuello, R. Elde, P. Emson, R. L. Eskey, J. Martin, R. J. Miller, J. Oliver, Y. Patel, S. Said, H. W. M. Steinbusch, A. J. Verhofstad, and J. H. Walsh. We are grateful for the excellent technical help from Venetta Esson and Pat Vilimas. We would like to thank Dr Ida Llewellyn-Smith for her useful criticisms of the manuscript, and to express appreciation to our colleagues who have participated in the development of the application of immunohistochemical techniques to whole mounts: Neil Della, Rony Franco, Ida Llewellyn-Smith, Andrew Miller, and Ray Papka. This work has been supported by grants from the Australian Research Grant Committee and from the National Health and Medical Research Council.

APPENDIX 1
PROTOCOL FOR IMMUNOHISTOCHEMISTRY IN WHOLE MOUNTS

(a) *Peptides immunofluorescence*
  (1) Pin the tissue flat on to a sheet of balsa wood.
  (2) Fix in picric acid–formaldehyde mixture (Zamboni's) at 4°C for 18 h.
  (3) Remove tissue from balsa.
  (4) Wash in 80% ethanol until clear of picric acid.
  (5) Dehydrate in 95% then 100% ethanol (30 min each).
  (6) Clear in 100% xylol (30 min).
  (7) Rehydrate through 100%, 80%, 50% ethanol (30 min each) toapbs.
  (8) If necessary store in PBS at 4°C.
  (9) Dissect different layers if necessary.
  (10) Incubate the thin laminae in diluted antiserum overnight at room temperature in a humid chamber.
  (11) Wash in PBS (3 × 5 min).
  (12) Incubate in FITC or rhodamine-labelled second layer antiserum at room temperature for 1 h (dilutions 1:10 to 1:80).
  (13) Wash in PBS.
  (14) Mount in PBS:glycerol (1:1 or 3:1) buffered at pH 8.6.

(b) *Peptides PAP immunohistochemistry*
  (1) to (11) as in method (a)
  (12) Incubate in second layer antiserum at room temperature for 1 h (dilutions 1:4 to 1:40). This second antibody can be labelled as in (a)12 and the tissue temporarily mounted and observed at the fluorescence microscope before proceeding.
  (13) Wash in PBS (3 × 5 min).
  (14) Incubate in peroxidase–antiperoxidase antiserum, 1:40 for 1 h at room temperature.
  (15) Wash in PBS (3 × 5 min).
  (16) Incubate in freshly prepared 4 chloro-1-naphthol–H_2O_2 mixture until immunoreactive sites are visible.
  (17) Wash in distilled water (3 × 5 min).
  (18) Mount in pure glycerol.

(c) *5-HT immunofluorescence*
 (1) Pin the tissue flat onto a sheet of balsa wood.
 (2) Fix in 4% formaldehyde for 2 h at 4 °C.
 (3) Remove tissue from balsa.
 (4) Wash in 80% ethanol (6 × 10 min).
 (5) If necessary store in PBS.
 (6) Dissect the tissue in thin laminae if necessary.
 (7) Incubate tissue in diluted antiserum overnight in a humid chamber.
 (8) Wash in PBS (3 × 5 min).
 (9) Incubate in FITC-labelled second layer antiserum at room temperature for 1 h.
 (10) Wash in PBS (3 × 5 min).
 (11) Mount in PBS:glycerol as in (a)14.

(d) *Dopamine β-hydroxylase immunofluorescence*
 (1) Pin the tissue flat onto a sheet of balsa wood.
 (2) Fix in 4% formaldehyde for 2 h.
 (3) Remove tissue from balsa.
 (4) Wash tissue in PBS overnight.
 (5) Dissect layers if necessary.
 (6) Incubate in dilute anti-DBH antiserum overnight at room temperature in a humid chamber.
 (7) Wash in PBS (3 × 5 min).
 (8) Incubate in FITC-labelled second layer antiserum for 1 h at room temperature.
 (9) Wash in PBS (3 × 5 min).
 (10) Mount in PBS:glycerol as in (a)14.

REFERENCES

Busch, E. (1929). *Studies on the Nerves of the Blood Vessels with Especial Reference to Periarterial Sympathectomy*, Levin & Munsgaard, Copenhagen.

Coons, A. H. (1954). 'Fluorescent antibody methods.' In Danielli, J. F. (ed.), *General Cytochemical Methods*, pp. 399–422. Academic Press, New York.

Costa, M., Buffa, R., Furness, J. B., and Solcia, E. L. (1980a). 'Immunohistochemical localization of polypeptides in peripheral autonomic nerves using whole mount preparations.' *Histochemistry*, **65**, 157–165.

Costa, M., Cuello, A. C., Furness, J. B., and Franco, R. (1980b). 'Distribution of enteric neurons showing immunoreactivity for substance P in the guinea-pig ileum.' *Neuroscience*, **5**, 323–331.

Costa, M. and Furness, J. B. (1973a). 'The simultaneous demonstration of adrenergic fibres and enteric ganglion cells.' *Histochem. J.*, **5**, 343–349.

Costa, M. and Furness, J. B. (1973b). 'Observations on the anatomy and amine histochemistry of the nerves and ganglia which supply the pelvic viscera and on the associated chromaffin tissue in the guinea-pig.' *Z. Anat. Entwick-Gesch.*, **140**, 85–108.

Costa, M., Furness, J. B., Buffa, R., and Said, S. I. (1980c). 'Distribution of enteric nerve cell bodies and axons showing immunoreactivity for vasoactive intestinal polypeptide (VIP) in the guinea-pig intestine.' *Neuroscience*, **5**, 587–596.

Costa, M., Furness, J. B., Cuello, A. C., Verhofstad, A. A. J., Steinbusch, H. W. W., and Elde, R. P. (1982). 'Neurons with 5-hydroxytryptamine-like immunoreactivity in the enteric nervous system; their visualization and reactions to drug treatment.' *Neuroscience*, **7**, 351–363.

Costa, M., Furness, J. B., Llewellyn-Smith, I. J., and Cuello, A. C. (1981). 'Projections of substance P neurons within the guinea-pig small intestine.' *Neuroscience*, **6**, 411–424.

Costa, M., Furness, J. B., Llewellyn-Smith, I. J., Davies, B., and Oliver, J. (1980d). 'An immunohistochemical study of the projections of somatostatin containing neurons in the guinea-pig intestine.' *Neuroscience*, **5**, 841–851.

Costa, M., Furness, J. B., and McLean, J. R. (1976). 'The presence of aromatic 1-amino acid decarboxylase in certain intestinal nerve cells.' *Histochemistry*, **48**, 129–143.

Costa, M. and Gabella, G. (1971). 'Adrenergic innervation of the alimentary canal.' *Z. Zellforsch.*, **122**, 357–377.

Costa, M., Patel, Y., Furness, J. B., and Arimura, A. (1977). 'Evidence that some intrinsic neurons of the intestine contain somatostatin.' *Neurosci. Lett.*, **6**, 215–222.

Costa, M., Rush, R. A., Furness, J. B., and Geffen, L. B. (1976). 'Histochemical evidence for the degeneration of peripheral noradrenergic axons following intravenous injection of antibodies to dopamine β-hydroxylase.' *Neurosci. Lett.*, **3**, 201–207.

Dogiel, A. S. (1899a). 'Über den Bau der Ganglion in den Geflechten des Darmes und der Gallenblase des Menschen und der Säugethiere.' *Arch. Anat. Physiol. Anat.*, pp. 130–158.

Dogiel, S. A. (1899b). 'Die sensiblen Nervenendigungen im Herzen, und in der Blutgefässen der Säugethiere.' *Arch. Mikrosk. Anat.*, **57**, 44–70.

Ellison, J. P. (1971). 'Cholinesterase-positive and catecholamine containing nerves in the guinea-pig pericardium.' *Am. J. Anat.*, **131**, 121–132.

Erlich, P. (1886). 'Über die Methylenblau reaktion der lebenden Nervensubstang.' *Deutsch Med. Wschr.*, **12**, 49–52.

Falk, B. (1962). 'Observations on the possibilities of the cellular localization of monoamines by a fluorescence method.' *Acta Physiol. Scand.*, **56** (Suppl. 197), 19–25.

Filogamo, G. (1960). 'Il plesso di Auerbach nella stenosi sperimentale dell'intestino studiato con il metado di Koelle per l'AChe nel coniglio.' *Giornale dell' Accademia de Medicina di Torino*, Fasc. **7–12**, 1–7.

Franco, R., Costa, M., and Furness, J. B. (1979). 'Evidence for the release of endogenous substance P from intestinal nerves.' *Naunyn-Schmied. Arch. Pharmacol.*, **306**, 195–201.

Furness, J. .B. (1971). 'The adrenergic innervation of the vessels supplying and draining the gastrointestinal tract.' *Z. Zellforsch.*, **113**, 67–82.

Furness, J. B. and Costa, M. (1972). 'Monoamine oxidase histochemistry of enteric neurones in the guinea-pig.' *Histochemie*, **28**, 324–336.

Furness, J. B. and Costa, M. (1975). 'The use of glyoxylic acid for the fluorescence histochemical demonstration of peripheral stores of noradrenaline and 5-hydroxytryptamine in whole mounts.' *Histochemistry*, **41**, 335–352.

Furness, J. B. and Costa, M. (1978) 'Distribution of intrinsic nerve cell bodies and axons which take up aromatic amines and their precursors in the small intestine of the guinea-pig.' *Cell Tissue Res.*, **188**, 527–543.

Furness, J. B. and Costa, M. (1979). 'Projections of intestinal neurons showing immunoreactivity for vasoactive intestinal polypeptide are consistent with these neurons being the enteric inhibitory neurons.' *Neurosci. Lett.*, **15**, 199–204.

Furness, J. B. and Costa, M. (1980). 'Types of nerves in the enteric nervous system.' *Neuroscience*, **5**, 1–21.

Furness, J. B. and Costa, M. (1982). 'Neurons with 5-hydroxytryptamine-like immunoreactivity in the enteric nervous system: their projections in the guinea-pig small intestine.' *Neuroscience*, **7**, 341–349.

Furness, J. B., Costa, M., and Howe, P. R. C. (1980a). 'Intrinsic amine-handling neurons in the intestine.' In Eranko, O. *et al.* (eds), *Histochemistry, Cell Biology of Autonomic Neurons, SIF cell and Paraneurons*. Raven Press, New York. pp. 367–372.

Furness, J. B., Costa, M., Llewellyn-Smith, I. J., and Franco, R. (1980b). 'Neuronal peptides in the intestine: distribution and possible functions.' *Adv. Biochem. Psychopharmacol.*, **5**, 601–617.

Furness, J. B. and Malmfors, T. (1971). 'Aspects of the arrangement of the adrenergic innervation in guinea-pig as revealed by the fluorescence histochemical method applied to stretched, air-dried preparations.' *Histochemie*, **25**, 297–309.

Furness, J. B., Costa, M., and Walsh, J. H. (1981a). 'Evidence for and significance of the projections of VIP neurons from the myenteric plexus to the taenia coli in the guinea-pig.' *Gastroenterology*, **80**, 1557–1561.

Furness, J. B., Costa, M., and Wilson, A. J. (1977). 'Water Stable fluorophores produced by reaction with aldehyde solutions, for the histochemical localization of catechol- and idolethylamines.' *Histochemistry*, **52**, 159–170.

Furness, J. B., Papka, R. E., Della, N. G., Costa, M., and Eskay, R. L. (1981b). 'Substance P-like immunoreactivity in nerves associated with the vascular system of guinea-pigs.' *Neuroscience*, **7**, 447–459.

Gabella, G. (1969). 'Detection of nerve cells by a histochemical technique.' *Experientia*, **25**, 218–219.

Hartman, B. K., Zide, D., and Udenfriend, S. (1972). 'The use of dopamine β-hydroxylase as a marker for the noradrenergic pathways of the central nervous system in the rat.' *Proc. Natl. Acad. Sci. USA*, **69**, 2722–2726.

Hill, C. J. (1927). 'A contribution to our knowledge of the enteric plexuses.' *Phil. Trans. Roy. Soc.*, **215**, 355–387.

Hillarp, N.-A. (1959). 'The construction and functional organization of the autonomic innervation apparatus.' *Acta Physiol. Scand.*, **46** (Suppl. 157), 1–38.

Hökfelt, T., Johansson, O., Ljungdahl, A., Lundberg, J. M., and Schultzberg, M. (1980). 'Peptidergic neurons.' *Nature*, **284**, 515–521.

Huber, G. C. (1899). 'Observations on the innervation of the intracranial vessels.' *J. Comp. Neurol.*, **9**, 1–25.

Larsell, O. (1922). 'The ganglia, plexuses, and nerve terminations of the mammalian lung and pleura pulmonalis.' *J. Comp. Neurol.*, **35**, 97–132.

Malmfors, T. (1965). 'Studies on adrenergic nerves.' *Acta Physiol. Scand.* **64**, (Suppl. 248), 1–93.

Meissner, G. (1857). 'Uber die Nerven der Darmwand.' *Z. Rationelle Med.*, **8**, 364–366.

Miller, A., Costa, M., Furness, J. B., and Chubb, I. W. (1981). 'Substance P immunoreactive sensory nerves supply the rat iris and cornea.' *Neurosci. Lett.* **23**, 243–249.

Mitchell, G. A. G. (1956). *Cardiovascular Innervation*. E. & S. Livingstone, Edinburgh and London.

Nakane, P. K. (1968). 'Simultaneous localization of multiple tissue antigens using the peroxidase labeled antibody method: a study on pituitary gland of the rat.' *J. Histochem. Cytochem.*, **16**, 557–560.

Owman, Ch., Edvinsson, L., and Nielsen, K. C. (1974). 'Autonomic neuroreceptor mechanisms in brain vessels.' In Fuxe, K., Olson, L., and Zotterman, Y. (eds), *Dynamics of Degeneration and Growth in Neurons*, pp. 535–560. Pergamon Press, Oxford and New York.

Rintoul, J. R. (1960). 'The comparative morphology of the enteric nerve plexuses.' Ph.D. thesis, University of St Andrews.

Sachs, C. (1970). 'Noradrenaline uptake mechanisms in the mouse atrium. A biochemical and histochemical study.' *Acta Physiol. Scand.* (Suppl. 341), 1–67.

Schabadasch, A. (1930a). 'Die Nerven des Magen der Katze.' *Z. Zellforsch. Mikroscop. Anat.*, **10**, 254–319.

Schabadasch, A. (1930b). 'Intramurale Nervengeflechte des Darmohrs.' *Z. Zellforsch. Mikroscop. Anat.*, **10**, 320–385.

Schultzberg, M., Hökfelt, T., Terenius, L., Elfvin, L.-G., Lundberg, J. M., Brandt, J., Elde, R. P., and Goldstein, M. (1979). 'Enkephalin immunoreactive nerve fibre and cell bodies in sympathetic ganglia of the guinea-pig and rat.' *Neuroscience*, **4**, 249–270.

Stach, W. (1971). 'Über die in der Dickdarmwand aszendierenden Nerven des Plexus pelvinus und die Grenze der vagalen und sakralparasympathischen Innervation', *Z. Mikrosk. Anat. Forsch.*, **84**, 65–90.

Stach, W. and Hung, N. (1979). 'Zur Innervation der Dünndarmschleimhaut von Laboratoriumstieren. I. Architektur, lichtmikroskopische Struktur und histochemische Differenzierung.' *Z. Mikrosk. Anat. Forsch.*, **93**, 876–887.

Stefanini, M., De Martino, C., and Zamboni, L. (1967). 'Fixation of ejaculated spermatozoa for electron microscopy.' *Nature (Lond.)*, **26**, 173–174.

Sternberger, L. A. (1974). *Immunocytochemistry*. Prentice-Hall, Englewood Cliffs, New Jersey.

Taxi, J. (1965). 'Contribution à l'étude des connexions des neurones moteurs du système nerveux autonome.' *Ann. des Sc. Nat. Zool.*, 12 ser, **7**, 413–674.

Zander, E. and Weddell, G. (1951). 'Observations on the innervation of the cornea.' *J. Anat. (Lond.)*, **85**, 68–99.

Immunohistochemistry
Edited by A. C. Cuello
© 1983 IBRO

CHAPTER 15

Immunohistochemistry and Immunocytochemistry of Neural Cell Types *in vitro* and *in situ*

M. SCHACHNER

Department of Neurobiology, University of Heidelberg, Im Neuenheimer Feld 504, 6900 Heidelberg 1, Fed. Rep. Germany

ABBREVIATIONS

BME	basal medium Eagle's
CMF	calcium and magnesium free
DAB	3,3'-diaminobenzidine · 4HCl
DPBS	Dulbecco's modified phosphate buffered saline
Fab'	fragment antibody binding
FITC	fluorescein isothiocyanate
GAM	goat anti-mouse immunoglobulin
GAR	goat anti-rabbit immunoglobulin
GFA	glial fibrillary acidic
HBSS	Hanks' balanced salt solution
HRPO	horseradish peroxidase
Ig	immunoglobulin
NS1	myeloma P3-NS1/1-Ag4-1
PBS	phosphate buffered saline
RAM	rabbit anti-mouse immunoglobulin
SAM	sheep anti-mouse immunoglobulin
TRITC	tetramethyl rhodamine isothiocyanate

I INTRODUCTION

Crucial to the investigation of cell–cell interactions in the nervous system is the availability of cell-type-specific markers which can be recognized by immunological reagents. These reagents would not only identify the particular cell types at various developmental stages, but also lead to the isolation of homogeneous cell populations or specific elimination of particular cell types *in situ* and *in vitro*.

In this chapter I wish to focus on the strategies and techniques that have led to the definition and characterization of cell-type-specific immunological probes, both in the intact tissue and in monolayer cultures of dissociated neural cells. Table 1 presents a list of markers that have been used in the author's laboratory. For a demonstration of strategies and techniques, the immunocytochemical analysis of monoclonal antibodies to cell surface constituents of oligodendrocytes will be discussed.

II IMMUNOCYTOCHEMICAL CHARACTERIZATION OF MONOCLONAL ANTIBODIES TO CELL SURFACES OF OLIGODENDROGLIA

II.1 Immunizations

BALB/c female mice (4–6 weeks old) were injected with homogenate of white matter dissected from corpus callosum of bovine brain. Homogenates were prepared from fresh tissue pieces at 0 °C. One gram of tissue was homogenized with 1 ml physiological saline in a Sorvall ultrasonicator set at

Table 1 List of immunologically detectable markers for neural cell types

Marker	Astroglial	Oligodendroglial	Neuronal	References
GFA protein	+			Eng et al. (1971) Bignami et al. (1972) Schachner et al. (1977b)
Vimentin	+			Franke et al. (1978) Paetau et al. (1979a) Schnitzer et al. (1980)
C1 antigen	+			Sommer et al. (1980)
M1 antigen	+			Lagenaur et al. (1980)
Corpus callosum antigen	+	+		Schachner et al. (1977a) Campbell et al. (1977)
NS-1 antigen		+		Schachner (1974) Schachner and Willinger (1979b)
Galactocerebroside		+		Schachner and Willinger (1979a,b) Raff et al. (1978)
O1 to O4 antigens		+		Sommer and Schachner (1980) Schachner et al. (1980)
NS-4 antigen			+	Schachner et al. (1975) Schachner and Willinger (1979a) Rohrer and Schachner (1980)
Tetanus toxin receptors			+	Dimpfel et al. (1977) Mirsky et al. (1978) Schachner and Willinger (1979a)

7.5, twice for 30 s (Schachner *et al.*, 1977a). Mice received seven subcutaneous injections at intervals of 2–4 weeks. Injections were placed at
several sites, in the neck region, on the back, and under the stomach. The
first injection was made with homogenate without adjuvant, the second with
complete Freund's adjuvant and 15 mg protein of homogenate in 0.5 ml
phosphate buffered saline (PBS), pH 7.3. Care was taken to obtain by
ultrasonication an emulsion of solid, almost stiff consistency. Subsequent
injections were made subcutaneously without adjuvant and with the same
amount of homogenate as the first two injections. The last injection was done
intraperitoneally 2 weeks after the previous injection, also with 15 mg protein
of homogenate in 0.5 ml PBS (for immunization of small rodents see also
Chapter 9). Three days after the last injection mice were sacrificed, their
spleen removed under sterile conditions and splenocytes recovered by
mincing the spleen with curved scissors and trituration of small tissue pieces at
room temperature in PBS with a Pasteur pipette. Tissue pieces were allowed
to settle for 5 min. Single spleen cells were collected from the supernatant by
centrifugation at 200 *g* for 5 min at room temperature and washed twice in
Dulbecco's PBS (DPBS). One million to two million splenocytes were usually
recovered from one spleen.

II.2   Cell Fusion and Cloning Procedures (see also Chapter 9)

Myeloma P3-NS1/1-Ag4-1 (NS1) cells were maintained in RPM I-1640
culture medium containing 10% fetal calf serum, 1.35 mg/l amphotericin,
200 mg/l streptomycin, 2 mM glutamine, and 2×10^{-5} M β-mercaptoethanol
in a humidified CO_2 incubator with 5% CO_2 and 95% air at 37 °C (Lagenaur
et al., 1980). Cell fusion with logarithmically growing NS1 myeloma cells and
washed splenocytes from immunized mice was carried out by a modification
of the methods of Lemke *et al.* (1978) and Galfré *et al.* (1977) as described by
Lagenaur *et al.* (1980). Myeloma cells were washed twice in DPBS by
centrifugation at 120 *g* for 5 min at room temperature. Washed myeloma cells
(2×10^7) and splenocytes (1×10^8) were then centrifuged together at 120 *g*
for 5 min at room temperature. The spleen cell–myeloma pellet was gently
and only partially resuspended in 1.5 ml DPBS containing 41.3% polyethylene glycol PEG 4000 (Roth, Karlsruhe, Fed. Rep. Germany) and 8.5%
dimethylsulphoxide (v/v) and gently shaken for exactly 1 min at 37 °C in a
water bath. Ten millilitres of DPBS were then added at room temperature in
a dropwise fashion, also under gentle shaking. The cell suspension was then
quickly transferred to a centrifuge and centrifuged at 120 *g* for 5 min at room
temperature. The pellet was resuspended in 4.5 ml of NS1 culture medium.
Cells were distributed among 48 wells of Linbro culture dishes (Greiner,
Nürtingen, Fed. Rep. Germany), each containing 0.5 ml of prewarmed NS1
culture medium. Cultures were fed daily starting 1 day after the fusion by

replacing the culture medium with HAT selective medium (Littlefield, 1964). Hybrid growth was detectable 5 to 10 days after fusion. Approximately two weeks after fusion HAT culture medium was replaced by HAT without aminopterin (HT medium). After several passages in HT medium hybridomas were grown in NS1 culture medium. Hybridoma cells were cloned twice by placing one or two cells in 20 µl of cloning medium in microtest plates (Greiner, Nürtingen, Fed. Rep. Germany). Cloning medium consisted of 50% freshly prepared and 50% myeloma conditioned culture medium, taken from logarithmically growing NS1 myeloma cultures. For conditioning and cloning, media were prepared containing 20% fetal calf serum instead of 10%.

II.3   Testing Antibodies by Immunofluorescence on Histological Sections

After detection of hybrid growth supernatants were taken from cultures in which the culture medium had turned from an orange to a yellow colour. Supernatants were either concentrated approximately 10-fold by precipitation with ammonium sulphate (Weir, 1979) or taken directly for immunofluorescence procedures.

Screening of hybridoma supernatants for antibodies binding to antigenic components in the nervous system was performed on 10 µm sections of fresh frozen adult mouse brain tissue (Goridis *et al.*, 1978). Fresh frozen rather than chemically fixed sections were used to prevent damage of antigens and resultant loss of antibody binding. However, if antigens are extremely soluble, they may be washed out of the section during the first incubation step with antibody and subsequent washing procedures. For each individual antibody and particular problem the type of treatment which the tissue undergoes will have to be determined.

After freezing, the brain was cut sagitally in the midline with a razor blade and the halves embedded and mounted separately in OTC (Miles Laboratories, Elkhart, Indiana, USA) which was quickly frozen down to −12 °C in a cryostat (Cryocut, Jung, Nussloch, Fed. Rep. Germany). Sections of 10 µm thickness were cut at −12 °C and melted onto glass slides or coverslips and allowed to dry for 1 h at room temperature. All further manipulations were carried out at room temperature. Incubations of sections with hybridoma supernatants were performed in Petri dishes with a humidified atmosphere created by moist filter paper lying at the bottom of the dish. Slides were exposed by covering them with supernatant (usually 30–50 µl) for 20 min. Supernatants were then washed off by draining the fluid with a filter paper and rinsing the slides or coverslips in PBS in glass slide holders or porcelain racks. Three washes were carried out for 5 min each. After the washes slides were dried with a filter paper around the sections leaving the section itself always in a moist condition to avoid non-specific reactions. Coverslips with sections were not dried around the section, but simply wiped on the back of the coverslip and placed immediately into the humidified Petri dishes. Fluorescein coupled goat anti-mouse immunoglobulin (1:50 diluted in PBS) from Antibodies Inc., Irvine, California, USA, was then applied to the sections so they were again fully covered and incubated for 20 min in the Petri dishes. Sections were again thoroughly washed three times and mounted in PBS:glycerol (1:1 v/v), either by covering with a coverslip or placing the section bearing coverslip onto a slide, face down. Sections were examined with a Zeiss fluorescence microscope equipped with Ploëm optics and epi-illumination, an Osram HBO 200 W mercury lamp, and BG 38 excitor, KP490 interference, and K530 barrier filters.

As controls for the immunofluorescence procedures normal mouse serum or supernatant from NS1 myeloma culture were used instead of the hybridoma supernatants.

Four hybridoma supernatants were obtained which stained white matter tracts in a diffuse pattern (Figure 1). Immunolabelling of white matter was prominent, but additional label was seen in the granular layer in round or oval membranous structures. This staining pattern was seen with three out of the four antibodies which were designated O2, O3, and O4. In addition, radially oriented processes in the molecular layer, the Bergmann glial cells, were readily visible with O2 and O3 antibodies, but less strongly stained by O1 and O4 antibodies.

Since in fresh frozen sections intracellular as well as extracellular antigens are accessible to antibody it is important to search the localization of the O antigens under conditions where cell surface constituents are unequivocally distinguished from intracellular ones. This is most readily achieved in monolayer cultures of neural cells, where cell surface constituents only are recognized, when antibody is applied to living cells, and intracellular antigens are recognized only after the cytoplasmic membrane has been made permeable to antibodies by fixation with protein denaturing agents and lipid extraction by organic solvents. Monolayer cultures were therefore established from early postnatal mouse cerebellum. At this age, dissociation of tissue into single viable cells is still possible using a combination of enzymatic and mechanical treatments. At later stages, from 10 days of age onwards, this type of dissociation does not yield intact cell bodies with a high degree of viability and little cellular debris, such that plating in monolayer cultures, where cellular processes should regenerate, becomes impossible. If antigens are expressed only on fully differentiated cell surfaces the use of monolayer cultures obtained by dissociation of immature brain tissue into single cells poses a problem. Even after prolonged culture periods cells may not attain their mature cell surface composition with the presently available methods. Explant cultures of intact tissue slices or reaggregate cultures which generally tend to support differentiation more readily than monolayer cultures are

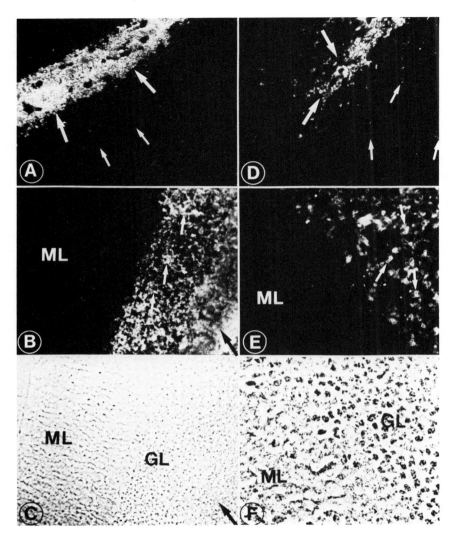

Figure 1 Immunolabelling for O antigens in fresh frozen sagittal sections of adult C57BL/6J mouse cerebellum. A and D: Antigen O1 is stained in white matter tracts (large arrows) Some labelling is also seen in the granular layer (small arrows) at the end of a cerebellar folium. B and E: Antigen O4 is stained in white matter (large arrow) and small vesicular structures in the granular layer (GL, small arrows). Molecular layer (ML) is not stained. C and F are phase contrast micrographs to B and E, respectively (A, D, E, and F ×360; B and C ×143.) (From Sommer and Schachner, 1980)

useless for the unambiguous detection of surface antigens, since these forms of culture material resemble more the original, compact tissue. Imperative for the detection of cell surface antigens is the availability of sparsely seeded cells in monolayers, where cell body and processes can be observed as distinct entities in isolation from other cells. Another important aspect is the need for cell cultures with little or no cellular debris attached to the intact cells. Once attached to a substrate, debris is generally difficult to get rid of, even by extensive washing procedures. Cellular debris often displays intense non-specific stain and specific immunoreactions may be obscured. If culturing dissociated cells from adult nervous tissue with a high degree of viability becomes possible, the analysis of adult cell surface antigens would be more readily feasible.

II.4   Monolayer Cultures of Neural Cells (Schnitzer and Schachner, 1981a,b,c)

The aim of the present procedure is to obtain cell cultures with a high degree of viability and yield by gentle dissociation of the intact tissue into single cells. This is best achieved by a combination of enzymatic, mostly proteolytic, loosening of cellular contacts and mechanical disruption. If these procedures are carried out in a carefully controlled fashion, cells remain viable, even though their processes are mostly torn off. The attachment of these cells to a solid substrate should be efficient and rapid so that morphological differentiation of cellular processes can readily be obtained.

II.4.1   *Enzymes, solutions and culture medium*

Enzymes: bovine pancreas trypsin (twice crystallized, dialysed salt free, lyophilized) and DNase I (purified, precrystalline, lyophilized) (Worthington Biochemical Corporation, Codes TRL and DP, respectively).

Buffers and culture media: all buffers and media are sterilized by filtration through Millipore filters (0.4 μm pore size).

Calcium and magnesium free Hanks' balanced salt solution (CMF-HBSS) is prepared with distilled water (deionized and quartz-distilled). A 3.0% trypsin and 0.15% DNase solution is prepared by diluting with Hanks' balanced salt solution (HBSS). The pH is adjusted at 7.3 with 1 M NaOH. The trypsin/DNase stock solution is stored at -70 °C and thawed only once for use. Directly before use the stock solution is thawed quickly and 1 ml diluted with 2 ml CMF-HBSS supplemented with 12 mM $MgSO_4$ (CMF-HBSS + Mg). A DNase solution (0.05%) is prepared with basal medium Eagle (BME) with Hanks' salts (Seromed, München, Fed. Rep. Germany), in powdered form and dissolved in distilled water and supplemented with

2.5 mg/ml glucose. It was stored at −70 °C, thawed only twice and directly before use. BME with Earle's salts (Seromed, in powdered form) are dissolved in distilled water. It is supplemented with 2.5 mg/ml glucose, 2 mm L-glutamine (Merck), 100 U/ml penicillin, 100 μg/ml streptomycin (both from Serva, Heidelberg, Fed. Rep. Germany), and 10% horse serum. This medium was designated culture medium and stored at −20 °C. It was thawed once and used within a week.

II.4.2 *Dissociation of cerebellar tissue into single cells*

This procedure is a modification of previously described methods (Barkley *et al.*, 1973; Messer, 1977; Trenkner and Sidman, 1977; Willinger and Schachner, 1980). All manipulations are carried out in sterile conditions.

Cerebellum is quickly removed from decapitated mice which had been dipped in 70% ethanol. Excess ethanol is wiped off with Kleenex. Cerebella are transferred into a drop of CMF-HBSS + Mg in a 35 mm diameter Petri dish. Meninges and choroid plexus are removed with pairs of fine forceps and the cerebellar tissue incubated in 1 ml of 1.0% trypsin and 0.05% DNase solution for various periods of time at room temperature. The incubation time depends on the age of the animals from which cerebella were taken. Cerebella from embryonic day 13 are incubated for 1 min, from embryonic day 15 for 2.5 min, from embryonic day 17 for 4.0 min, from neonatal ages for 5 min, from postnatal day 3 for 8 min, from postnatal day 6 for min, and from postnatal day 9 for 17 min. Cerebella from all embryos (usually 7–12) of a pregnant NMRI female are incubated together in 1 ml of trypsin/DNase solution. DNase is added during tryptic or mechanical dissociation to avoid formation of chromatin clumps which are released by dead cells. Such clumps entangle living cells in solid clots which are often difficult to dissociate again mechanically (i.e. by pipetting up and down).

Postnatal cerebella are cut sagitally into three pieces. Five cerebella from neonatal animals, or three cerebella from 3-day-old animals, or one cerebellum from 6- and 9-day-old animals are incubated in 1 ml of trypsin/DNase solution. Tissue pieces are then washed three times with CMF-HBSS and resuspended in 1 ml 0.05% DNase solution, at room temperature. The tissue pieces are then triturated at room temperature through fire-polished Pasteur pipettes, first with ten passes (in and out) of a relatively wide bore (approximately 1.0 mm diameter) and then with twenty passes of a narrower bore (0.1–0.2 mm diameter). Suspensions are allowed to stand in a conical 12 ml glass centrifuge tube for 5 min at room temperature to allow small clumps to settle. The upper nine-tenths of the suspension are transferred to another conical tube and centrifuged for 5 min at 4 °C in a Heraeus–Christ centrifuge at 60 g. The pelleted cells are resuspended in 1 ml of culture medium and counted in a haemocytometer or Coulter counter. Cell concentrations are adjusted as needed.

Cell viability is determined by trypan blue uptake with a freshly prepared solution of 0.16% trypan blue in physiological saline. Viability always amounted to more than 90%, usually to more than 98%. Cell yields from one cerebellum were 1.0–3.2 × 10^5 for embryonic day 13, 2.8–4.0 × 10^5 for embryonic day 15, 5.4–8.8 for embryonic day 18, 6.6–10.0 × 10^5 for postnatal day 0, 1.7–2.4 × 10^6 for postnatal day 3, 7.5–8.9 × 10^6 for postnatal day 6, and 8.0–9.9 × 10^6 for postnatal day 9.

II.4.3 *Plating and maintenance of cerebellar cells in monolayer culture*

Single cell suspensions prepared as described in the previous paragraphs were plated on poly-L-lysine coated coverslips (16 mm diameter). These are prepared by dry heat sterilization, incubation in 0.01% poly-L-lysine · HBr (Type I-B from Sigma Chemie GmbH, München, Fed. Rep. Germany) in distilled water for 1 h at 35.5 °C in a CO_2 incubator and washed by three short rinses in PBS. Coverslips are then equilibrated with culture medium in a CO_2 incubator with a humidified atmosphere containing 2.2% CO_2 and 97.8% air before addition of cells. Alternatively, sterilized coverslips are incubated with 0.001% poly-L-lysine in distilled water for 0.5–1 h at room temperature. The poly-L-lysine solution is then completely removed and coverslips are dried under a laminar-flow tissue culture hood without further washing or incubation with culture medium. The use of poly-L-lysine (a highly charged compound) greatly facilitates the attachment of cerebellar cells to plastic or glass surfaces. Without this or a comparable treatment attachment of cells is negligible when horse serum is used in culture media. Precoating of culture vessels with poly-L-ornithine has not yielded better plating efficiencies for mouse cerebellum in our hands. For cultures which have to be maintained for more than 2 weeks collagen coating (Bornstein, 1958) has been used to avoid detachment of cells which is thought to result from proteolytic degradation of the poly-L-lysine. We have found it useful to coat with poly-D-lysine, if more prolonged culture periods are required.

Cells are plated directly onto dried coverslips at concentration of 1.5–2.0 × 10^6 cells in 2 ml of culture medium into a 35 mm diameter plastic Petri dish (Greiner, Nürtingen, Fed. Rep. Germany) containing three coverslips. Alternatively, 2.5 × 10^5 cells in 0.1 ml of culture medium are pipetted into the centre of a coverslip. Cells in small volumes of culture medium attach generally more rapidly to the substrate. Fifteen of such coverslips are usually contained in a 100 mm diameter plastic Petri dish. After a 2–24 h period in the CO_2 incubator coverslips are flooded with 5 ml of culture medium and maintained in the incubator for various time periods.

Culture medium is changed twice per week by replacing half of the culture supernatant medium by fresh medium. Culture medium is changed for the first time 5 days after plating. Plating efficiency should amount to 70–90% of the original cell counts.

After the first week *in vitro* neurons with small cell bodies, the granule, basket, and stellate cells, begin to degenerate and disappear from the cultures. At the same time an increase in fibroblasts of fibroblast-like cells and astrocytes becomes apparent. There is a very slow rate of proliferation of oligodendrocytes. After 3–4 weeks in culture neurons with small cell bodies have generally disappeared from the cultures. An almost confluent layer of epithelioid astrocytes has formed with areas of underlying patches of fibroblasts or fibroblast-like cells. The frequency of these patches varies from culture to culture. Oligodendrocytes with round cell bodies and an elaborate system of cellular processes are found on top of the layer of epithelioid cells. Neurons with large cell bodies, the Purkinje and Golgi type II cells, are rarely present in cerebellar cultures, but tend to appear more frequently in cerebellar cultures of late embryonic rather than postnatal mice. These cells have occasionally been found to extend rudimentary cellular processes, but generally survive only for a few days as round cell bodies without processes.

II.5 Immunofluorescence on Monolayer Cultures (Schnitzer *et al.*, 1980; Schnitzer and Schachner, 1981a)

II.5.1 *Antibodies*

Rabbit antibodies to fibronectin, GFA protein, and tetanous toxin were obtained from R. O. Hynes (Massachusetts Institute of Technology, Cambridge, USA), L. F. Eng (Stanford University, Palo Alto, USA), and V. R. Zurawsky (Harvard University Medical School, Boston, USA), respectively. Tetanus toxin was obtained from E. Habermann (University of Giessen, Fed. Rep. Germany). Antiserum to neurofilament (NF) protein has been raised in C57BL/6J mice and its specificity has been described (Schachner *et al.*, 1978b).

Fluorescein isothiocyanate (FITC) conjugated goat anti-mouse immunoglobulins were purchased from Antibodies Incorporated and used at a dilution of 1:200. Tetramethylrhodamine isothiocyanate (TRITC) conjugated goat anti-rabbit immunoglobulins were obtained from Nordic Immunology (Byk Mallinckrodt, Dietzenbach-Steinberg, Fed. Rep. Germany) and used at a dilution of 1:300. Rabbit anti-mouse immunoglobulins conjugated with tetramethylrhodamine were obtained from N. L. Cappel Laboratories (Cochranville, Pa, USA) and used at a dilution of 1:500.

II.5.2   *Immunocytochemical procedures*

Indirect immunofluorescence on coverslips with monolayer cultures is performed on live cultures to detect cell surface antigens only, while fixed cultures are used to detect intracellular antigens.

For immunolabelling of live cells, coverslips are washed first with culture medium by taking off the culture medium supernatant in the Petri dish and adding fresh medium, all at room temperature. Coverslips are then transferred to a humidified Petri dish (see Section II.3) and incubated with first antibody (in this case, monoclonal O antibodies) diluted in culture medium. After 20 min incubation at room temperature, coverslips are washed three times in culture medium in a manner as described in Section II.3 for histological sections. Coverslips are then transferred to a freshly prepared 4% paraformaldehyde solution in PBS for 5 min at room temperature.

Coverslips are washed again three times with PBS and incubated with GAM-FITC as described in Section II.3. Fixation after application of first antibody is important for preserving integrity of cells during subsequent manipulations. Without fixation, cells tend to detach from the coverslip or deteriorate morphologically. Furthermore, fixation prevents alterations in distribution of cell surface components in the plasma membrane.

For immunolabelling of intracellular antigens, cells have to be fixed and the plasma membranes made permeable to antibody. Coverslips are taken from the incubator and washed once in DPBS containing 0.1% BSA. Coverslips are then transferred to a 4% paraformaldehyde solution in PBS for 5 min at room temperature. They are washed again three times with 0.1% BSA in DPBS and treated with a mixture of acetone and water (1:1, v/v), or with 96% ethanol for 2 min at -20 °C. Acetone–water-treated cells are then further incubated for 5 min with pure acetone and then again with the acetone–water mixture for 2 min, all at -20 °C. Ethanol and acetone-treated cells are then washed three times in 0.1% BSA in DPBS at room temperature. Incubations with first and second antibodies are then carried out in 0.1% BSA in DPBS as described for histological sections and live monolayer cultures (Section II.3 and above). The result of immunolabelling of live monolayer cells and O antibodies is shown in Figure 2. There, cells of various forms were labelled with fluorescein, while others were clearly unstained. To identify the cell type of the antigen-positive cells double immunolabelling experiments were performed in which O antigens were labelled with fluorescein, and other, more established markers for several neural cell types (see Table 1) were labelled with rhodamine.

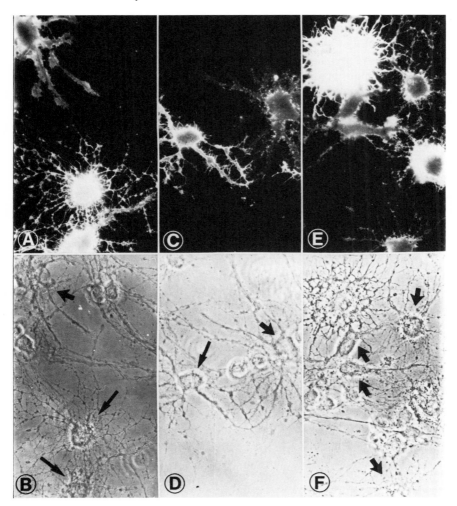

Figure 2 Immunolabelling for O antigens in cerebellar cultures from 6-day-old Sprague-Dawley rats after 4 days *in vitro*. A and C: O3 antigen with corresponding phase contrast micrographs B and D, respectively. E: O4 antigen with corresponding phase contrast micrograph F. Immunolabelled cells display various degrees of fluorescence intensities. More heavily fluorescent cells are marked by long arrows, the faintly fluorescent cells by short arrows, (B, D, F). Culture areas with high densities of O antigen-positive cells were chosen for these photographs (×570) (From Sommer and Schachner, 1980)

II.5.3   *Double immunolabelling procedures* (Sommer and Schachner, 1980)

Here we describe experiments where live cells were incubated first with antibodies to cell surfaces (antibodies to O antigens and galactocerebroside) or tetanus toxin either singly or simultaneously for 20 min at room temperature in culture medium. Cells were then washed three times in culture medium and fixed with 4% paraformaldehyde in PBS as described in the previous paragraphs. Treatment with acetone or ethanol was performed, also as described, for the detection of intracellular antigens. Cells were incubated with antibodies to GFA protein, tetanus toxin, or fibronectin (Schachner *et al.*, 1978a; Schachner and Willinger, 1979a) and washed again three times. Fluorochrome-labelled immunoglobulins to mouse and rabbit Ig (GAM-FITC and GAR-TRITC) were then added simultaneously and incubated for 20 min at room temperature. No reactivities of GAM with rabbit Ig nor GAR with mouse Ig were observed under these conditions.

Double labelling experiments by indirect methods are successful only when first antibodies are derived from different species or different Ig subclasses, such that the second antibodies carrying the different fluorochromes are completely specific for a single first antibody. If cross-reactivity of Ig molecules among species and subclasses becomes apparent with commercially available second antibodies, these have to be made specific by immuno-adsorption using affinity chromatography to remove the unwanted reactivities. For example, GAM-FITC which reacts not only with immunoglobulins from mouse, but also from rabbit, are passed through a Sepharose–rabbit Ig column (Weir, 1979). The fraction of the original GAM-FITC which is not retained by the column can be considered specific for mouse Ig.

Double immunolabelling experiments in which both first antibodies are derived from the same species or immunoglobulin subclass cannot be carried out by indirect methods. For these experiments first antibodies have to be conjugated directly to their fluorochromes.

Figures 3 to 8 show the results of double immunolabelling experiments for O antigens and GFA protein (Figure 3), tetanus toxin receptors (Figures 4 and 5), fibronectin (Figure 6), and galactocerebroside (Figures 7 and 8). Coincident labelling of O1 or O2 with galactocerebroside, but exclusive labelling for GFA protein, tetanus toxin receptors, and fibronectin supports the notion that O1 and O2 antigens are localized on the cell surfaces of oligodendrocytes. Cells which are labelled by O4 antibodies, but are un-

---

Figure 3   Double immunolabelling for GFA protein and O antigens in 10-day-old cultures of optic nerve from 3-day-old C57BL/6J mice. GFA protein was visualized by rhodamine (GAR-TRITC) (A and D) and O4 (B) and O3 (E) antigens by fluorescein (GAM-FITC) labels. O antibodies were applied first to live, unfixed cultures. After washing, cultures were treated with 4% paraformaldehyde in PBS, pH 7.3 (5 min at room temperature) and then with acetone (3 min in acetone–water, 1:1, 2 min in

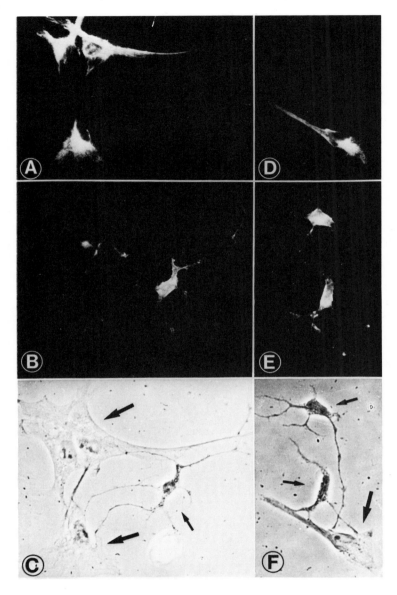

acetone, and again 3 min in the water–acetone mixture all at −20 °C). After washing, GAR-TRITC (1 : 300 diluted) and GAM-FITC (1 : 50 diluted) are added simultaneously. C and F are phase contrast micrographs belonging to A and B, and D and E, respectively. Flat, epithelioid cells (large arrows) are GFA protein-positive. O antigen-positive cells (small arrows) have few slender processes and a small dark cell body with scanty cytoplasm (×360). (From Sommer and Schachner, 1980)

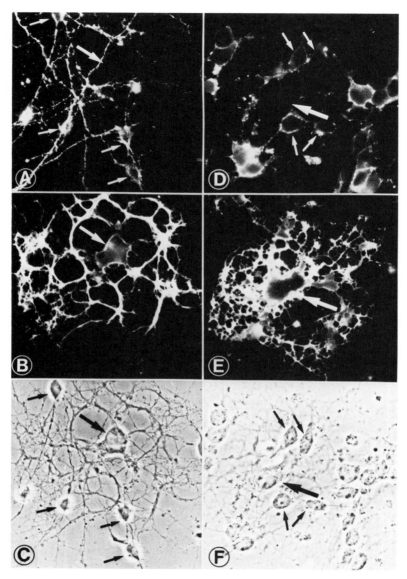

Figure 4 Double immunolabelling for tetanus toxin receptors and O antigens in 5-day-old cultures of cerebellum from 7-day-old C57BL/6J mice. Tetanus toxin cell surface receptors were visualized by application of tetanus toxin followed by rabbit antiserum to tetanus toxin and GAR-TRITC (A and D). Antigens O1 (B) and O2 (E) were visualized with GAM-FITC. Phase contrast pictures C and F correspond to A and B, and D and E, respectively. Micrographs A, B, and C were focussed in the plane of the O antigen-positive cell (large arrow); tetanus toxin-positive cell bodies (small

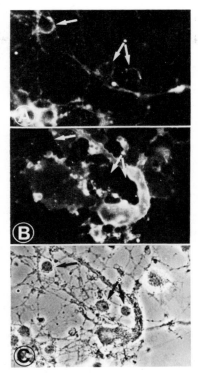

Figure 5 Double immunolabelling for tetanus toxin receptors and O4 antigen in 5-day-old cultures of cerebellum from 7-day-old C57BL/6J mice. Tetanus toxin receptors (A) and O4 antigen (B) were visualized as described in legend to Figure 2. Phase contrast micrograph of the same field (C). Tetanus toxin-positive cell bodies (arrows) in A are not positive for O4 antigen (×360). (From Sommer and Schachner, 1980)

stained by all other antibodies, could be shown to be precursors to galacto-cerebroside and O1 antigen-positive cells (Sommer and Schachner, 1982.)

Further proof came from the following experiment: O1 negative, but O4 antigen positive cells were selected for in single cerebellar cell suspensions by complement-dependent immunocytolysis. Residual O4 antigen positive cells were labelled with O4 antibodies which had been conjugated directly with rhodamine. Excess antibodies were washed away before cells were plated in monolayer cultures. The appearance of O1 antigen on rhodamine-labelled

arrows) in A and C therefore appear out of focus. Micrographs D and F were focussed in the plane of tetanus toxin-positive cell bodies (small arrows); O2 antigen- and tetanus toxin-positive processes appear out of focus (A, B, and C ×360; D, E, and F ×570). (From Sommer and Schachner, 1980)

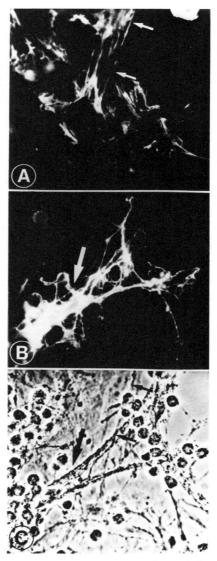

Figure 6 Double immunolabelling for fibronectin and O1 antigen in 4-day-old cultures of cerebellum from 7-day-old C57BL/6J mice. Fibronectin (A) and O1 antigen (B) were visualized by labelling with GAR-TRITC (A) and GAM-FITC (B), respectively. A typical fibronectin staining pattern on epithelioid background fibroblasts is visible (small arrows). O1 antigen-positive cell (large arrows) is not fibronectin-positive (×360). (C) represents a phase contrast image of B (×360). (From Sommer and Schachner, 1980

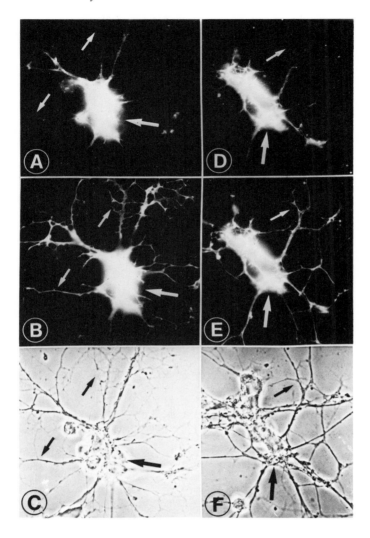

Figure 7 Double immunolabelling for galactocerebroside and O antigens in 4-day-old cultures of cerebellum from 7-day-old C57BL/6J mice. Galactocerebroside (A and D) and antigens O3 (B) and O2 (E) were visualized on live cultured cells by simultaneous application of the fluorochrome labelled second antibodies. Cellular processes are more distinctly stained by O antibodies (small arrows) than by anti-galactocerebroside serum which mostly labels cell bodies (large arrows). C and F are phase contrast micrographs of fields represented in A and B, and D and E, respectively (×360). (From Sommer and Schachner, 1980)

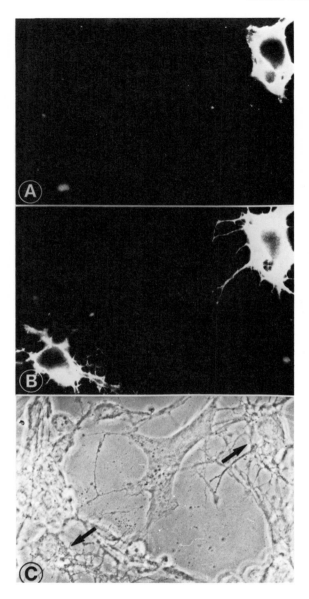

Figure 8   Double immunolabelling for galactocerebroside (A) and O4 antigen (B) in 4-day-old cultures of cerebellum from 7-day-old C57BL/6J mice. Galactocerebroside (A) and O4 antigen (B) were visualized on live cultured cells as described in Figure 5. C is the corresponding phase contrast micrograph. Arrows point to two O4 antigen-positive cells; only one of them is positive for galactocerebroside (×360). (From Sommer and Schachner, 1980)

cells was then detected by fluorescein-conjugated antibodies to O1 antigen. After 1 day *in vitro*, cells which had started to internalize the rhodamine label became positive for O1 antigen. These experiments suggest that O antibodies react with oligodendroglia and precursors to oligodendroglia, which have not been recognized by means of the previously available markers.

It should be mentioned here that fixation of cerebellar cultures with paraformaldehyde and ethanol leads to immunolabelling of astrocytes by O antibodies. The cytoplasmic labelling pattern is very similar to the one with antiserum to GFA protein as can be shown in double labelling experiments. Specificity of O antibodies for oligodendrocytes is, therefore, guaranteed only when intact cells are taken for immunolabelling. These results suggest that labelling of Bergmann glial cells in histological sections, which is particularly prominent with O2 and O3 antibodies, is due to intracellularly localized cross-reactive components. Whether these are identical or just similar to the ones present on the surfaces of oligodendrocytes will have to await the characterization of the antigens' molecular nature in isolated populations of oligodendroglia and astroglia.

II.6   Immunoperoxidase on Monolayer Cultures and Electron Microscopy
(Berg and Schachner, 1982)

The aim of an immunoelectron microscopic examination is to confirm the identity of cell types established by ultrastructural criteria and to try to recognize particular ultrastructural features which may correlate with the maturational stage of cell types defined by the monoclonal antibodies. Immunoperoxidase studies are therefore performed with monolayer cultures of early postnatal mouse cerebellum in which surface antigenic sites are freely accessible to antibody, and cellular integrity is preserved to assure immuno-labelling of cell surfaces, but not intracellular structures.

II.6.1   *Materials and antibodies*

Glutaraldehyde (EM grade) and 3,3'-diaminobenzidine · 4HCl (DAB) were obtained from Serva, Heidelberg, Fed. Rep. Germany. Paraformalde-hyde was obtained from Merck, Darmstadt, Fed. Rep. Germany. Parafor-maldehyde and glutaraldehyde solutions in PBS, pH 7.3 were prepared freshly and filtered before use. Peroxidase-conjugated rabbit anti-mouse Ig (RAM-HRPO) was obtained from Dako-Immunoglobulins, Copenhagen, Denmark. These were used at dilutions of 1 : 20.

II.6.2   *Cell cultures*

Primary monolayer cultures of late embryonic or early C57BL/6J mouse cerebellum are prepared essentially as described in Section II.4 with a few exceptions: cells are not grown on glass coverslips, but on Aclar discs (Allied Chemicals, Morristown, NJ, USA). Aclar is a plastic material which can be more readily removed from Epon–Araldite-embedded cells than from glass. Prior to use the Aclar discs are soaked in 70% ethanol and sonicated for 30 min followed by three rinses of sterile, distilled water. Cerebellar cultures do not appear as healthy on Aclar as they do on glass. To improve cell attachment to Aclar discs and to obtain a more even cell distribution, discs are soaked in 0.1% poly-L-lysine for 1 h, dried for 1 h and equilibrated in culture medium at 37 °C in a CO_2 incubator for 1 h before seeding the single cell suspension.

II.6.3 *Immunocytological procedures*

Monolayer cultures are rinsed twice at room temperature. These and all rinses up to the DAB reaction are performed using BME–Earle's containing 10% horse serum. Cells are fixed for 5 min in 4% paraformaldehyde, 0.25% glutaraldehyde in PBS and rinsed twice before application of antibody. Fixation with aldehydes under the described conditions does not generally lead to accessibility of intracellular antigens. Penetration of plasma membranes requires treatment with lipid solvents such as acetone or ethanol. After the removal of aldehydes, cells are incubated with O antibodies for 20 min at 4 °C, rinsed three times, and fixed again for 20 min at room temperature with 4% paraformaldehyde, 1.25% glutaraldehyde in PBS. After two washes the cells are then incubated with RAM-HRPO for 1 h at 4 °C. They are rinsed twice in 0.04 M Tris buffer, pH 7.6. The DAB is then performed using a modified procedure of Graham and Karnovsky (1966) and Schachner *et al.* (1977b). Cultures are exposed to DAB (0.4 mg/ml) in 0.04 M Tris buffer, pH 7.5 for 10 min at room temperature in the dark. Hydrogen peroxide (Merck, Darmstadt, Fed. Rep. Germany) is then added at a final concentration of 0.005% to the DAB solution. After 15 min incubation cultures are washed twice for 5 min in PBS and osmicated (2% OsO_4 in PBS at room temperature).

II.6.4 *Electron microscopy*

After osmication, cells are rinsed in distilled water, dehydrated in a series of ethanol, and embedded in Araldite–Epon contained in a plastic capsule. The Aclar disc easily peels off the polymerized Araldite–Epon, leaving the cells at the surface of the block to be thin-sectioned parallel to their plane of attachment. Sections are contrasted in uranyl acetate and examined by electron microscopy.

Figure 9 shows an O4 antigen-positive cell in which the characteristic features of a more mature oligodendrocyte are distinguishable (Imamoto *et*

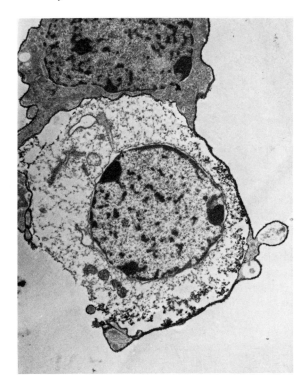

Figure 9 Transmission electron micrograph of an O4 antigen-positive cell labelled by indirect immunoperoxidase procedures in cell culture. Granular, electron-dense DAB reaction product is seen at the surface of an oligodendrocyte characterized by its scanty and dark cytoplasm, filled with ribosomes. The rough endoplasmic reticulum is found in short stacks of cisternae. Mitochondria are also present. Cellular processes surround the cell body of a granule cell which is devoid of reaction product (×5270). (From Berg and Schachner, 1982)

al., 1978; Privat, 1975; Skoff *et al.*, 1976; Sturrock, 1974). A neighbouring granule cell neuron is seen devoid of DAB reaction product.

II.7   Immunoperoxidase and Electron Microscopy on Tissue Sections
(Schachner *et al.*, 1977b, 1978a,b; Hedley-Whyte *et al.*, 1978; Füchtbauer and Schachner, unpublished observations)

To identify oligodendroglial cells and localize O antigen-positive sites on myelin in the intact brain tissue *in situ*, attempts were made to apply antibodies to histological sections in indirect immunoperoxidase procedures and recognize O antigens at the electronmicroscopic level. The methods used were essentially those described for the detection of intracellular antigens, such as GFA and neurofilament proteins (Schachner *et al.*, 1977b, 1978b).

II.7.1   *Preparation of tissue for immunohistology*

C57BL/6J mice (about 4 weeks old) are anaesthetized by intraperitoneal injection of avertin (0.02 ml/g body weight) and perfused through the heart with freshly prepared 4% paraformaldehyde in PBS. For some experiments, solutions containing 4% paraformaldehyde and 0.1% or 0.25% glutaraldehyde were used. After perfusion, the brains are removed and immersed in the fixative at 4 °C for 2–4 h. Mid-sagittal slices of cerebellum 60 μm in thickness are cut on an Oxford Vibratome (Ted Pella, Inc., Tucson, Calif., USA) and rinsed overnight with six changes of PBS at 4 °C. The slices are then treated with 0.01 M $NaIO_4$ in PBS for 15 min, rinsed with three changes of PBS for 15 min, and incubated with a solution of $NaBH_4$ (10 mg/ml PBS) for 10 min, all at room temperature. After four changes of PBS, sections are further incubated at room temperature with 5% dimethylsulphoxide in PBS for 10 min. After two further changes of PBS, the slices are ready for the immunoperoxidase reaction.

II.7.2   *Immunocytological procedures*

The 60 μm slices are incubated for 1 h at room temperature in Linbro plates (Greiner, Nürtingen, Fed. Rep. Germany) in 0.3 ml of appropriately diluted antibodies. Slices are rinsed with six changes of PBS at room temperature over a 2-h period and then incubated with Fab' fragments coupled to HRPO (SAM Fab'-HRPO, from Institut Pasteur Production, Paris, France) or with RAM-HRPO (Dako-Immunoglobulins, Copenhagen, Denmark) for 1 h at room temperature. Slices are again rinsed for 2 h with six changes of PBS at room temperature. Some slices are post-fixed for 30 min in 1% glutaraldehyde in 0.01 M phosphate buffer, pH 7.2. After two 10-min rinses with PBS, slices are incubated with 3,3'-diaminobenzidine · 4HCl (DAB) at a concentration of 0.2 or 0.4 mg/ml in Tris buffer, pH 7.6 for 30 min in the dark at room temperature with constant agitation. Slices were then further treated with a DAB solution containing 0.005% H_2O_2 for 15 min, also in the dark with constant agitation. The reaction is terminated by two changes of PBS, 5 min each.

II.7.3   *Electron microscopy*

Slices are post-fixed for 45 min at room temperature, either in 2% OsO_4 in 0.12 M phosphate buffer, or 1% Dalton's chrome–osmium, pH 7.2, rinsed and dehydrated in acetone and propylene oxide, and embedded in Epon, or an Epon–Araldite mixture. One micrometre sections are examined for localization DAB reaction product at the light microscopic level. Sections 500–600Å in thickness are then cut with a diamond knife parallel and perpendicular to the sagittal block face, from areas with reaction product, and collected on grids.

In our studies with O antibodies, myelin turned out to be a particularly difficult tissue element for immunoelectron-microscopic studies. Not only was myelin difficult to preserve ultrastructurally under the mild fixation conditions used to preserve antigenic sites, but penetration of antibody into the intact myelin lamellae was practically impossible to achieve. Penetration of antibody, and hence presence of DAB reaction product, was found at depths of 5–10 μm for intracellular antigen such as neurofilament. Penetration depended, however, on the orientation of axons with respect to the Vibratome block face of the tissue slice. When the cut through the axon was perpendicular to the cut of the Vibratome section (i.e. the microtome section was perpendicular to the Vibratome block face) immunolabelled intracellular structures were seen at depths of several micrometres (Figure 10). Dimethylsulphoxide slightly enhanced penetration of antibody, but addition of Triton X-100 at concentrations of 0.1% to all reaction mixtures and rinses did not increase penetration. Fab' fragments penetrated better than whole Ig molecules, but never was more than 10 μm of penetration achieved under the described conditions. When axons were not cut in cross-section, but ran parallel to the block face of the Vibratome section, only axons situated directly at the section surface were immunolabelled. These axons often appeared damaged (Figure 11).

Control sections treated with normal mouse serum and several monoclonal antibodies are devoid of reaction product. Non-specific peroxidase deposition was markedly decreased by treating tissue slices with $NaIO_4$ and $NaBH_4$ before antibody reactions. This non-specific deposition occurred at the cut surface of the Vibratome section.

Treatment with $NaIO_4$ and $NaBH_4$ was omitted in some experiments with O antibodies, since modification of the sugar moieties by this treatment might destroy the antigenic sites. However, with or without this treatment no significant immunolabelling of myelin or oligodendrocytes was observed with O antibodies. Membrane fragments of myelin labelled specifically with O4 antibody. It reacted with loosely packed membranous structures, but not with the adjacent more compact myelin. It is possible that these membranous structures visible with the electron microscope are similar to those which are seen at the light microscopic level in the granular layer using fresh frozen sections (see Section II.3). Disruption of myelin can be prevented to some extent by pretreatment of tissue with fixatives before the sections are cut. Membranous vesicle-like structures are not seen in the granular layer at the

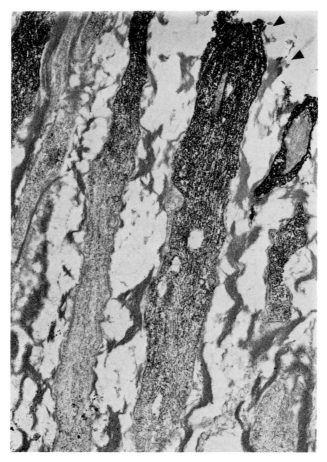

Figure 10 Transmission electron micrograph of neurofilament-positive axons labelled by indirect immunoperoxidase procedures in tissue slices of white matter of adult
mouse cerebellum. Longitudinal section through axons which were cut in cross-section
by the Vibratome. Block face of Vibratome slice is indicated by arrowheads. DAB
reaction product is seen up to approximately 3–5 μm in depth. Myelin is badly
preserved under the mild fixation conditions used to retain antigenicity (×11,250)

light microscopic level when fresh frozen sections are avoided and the tissue is
fixed prior to sectioning.

Astrocytes were prominently labelled by O antibodies not only at light
microscopic, but also at electron microscopic, levels. The reaction product
was diffusely distributed over the cytoplasma.

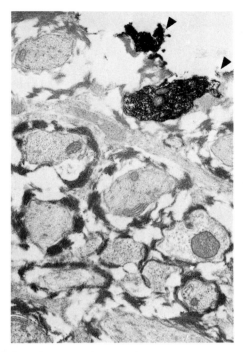

Figure 11 Transmission electron micrograph of neurofilament-positive axons labelled by indirect immunoperoxidase procedures in tissue slices of white matter of adult mouse cerebellum. Ultra-thin section is perpendicularly oriented to the face of the Vibratome block (arrows). Axons run parallel to the Vibratome cut. DAB reaction product is seen only in the most superficial axons which appear damaged by the cut. Myelin is badly preserved. Immunolabelling procedures were identical to the ones of Figure 10 (×11,250)

II.8   Combined Autoradiography and Immunocytochemistry (Leutz and Schachner, 1981). (For other combined autoradiography–immunocytochemistry procedures see also Chapters 9 and 17.)

To determine whether O antigen-positive oligodendroglia are capable of DNA synthesis and mitosis, the ability of these cells to incorporate radioactive thymidine was measured in monolayer cultures of early postnatal C57BL/6J mouse cerebella. The incorporation of radioactivity was monitored by autoradiography, while indirect immunofluorescence procedures served to identify the O antigen-positive cells (see procedure below).

II.8.1   *Cell culture and thymidine incorporation*

Primary cultures of early postnatal cerebella are prepared as described in
Section II.4. At the time of plating cells on coverslips ³H-thymidine (18–
28 Ci/mmol, from Amersham) is added to the culture medium at 4 μCi per
2 ml of 35 mm diameter Petri dish. Thymidine incorporation is terminated
after 2–48 h by removal of culture medium containing radioactive precursor.
Coverslips are then washed three times with culture medium, fixed with 4%
paraformaldehyde and 0.01% glutaraldehyde in PBS for 20 min, and washed

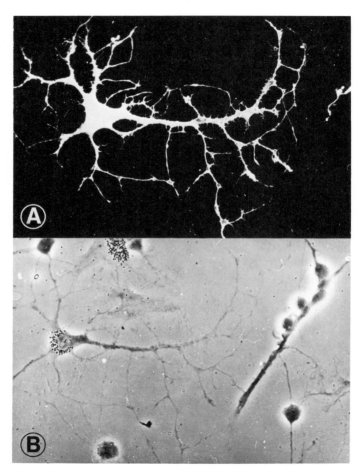

Figure 12   Combined immunofluorescence and autoradiography for O4 antigen and
incorporated ³H-labelled thymidine. A: O4 antigen in indirect immunofluorescence.
B: Autoradiograph of same visual field demonstrating grains over nuclei of cultured
cerebellar cells from 4-day-old C57BL/6J mice maintained *in vitro* for 3 days (×420)

again three times in PBS, all at room temperature. Coverslips are stained for O antigens as described in Section II.5. After immunolabelling, cells are washed twice in distilled water, dried in a desiccator at 4 °C in the dark, and dipped in autoradiographic emulsion (Kodak NTB-2, 2:1 diluted with water). After 3 days at 4 °C in the dark, coverslips are developed with Amidol, mounted in Elvanol (Hoechst Farbenwerke, Frankfurt, Fed. Rep. Germany) or glycerol–PBS (1:1, v/v) face down, on slides. Cells are scored as positive when cell body, nucleus, and processes could easily be distinguished and when more than 10 grains appeared over the nucleus.

Figure 12 shows that an O4 antigen-positive cell is able to incorporate thymidine. Thymidine incorporation in O antigen-positive cells is seen at 2, 24, and 48 h of labelling periods. The percentage of thymidine-labelled cells is low and generally in the range of 1% of all O antigen-positive cells in early postnatal cerebellar monolayer cultures. O1 as well as O4 antigen-positive cells were found to incorporate thymidine.

ACKNOWLEDGEMENTS

The author wishes to express her gratitude to her colleagues and students who have participated in this work. Support from Land Baden-Württemberg, Deutsche Forschungsgemeinschaft, Stiftung Volkswagenwerk, and Gemeinnützige Hertie Stiftung is gratefully acknowledged.

REFERENCES

Barkley, D. S., Rakic, L. L., Chaffee, J. K., and Wong, D. L. (1973). 'Cell separation by velocity sedimentation of postnatal mouse cerebellum.' *J. Cell Physiol.*, **28**, 271–280.

Berg, G. and Schachner, M. (1982). 'Immunoelectronmicroscopic identification of O antigen bearing oligodendroglial cells *in vitro*.' *Cell and Tissue Research*, **219**, 313–325.

Bignami, A., Eng, L. F., Dahl, D., and Uyeda, C. T. (1972). 'Localization of the glial fibrillary acidic protein in astrocytes by immunofluorescence.' *Brain Res.*, **43**, 429–435.

Bornstein, M. B. (1958). 'Reconstituted rat-tail collagen used as a substrate for tissue cultures on coverslips in Maximow slides and roller tubes.' *Lab. Inv.*, **7**, 134–137.

Campbell, G. LeM., Schachner, M., and Sharrow, S. (1977). 'Isolation of glial cell-enriched and -depleted populations from mouse cerebellum by density gradient centrifugation and electronic cell sorting.' *Brain Res.*, **127**, 69–86.

Dimpfel, W.; Huang, R. T. C., and Habermann, E. (1977). 'Gangliosides in nervous tissue and binding of ^{125}I-labelled tetanus toxin, a neuronal marker.' *J. Neurochem.*, **29**, 329–334.

Eng, L. F., Vanderhaeghen, J. J., Bignami, A., and Gerstl, B. (1971). 'An acidic protein isolated from fibrous astrocytes.' *Brain Res.*, **28**, 351–354.

Franke, W. W., Schmid, E., Osborn, M., and Weber, K. (1978). 'Different intermediate-sized filaments distinguished by immunofluorescence microscopy.' *Proc. Natl. Acad. Sci. USA*, **75**, 5034–5038.

Galfré, G., Howe, S. C., Milstein, D., Butcher, G. W., and Howard, J. C. (1977). 'Antibodies to major histocompatibility antigens produced by hybrid cell lines.' *Nature (London)*, **266**, 550–552.

Goridis, C., Martin, J., and Schachner, M. (1978). 'Characterization of an antiserum to synaptic glomeruli from rat cerebellum.' *Brain Res. Bulletin*, **3**, 45–52.

Graham, Jr., R. C. and Karnovsky, M. T. (1966). 'The early stages of absorption of injected horseradish peroxidase in the proximal tubules of mouse kidney.' *J. Histochem. Cytochem.*, **14**, 291–302.

Hedley-Whyte, E. T., Schachner, M., Hsu, D. W., and Schoonmaker, G. (1978). 'Ultrastructural localization of nervous system cell surface antigen-2 (NS-2) in a murine glioblastoma.' *Brain Res.*, **148**, 260–264.

Imamoto, K., Paterson, J. A., and Leblond, C. P. (1978). 'Radio autographic investigation of gliogenesis in the corpus callosum of young rats. 1. Sequential changes in oligodendrocytes.' *J. Comp. Neurol.*, **180**, 115–138.

Lagenaur, C., Sommer, I., and Schachner, M. (1980). 'Subclass of astroglia recognized in mouse cerebellum by monoclonal antibody.' *Devel. Biol.*, **79**, 367–378.

Lemke, H., Hämmerling, G. J., Höhmann, C., and Rajewsky, D. (1978). 'Hybrid cell lines secreting monoclonal antibody specific for major histocompatibility antigens of the mouse.' *Nature (London)*, **271**, 249–251.

Leutz, A. and Schachner, M. (1981). 'Epidermal growth factor stimulates DNA synthesis of astrocytes in primary cerebellar cultures.' *Cell and Tissue Research*, **220**, 393–404.

Littlefield, J. W. (1964). 'Selection of hybrids from matings of fibroblasts *in vitro* and their presumed recombinants.' *Science*, **145**, 709.

Messer, A. (1977). 'The maintenance and identification of mouse cerebellar granule cells in monolayer culture.' *Brain Res.*, **130**, 1–12.

Mirsky, R., Wendon, L., Black, P., Stolkin, C., and Bray, D. (1978). 'Tetanus toxin: a cell surface marker for neurones in culture.' *Brain Res.*, **148**, 251–259.

Paetau, A., Virtanen, I., Stenman, S., Kurki, P., Linder, E., Vaheri, A., Westermark, B., Dahl, D., and Haltia, M. (1979). 'Glial fibrillary acidic protein and intermediate filaments in human glioma cells.' *Acta Neuropathol.*, **47**, 71–74.

Privat, A. (1975). 'Postnatal gliogenesis in the mammalian brain.' *Int. Rev. Cytol.*, **40**, 281–323.

Raff, M. C., Mirsky, R., Fields, K. L., Lisak, R. P., Dorfmann, S. H., Silberberg, D. H., Gregson, N. A., Liebowitz, S., and Kennedy, M. (1978). 'Galactocerebroside: a specific cell surface antigenic marker for oligodendrocytes in culture.' *Nature (London)*, **274**, 813–816.

Reynolds, E. S. (1963). 'The use of lead citrate at high pH on electron-opaque stain in electron microscopy.' *J. Biophys. Biochem. Cytol.*, **17**, 208–212.

Rohrer, H. and Schachner, M. (1980). 'Surface proteins of cultured mouse cerebellar cells.' *J. Neurochem.*, **35**, 792–803.

Schachner, M. (1974). 'NS-1 (nervous system antigen-1), a glial cell specific antigenic component of the surface membrane.' *Proc. Natl. Acad. Sci., USA*, **71**, 1795–1799.

Schachner, M. (1979). 'Cell surface antigens of the nervous system.' *Current Topics in Developmental Biology*, **13**, Teil 1, 259–279.

Schachner, M., Hedley-Whyte, T., Hsu, D., Schoonmaker, G., and Bignami, A. (1977b). 'Ultrastructural localization of glial fibrillary acidic protein in mouse cerebellum by immunoperoxidase labeling.' *J. Cell Biol.*, **75**, 67–73.

Schachner, M., Kim, S. K., and Zehnle, R. (1981). 'Developmental expression in central and peripheral nervous system of oligodendrocyte cell surface antigens (O antigens) recognized by monoclonal antibodies.' *Devel. Biol.*, **83**, 328–338.

Schachner, M., Schoonmaker, G., and Hynes, R. O. (1978a). 'Cellular and subcellular localization of LETS protein in the nervous system.' *Brain Res.*, **158**, 149–158.

Schachner, M., Smith, C., and Schoonmaker, G. (1978b). 'Immunological distinction between neurofilament and glial fibrillary acidic protein by mouse antisera and their immunohistological characterization.' *Develop. Neurosci.*, **1**, 1–14.

Schachner, M. and Willinger, M. (1979a). 'Cell type specific cell surface antigens in the cerebellum.' *Prog. Brain Res.*, **51**, 23–44.

Schachner, M. and Willinger, M. (1979b). 'Developmental expression of oligodendrocyte specific cell surface markers: NS-1 (nervous system anti-1), cerebroside, and basic protein of myelin.' In Miescher, P. A. *et al.* (eds), *The Menarini Series on Immunopathology*, **2**, 37–60.

Schachner, M., Wortham, K. A., Carter, L. D., and Chaffee, J. K. (1975). 'NS-4 (nervous system antigen-4), a cell surface antigen of developing and adult mouse brain and sperm.' *Devel. Biol.*, **44**, 313–325.

Schachner, M., Wortham, K. A., Ruberg, M. Z., Dorfman, S., and Campbell, G. LeM. (1977a). 'Brain cell surface antigens detected by anti-corpus callosum antiserum.' *Brain Res.*, **127**, 87–97.

Schnitzer, J., Franke, W. W., and Schachner, M. (1980). 'Immunocytochemical demonstration of vimentin in astrocytes and ependymal cells of developing and adult mouse nervous system.' *J. Cell Biol.*

Schnitzer, J. and Schachner, M. (1981a). 'Expression of Thy-1, H-2 and NS-4 cell surface antigens and tetanus toxin receptors in early postnatal and adult mouse cerebellum.' *J. Neuroimmunology*, **1**, 429–456.

Schnitzer, J. and Schachner, M. (1981b). 'Characterization of isolated mouse cerebellar cell populations *in vitro*.' *J. Neuroimmunology*, **1**, 457–470.

Schnitzer, J. and Schachner, M. (1981c). 'Developmental expression of cell type specific markers in mouse cerebellar cortical cells *in vitro*.' *J. Neuroimmunology*, **1**, 471–487.

Skoff, R. P., Price, D. L., and Stocks, A. (1976). 'Electron microscopic autoradiographic studies of gliogenesis in rat optic nerve 1. Cell proliferation.' *J. Comp. Neurol.*, **169**, 291–312.

Sommer, I., Lagenaur, C., and Schachner, M. (1981). 'Recognition of Bergmann glial and ependymal cells in the mouse nervous system by monoclonal antibody.' *J. Cell Biol.*, **90**, 448–458.

Sommer, I. and Schachner, M. (1982). 'Cells that are O4 antigen positive and O1 antigen negative differentiate into O1 antigen positive oligodendrocytes.' *Neuroscience Letters*, **29**, 183–188.

Sommer, I. and Schachner, M. (1981). 'Monoclonal antibodies (O1 to O4) to oligodendrocyte cell surfaces: an immunocytological study in the central nervous system.' *Devel. Biol.*, **83**, 311–327.

Sturrock, R. R. (1974). 'Histogenesis of the anterior limb of the anterior commissure of the mouse brain. 3. An electron microscopic study of gliogenesis.' *J. Anat.*, **117**, 37–53.

Trenkner, E. and Sidman, R. L. (1977). 'Histogenesis of mouse cerebellum in microwell cultures. Cell reaggregation and migration, fiber and synapse formation.' *J. Cell Biol.*, **75**, 915–940.

Weir, D. M. (ed.) (1979). *Handbook of Experimental Immunology*, 3rd edn, vol. I. Blackwell Scientific Publications, Oxford.

Willinger, M. and Schachner, M. (1980). 'G_{MI} ganglioside as a marker for neuronal differentiation in mouse cerebellum.' *Devel. Biol.*, **74**, 101–117.

Immunohistochemistry
Edited by A. C. Cuello
© 1983 IBRO

CHAPTER 16

Golgi-like Immunoperoxidase Staining of Neurons Producing Specific Substances or of Neurons Transporting Exogenous Tracer Proteins

MICHAEL V. SOFRONIEW

Neuroanatomy-Neuropharmacology Group, Department of Human Anatomy, University of Oxford, South Parks Road, Oxford OX1 3QX, UK

I INTRODUCTION

The Golgi impregnation staining procedure (Golgi, 1894) has been one of the fundamental morphological techniques used to study the structure and function of the nervous system for over 100 years. Cajal (1909–1911; 1954) used findings obtained from Golgi preparations to pioneer the theory of the neuron; and with relatively minor modification the Golgi impregnation procedure is still being used, and is still of great value, today. One of the unique features of this procedure is that it enables examination of the three-dimensional morphology of neurons and their processes, as well as of the local interconnectivity of neurons. However, the procedure is in a sense non-specific in that it stains various types of neurons and glial cells indiscriminately, and yields no information regarding the nature of the substance or

431

substances produced by the stained neurons. During the past decade, immunohistochemical techniques have been successfully applied to identifying the substances produced by individual neurons (see Cuello, 1978). Such immunohistochemical procedures have become increasingly important as the number of substances thought to be produced by neurons (and used in interneural communication) has increased. At present, probably 50 or more different substances can be identified immunohistochemically within neurons of the central nervous system, and the number is steadily increasing. These substances include amines, amino acids, peptides, proteins, and enzymes produced by neurons.

Conventional light microscopic immunohistochemical (immunofluorescent or immunoperoxidase) staining has been generally conducted in relatively thin (5–10 µm) sections for light microscopy, allowing only minor analysis of the three-dimensional morphology of the stained neurons. Nevertheless, thicker (40–100 µm) sections can be stained positively using the immunoperoxidase procedure, and such thick sections are routinely used in the so-called pre-embedding immunoperoxidase staining procedure for ultrastructural study (Sternberger, 1974; see also Chapter 11). In many cases the stained neurons and their processes can be examined in these thick sections, and Grzanna *et al.* (1978) were the first to report that this procedure may be of value in studying the morphology of neurons specifically identified as producing a given substance, in their case the enzyme dopamine-β-hydroxylase. Subsequently, it has been shown that this procedure can also be used to study the morphology of immunospecifically identified neurons using antibodies directed against peptides (Burchanowski *et al.*, 1979; Sofroniew and Glasmann, 1981) or amines (Steinbusch *et al.*, 1981) produced by the neurons. In addition, this procedure can also be used to study the morphology of neurons transporting tracer proteins (Sofroniew and Schrell, 1980). In this chapter, several different procedures used to achieve this so-called Golgi-like immunoperoxidase staining, either of neurons producing specific antigens, or of neurons transporting exogenous tracer proteins, will be described.

II THE EXPERIMENTAL PROCEDURES

The basic principle of Golgi-like immunoperoxidase staining is essentially that of conventional unlabelled antibody–enzyme bridge immunoperoxidase staining as described by Sternberger (1974) (see also Chapters 4 and 11). However, instead of staining sections mounted on glass slides, the frozen or Vibratome sections 40–200 µm in thickness are stained free-floating. These are incubated with a primary antibody, followed by the various components of the antibody–enzyme bridge. The final enzyme, peroxidase, is then used to catalyse the polymerization of diaminobenzidine, yielding a visible reaction product. Neurons containing the substance against which the primary antibody is directed are stained dark brown or black and often appear similar to

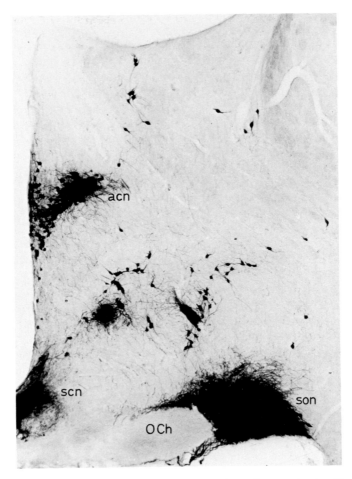

Figure 1 *Rat.* Golgi-like immunoperoxidase staining of neurophysin. Fixation with Bouin's solution. Survey of a frontal section through the rostral hypothalamus. Magnocellular neurophysin-containing neurons are present in the supraoptic nucleus (son), anterior commissural nucleus (acn), as well as scattered in various other accessory groups. Parvocellular neurophysin-containing neurons are present in the suprachiasmatic nucleus (scn). Och, optic chiasm. (×31)

Golgi impregnated neurons (Figures 1–6). The primary antibody can either be directed against an endogenous substance produced by the neurons (Figures 1–3), or against an exogenous tracer protein which has been retrogradely transported by the neurons from a known injection site (Figures 4–6). Depending on the substance to be stained, various modifications in the fixation are used. For simplicity, the following description of the various modifications of the Golgi-like immunoperoxidase procedure has been di-

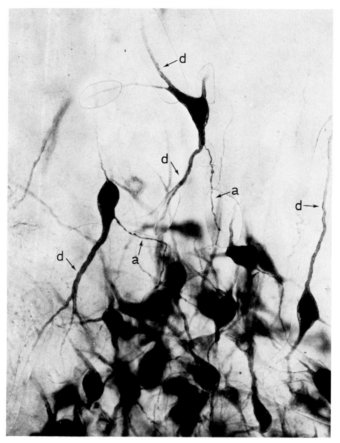

Figure 2 *Rat.* Golgi-like immunoperoxidase staining of neurophysin. Fixation with Bouin's solution. Horizontal section through the caudal, dorsal portion of the hypothalamic paraventricular nucleus. Note that beaded axons (a) can be distinguished from non-beaded, more transparently stained dendrites (d). (×360)

vided into: production of antisera, injection of tracers, fixation, sectioning, and staining. Special attention is given to modifications for staining of different substances.

II.1 Production of Antisera

Golgi-like immunoperoxidase staining can be conducted either using antisera produced by immunizing animals against a given substance, or using monoclonal antibodies. Production of monoclonal antibodies for use in neuroimmunocytochemistry has been described in detail (Cuello *et al.*, 1979; see also Chapters 11 and 15). For our studies, antisera against small peptides

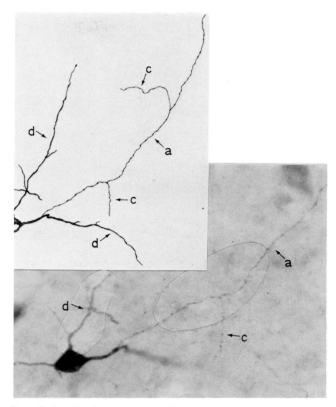

Figure 3 *Rat.* Golgi-like immunoperoxidase staining of somatostatin. Fixation by perfusion with 4% paraformaldehyde, 0.1% glutaraldehyde followed by immersion in 4% paraformaldehyde (4 h total). Somatostatin neuron in the cortical amygdaloid nucleus. (a) Camera lucida drawing. (b) Photomicrograph (×560). Note the beaded axon (a) which gives rise to two axon collaterals (c) and the long peptide-containing dendrites (d).

such as somatostatin, vasopressin or oxytocin were produced by conjugation of the peptide to thyroglobulin and injected as described elsewhere (Sofroniew *et al.*, 1978). Antisera against larger polypeptides or proteins were produced according to Vaitukaitis *et al.* (1971), as described previously for neurophysin* (Sofroniew and Glasmann, 1981), horseradish peroxidase (Sofroniew and Schrell, 1980), and wheat germ agglutinin (Sofroniew, 1983). Production of antisera against choline acetyltransferase (Eckenstein and Thoenen, 1982) or against tyrosine hydroxylase (Joh *et al.*, 1973), or of monoclonal antibodies against serotonin (Consolazione *et al.*, 1982) have been described elsewhere,

---

* Neurophysins are portions of precursor proteins produced (Gainer *et al.*, 1977; Russell *et al.*, 1980) and found by immunohistochemical methods (Vandesande *et al.*, 1975) in association with vasopressin or oxytocin within hypothalamic magnocellular neurons.

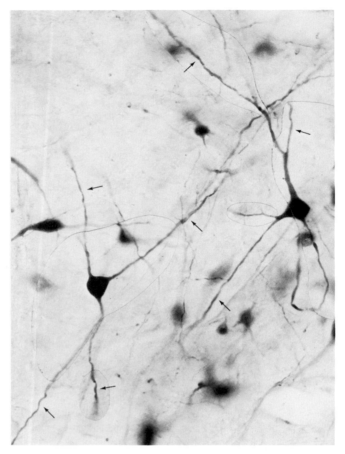

Figure 4 *Rat.* Golgi-like immunoperoxidase staining of horseradish peroxidase (HRP). Fixation with Bouin's solution. HRP-labelled neurons in the medial vestibular neucleus following HRP injection into the caudal medulla oblongata. Note that HRP has been transported secondarily for long distances away from the perikaryon, to fill various dendritic processes (arrows). (×260)

II.2 Injection of Tracer Proteins

The enzyme horseradish peroxidase (HRP) has found wide application as a neuroanatomical tracer. HRP combines the unique features of being both taken up and retrogradely transported by neurons, with an enzymatic activity that can readily be used to visualize the location of the enzyme. Although tracing techniques utilizing the enzymatic activity of HRP have been highly refined (Mesulam, 1978), generally the staining obtained yields little information concerning the morphology of labelled neurons, prompting Somogyi *et al.* (1979) to develop an elegant but complex procedure for combining HRP

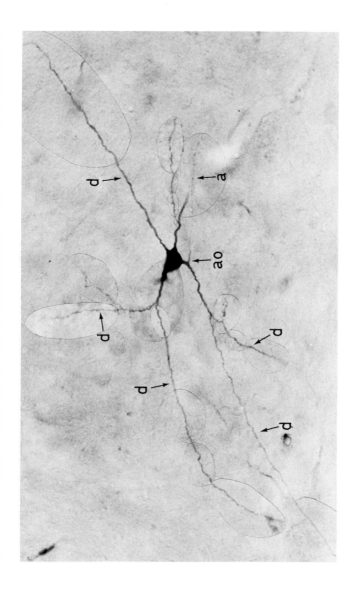

Figure 5 *Rat.* Golgi-like immunoperoxidase staining of horseradish peroxidase (HRP). Fixation with Bouin's solution. HRP-labelled neuron in the posterior hypothalamus following hrp injection into the caudal medulla oblongata. Note that even relatively small neurons located considerable distances away from the injection site can be stained well enough to clearly identify the size of the perikaryon, the orientation and extent of arborization of the dendrites (d), and the origin (ao) of the axon (a). (×315)

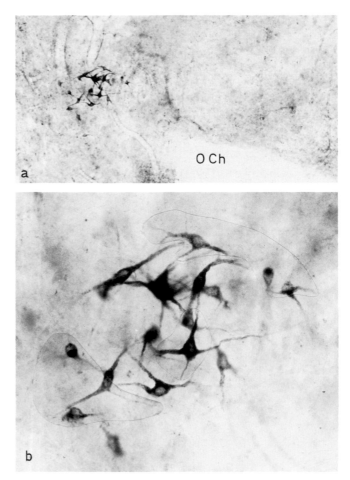

Figure 6 *Rat.* Golgi-like immunoperoxidase staining of wheat germ agglutinin (WGA). Fixation with Bouin/sublimate solution. (a) Survey of WGA-labelled neurons in the lateral hypothalamus following WGA injection into the caudal medulla oblongata. (b) Detail of (a): Och, optic chiasm. (×260)

transport studies with Golgi impregnation. HRP is also an excellent antigen, and antibodies can be raised against it without difficulty. Using these antibodies, HRP which has been transported by neurons can be visualized utilizing the immunoperoxidase procedure (Sofroniew and Schrell, 1980). Since the antigenic structure of the HRP is more stable against fixation than is the enzymatic activity, the immunoperoxidase staining of transported HRP appears to be more sensitive than the enzymatic staining. In many cases, processes into which the HRP has been secondarily transported are stained, yielding images of the transporting neurons very similar to Golgi impregnation.

In order to improve retrograde filling of neurons with HRP, and thereby improve the quality of the Golgi-like immunoperoxidase staining, various modifications of the injection techniques can be employed. Increasing the concentration of the HRP solution injected appears to improve the filling of transporting neurons and yields more intense staining. Also, addition of 5% Nonidet-P40 (Sigma) as described by Lipp and Schwegler (1980) to the injected HRP also appears to improve the staining. Thus, we have obtained very good results using 30% HRP (Sigma type VI) dissolved in 5% Nonidet-P40 in Ringer's solution. This solution is rather viscous and can only be injected mechanically, nevertheless, 0.05–0.1 µl injections are small and appear adequate for many cases. We have also used 7.5% HRP in water for iontophoresis, and have obtained in some cases excellent secondary filling of processes. However, as distance from the injection site increases, the filling of neurons appears to drop off as opposed to the 30% HRP injections. (For more detailed information on uses of HRP tracing consult Mesulam, 1982.)

Recently Schwab *et al.* (1978) have introduced a new protein to neuroanatomical tracing: lectin from wheat germ or wheat germ agglutinin (WGA) (Miles or Sigma). This protein is actively and specifically taken up and retrogradely transported by neurons. However, WGA has no enzymatic activity which can be used to visualize its location, and Schwab *et al.* (1978) radioactively labelled the WGA and detected its location using autoradiography. WGA is also a good antigen, and transported WGA can be visualized using the immunoperoxidase procedure (Figure 6) (Sofroniew, 1983). We have obtained good results by injecting the 0.25% WGA solution in phosphate buffer pH 7.4 as it is delivered by Miles-Yeda Ltd, or using 0.5% WGA in 0.01 M phosphate buffer pH 7.4 prepared from lyophilized WGA (Sigma).

II.3 Fixation

Normal animals, or animals 48 h following injection of a tracer protein, are anaesthetized using pentobarbital, the heart is exposed, and heparin injected followed immediately by transcardial perfusion with Ringer's solution, followed by one of the fixatives listed below. If possible, it is recommended that animals be tracheotomized and respirated with 95% O_2/5% CO_2 (Palay *et al.*, 1962; Sofroniew, 1983) prior to and during thoracotomy to expose the heart and prepare the perfusion. Following the perfusion, the brains are removed and stored in fixative for 4–18 h and thereafter in buffer at 4 °C. Some antigens are extremely sensitive to over-fixation, and should not be left in fixative more than 2–4 h at most.

Different fixatives are used for different substances. It is critical that fixations be optimal. We perfuse rats with a pressure of 150 cm H_2O, allow the Ringer's solution to flow for 10 s, and then switch to the fixative. We generally perfuse with fixatives which are at room temperature.

II.3.1 *Fixatives*

Bouin's solution. This consists of aqueous saturated picric acid:concentrated (37%) formaldehyde (Merck):glacial acetic acid, in ratios of 150:50:10. It is essential that the aqueous picric acid be truly saturated. It is best prepared by adding 1 litre of boiling distilled water to 200 g picric acid. When properly prepared, long crystals are formed as the solution cools. The picric acid solution and formaldehyde should be filtered separately shortly before use (within several hours), and can then be mixed. We recommend a 0.22 μm Millipore filter. The acetic acid (which need not be filtered) should be added immediately before use.

Bouin/sublimate solution. This consists of aqueous saturated picric acid:concentrated (37%) formaldehyde:saturated aqueous sublimate (mercuric chloride, $HgCl_2$):glacial acetic acid, in ratios of 150:50:20:10. The saturated sublimate solution is prepared by dissolving 60 g $HgCl_2$ in 1 litre boiling distilled water and allowing it to cool. Similar to Bouin's solution, the picric acid, formaldehyde, and sublimate solutions should be filtered separately before use, and the acetic acid added immediately before use. Sublimate is an excellent fixative for proteins (Romeis, 1968) and appears to greatly enhance the immunoreactivity of various peptides and proteins when added to the Bouin's solution.

4% paraformaldehyde in 0.1 M sodium phosphate buffer. Prepared by mixing 8% paraformaldehyde in water with 0.2 M sodium phosphate buffer pH 7.3 in 1:1 ratios.

4% paraformaldehyde, 0.5% glutaraldehyde. To 100 ml of 4% paraformaldehyde described above add 2 ml of 25% glutaraldehyde.

4% paraformaldehyde, 0.1% glutaraldehyde. To 100 ml of 4% paraformaldehyde add 0.4 ml of 25% glutaraldehyde.

2% paraformaldehyde, 0.1% glutaraldehyde. To 100 ml of 2% paraformaldehyde in phosphate buffer pH 7.4 add 0.4 ml of 25% glutaraldehyde.

The fixation procedure of perfusion with 4% paraformaldehyde, 0.1% glutaraldehyde for 15–30 min followed by immersion of tissue blocks in 4% paraformaldehyde without glutaraldehyde for a total time of about 4 h has yielded excellent results with a variety of antigens including amines, peptides and enzymes, and is highly recommended.

II.3.2 *Selection of fixative*

For endogenous peptides. We have obtained good staining of neurons containing various peptides such as vasopressin, oxytocin, and neurophysin (Sofroniew and Glasmann, 1981) using both Bouin's solution (Figures 1 and 2) and more recently Bouin/sublimate solution. The Bouin/sublimate solution yields a much more intense staining of the neurons and their processes than Bouin alone, but also gives a higher background staining. This background staining may be substantially reduced by pretreatment of the sections with iodine/potassium iodide solution as described below. Either fixative has advantages for different types of analysis, and both can be highly recommended. We have also obtained excellent staining of neurons producing other peptides such as somatostatin (Fig. 3) or enkephalin using the fixation procedure of perfusion with 4% paraformaldehyde, 0.1% glutaraldehyde followed by immersion in 4% paraformaldehyde only. Somatostatin neurons also stain well with Bouin's solution.

For exogenous tracer peptides. Here we also have obtained excellent results staining transported HRP (Sofroniew and Schrell, 1980) or WGA (Sofroniew, 1983) using both Bouin's solution (Figures 4 and 5) or Bouin/sublimate solution (Figure 6). Again, the Bouin/sublimate solution yields a much more intense staining of neurons and processes, but also gives a higher background staining (Figure 6). Both fixatives have advantages for different types of analysis and both are recommended.

For endogenous enzymes. The immunoreactivity of various endogenous enzymes appears to be quite sensitive to fixations which are too strong and alter their large and complex tertiary structure. Grzanna *et al.* (1978) and Grzanna and Molliver (1980) have achieved excellent staining of neurons containing the enzyme dopamine-β-hydroxylase by fixation with ice-cold 2% paraformaldehyde plus 0.1% glutaraldehyde at pH 7.4. We have obtained excellent Golgi-like staining of neurons containing the enzymes choline acetyltransferase (Sofroniew *et al.*, 1982) or tyrosine hydroxylase with the fixation procedure of perfusion with 4% paraformaldehyde, 0.1% glutaraldehyde followed by immersion in 4% paraformaldehyde.

For endogenous amines. For visualization of amines, Steinbusch *et al.* (1981) have obtained excellent results using fixation with ice-cold 4% paraformaldehyde at pH 7.3 for serotonin staining, or 4% paraformaldehyde plus 0.5% glutaraldehyde at pH 7.3 for noradrenaline staining, using their antisera. We have had very good results staining neurons containing serotonin using a monoclonal antibody and the fixation procedure of perfusion with 4% paraformaldehyde, 0.1% glutaraldehyde followed by immersion in 4% paraformaldehyde.

II.4 Sectioning

Either Vibtatome or frozen sections of 50–200 µm thickness may be used. Storage of blocks prior to sectioning is best done in fixative for 4–18 h at 4 °C following perfusion and thereafter in buffer at 4 °C. In general it is recommended that blocks be exposed to fixative for a total time of 2–5 h and that sections be prepared and incubation in the primary antibody is begun within

48 h of fixation. A useful protocol is: fixation followed by immersion of blocks in buffer overnight followed by sectioning and washing of sections overnight followed by incubation in primary antibody as discussed below.

Vibratome sections

Vibratome sections can be prepared from blocks taken out of fixative and washed in buffer. Vibratome sections are stable and give excellent preservation of morphology.

Frozen sections

Blocks fixed with Bouin's or Bouin/sublimate solution can be frozen directly out of the fixative. These blocks yield very stable 50–200 μm frozen sections when sectioned at temperatures from -18 to $-25\,°C$, and the preservation of light microscopic morphology is excellent (Figures 1–6).

Blocks fixed in 4% paraformaldehyde or paraformaldehyde/glutaraldehyde mixtures are best incubated in 10–25% sucrose solutions for 24 h prior to frozen sectioning to reduce brittleness and breakage of sections.

Collection of sections

Sections should be collected free-floating in containers of buffer. Depending on whether or not strict preservation of sequence is desired, single or multiple sections may be put in a container. The sections are then washed repeatedly in buffer, to remove the fixative prior to staining.

II.5   Staining

Solutions

Buffer. The same buffer, consisting of 1.48 g $Na_2HPO_4 \cdot 2H_2O$, 0.43 g KH_2PO_4, 7.0 g NaCl, and 5.0 g Tris (hydroxymethyl)-aminomethane in 1 litre of deionized water and adjusted to a pH of 7.8, is recommended to wash the sections, as well as to prepare other solutions described below. As a preservative, 0.05% NaN_3 may be used in buffer for all steps except for the DAB reaction and washes immediately prior to this.

Iodine/potassium iodide solution. The stock solution consists of 2 g iodine (I_2) plus 3 g potassium iodide (KI) dissolved in 100 ml of 90% ethyl alcohol. For use in washing sections fixed with Bouin/sublimate solution, the stock solution is diluted 1 ml per 100 ml in 70% ethyl alcohol.

Triton/carrageenan solution. This solution consists of 1.0% (by weight) Triton X-100 (Sigma) plus 0.5% (by weight) lambda carrageenan (Sigma) and 0.1% NaN_3 (as a preservative) dissolved in the buffer (freshly prepared) described above. Triton X-100 is a detergent added to facilitate penetration of antisera into the tissue. Lambda carrageenan is a non-gelling seaweed gelatin added to reduce non-specific staining (Sofroniew and Glasmann, 1981). All antisera used in the immunoperoxidase procedure should be diluted with this solution.

Primary antisera. Primary antisera (i.e. antisera directed against the substance contained within the neurons to be stained) are diluted in the Triton/carrageenan solution described above. The dilution yielding the best staining with any given antiserum must be determined empirically in initial staining tests using several dilutions. All of the antisera we have used are diluted within the range of 1:200–1:2000. Diluted primary antisera can be stored at 4 °C, and can in our experience be repeatedly re-used over a period of several years with no loss of activity.

Second antiserum. We use donkey anti-rabbit IgG (Wellcome Ltd) diluted at 1:50 in the Triton/carrageenan solution described above, although any other good anti-IgG directed against IgG of the species of the primary antisera can be used. Diluted second antiserum can also be stored at 4 °C and repeatedly re-used over a period of 10–12 months with no loss of activity.

Peroxidase–antiperoxidase (PAP). We use PAP complex (UCB Bioproducts), diluted 1:75 in the Triton/carrageenan solution described above. PAP must be diluted fresh from lyophilized vials or from concentrated frozen stock solution, not more than 1–2 h before use. Diluted PAP stored unfrozen for longer than 1–2 weeks was found to lose activity.

3,3'diaminobenzidine (DAB). DAB (Sigma) is diluted from 25–100 mg/ 50 ml in the buffer (without NaN_3) described above. Less concentrated solutions seem to give less intense staining. Immediately before use 10 or 20 µl/50 ml concentrated (30%) H_2O_2 are added.

Staining procedure

The sections collected in containers of buffer after sectioning are repeatedly washed with fresh changes of buffer over a period of several hours until all of the fixative has been completely removed. With the fixatives containing picric acid this is readily seen, as the sections become white. At this stage, sections which have been fixed with Bouin/sublimate solution may be treated to remove sublimate residues and reduce the background staining. This treatment consists of washing the sections for 30 min in the diluted iodine/ potassium iodide solution (Romeis, 1968). Subsequently the sections are washed again briefly in 70% ethyl alcohol followed by several changes of buffer over 30 min. Thereafter, the procedure for sections fixed in different manners is identical. The buffer is decanted, and diluted primary antiserum added for an incubation time of 24–72 h and in some cases up to 7 days, at 4 °C. Incubation time should be selected empirically, although 48 h is adequate for most antisera. Following incubation, the primary antiserum is decanted and saved, and sections are washed in 6–8 fresh changes of buffer over a 3 h period. Then diluted second antiserum is added to each container and incubated for 24 h at 4 °C. Following incubation, the second antiserum is decanted and saved, and sections are again washed in 6–8 fresh changes of buffer over a 3 h period. Then diluted PAP solution (prepared fresh) is added to each container and incubated for 24 h at 4 °C. Following incubation, the PAP solution is decanted and discarded, and sections washed in 10–12 fresh changes of buffer over a 4–5 h period. Then freshly prepared DAB solution (concentration should be selected empirically) is added to each test tube, and incubated for 5–15 min at room temperature under constant gentle shaking. DAB is then decanted, and sections washed briefly in buffer. Sections are best mounted from buffer onto gelatinized glass slides and allowed to air dry. Completely dried sections can then be placed directly into 100% alcohol, brought into xylene and coverslipped.

Note: primary and second antisera were always decanted into bottles and stored at 4 °C for repeated use. PAP solution should be discarded after use.

II.6   Analysis of Results

The appearance of the immunoperoxidase staining, obtained using the procedures outlined, is often quite similar to that of Golgi preparations and allows detailed morphological analysis of neurons identified as producing a specific substance (Figures 1–3) or identified as transporting an exogenous tracer protein injected into a known site (Figures 4–6). Figures 2 and 3 show peptidergic neurons in which the beaded axons can easily be distinguished from dendrites. This type of staining enables a detailed analysis of these neurons, revealing complex aspects of their morphology.

The morphology of neurons retrogradely transporting tracer proteins can also be examined in detail, since the tracer proteins are apparently transported secondarily throughout the various processes of the neuron (Figures 4–6). Thus, one can determine the number and extent of arborization of the dendrites (Figures 4 and 5); and one can identify beaded dendrites, axons (Figure 5) and occasionally collaterals. In general, although more neurons are retrogradely labelled using WGA, the Golgi-like staining of individual neurons is better using HRP.

III GENERAL CONSIDERATIONS

III.1 Specificity

The specificity of staining is determined primarily by the specificity of the primary antiserum. Therefore it is important to establish the extent of cross-reaction of every primary antiserum used, with various possibly interfering antigens. Although absorption control studies do not verify absolute specificity, they do allow discrimination between reaction of the antisera with closely related substances, and such controls should be conducted with every antiserum used (for serum specificity see Chapter 1, Section VII).

III.2 Resolution

The resolution of the procedure is such that in many cases it allows a detailed morphological analysis and comparison of various types of neurons producing the same substance (Sofroniew and Glasmann, 1981), or of different types of neurons projecting to the same area (Sofroniew and Schrell, 1980). Most neural processes, including fine collaterals, can be identified (Sofroniew and Glasmann, 1981). In general, the morphology of the neurons observed with Golgi-like immunoperoxidase staining appears to correlate well with the morphology observed with true Golgi impregnation. Some caution must be advised when using Bouin-fixed material. Although this appears to be a superior fixative for preserving the antigenicity of peptides and proteins, it is not a good fixative for preserving the integrity of membranes, and yields very poor ultrastructure. For this reason unusually appearing light microscopic structures should be interpreted with caution.

Another point to be considered is the possibility of dislocation of the antigen or staining product as a result of the procedure, giving the false impression that the antigen is located within processes in which it is not natively present. For example, the staining of peptides in processes which are considered dendrites. This has been discussed in detail elsewhere (Sofroniew and Glasmann, 1981). Briefly, dislocation of the antigen or staining product does not seem to occur to any major degree. This is based on the observation that all types of stained processes could be found in sections where such processes had been severed from their parent perikaryon, indicating that they contained the antigen at the time of sectioning (i.e. immediately after fixation and prior to staining), since the only source for diffusion, the perikaryon, had been eliminated.

In conclusion, the Golgi-like immunoperoxidase staining procedure appears to be a valuable new tool for examining the morphology of neurons identified as producing a specific substance or identified as transporting a tracer protein from a known site. Direct comparison with Golgi-impregnated material should yield new information concerning the chemical nature as well as interconnectivity of identified neurons in various neural systems.

ACKNOWLEDGEMENTS

The technical assistance of J. Werner and the editorial assistance of P. Campbell are gratefully acknowledged.

REFERENCES

Burchanowski, B. J., Knigge, K. M., and Sternberger, L. A. (1979). 'Rich ependymal investment of luteoliberin (LHRH), fibers revealed immunocytochemically in Golgi-like image.' *Proc. Natl. Acad. Sci. USA*, **76**, 6671–6674.

Cajal, S. Ramon y (1909–1911). *Histologie du Système Nerveux de l'Homme et des Vertébrés*, Parts 1, 2. A. Maloine, Paris.

Cajal, S. Ramon y (1954). *Neuron Theory or Reticular Theory?* (trans. W. U. Purkiss and C. A. Fox). Consejo Superior de Investigaciones Cientificas Instituto 'Ramon y Cajal', Madrid.

Cuello, A. C. (1978). 'Immunocytochemical studies of the distribution of neurotransmitters and related substances in CNS.' In Iversen, L. L. *et al.* (eds), *Handbook of Psychopharmacology*, vol. 9, pp. 69–137. Plenum Press, London.

Cuello, A. C., Galfre, G., and Milstein C. (1979). 'Detection of substance P in the central nervous system by a monoclonal antibody.' *Proc. Natl. Acad. Sci. USA*, **76**, 3532–3536.

Eckenstein, F. and Thoenen, H. (1982). 'Production of specific antisera and monoclonal antibodies to choline acetyltransferase: characterization and use for identification of cholinergic neurons.' *EMBO J.*, **1**, 363–368.

Gainer, H., Sarne, Y., and Brownstein, M. J. (1977). 'Biosynthesis and axonal transport of rat neurohypophysial proteins and peptides.' *J. Cell. Biol.*, **73**, 366–381.

Golgi, C. (1894). *Untersuchungen über den feineren Bau des centralen und peripherischen Nervensystems.* Fischer, Jena.

Grzanna, R. and Molliver, M. E. (1980). 'The locus coeruleus in the rat: an immunohistochemical delineation.' *Neuroscience*, **5**, 21–40.

Grzanna, R., Molliver, M. E., and Coyle, J. T. (1978). 'Visualization of central noradrenergic neurons in thick sections by the unlabeled antibody method: a transmitter-specific Golgi image.' *Proc. Natl. Acad. Sci. USA*, **75**, 2502–2506.

Joh, T. H., Gegham, C., and Reis, D. J. (1973). 'Immunochemical demonstration of increased tyrosine hydroxylase protein in sympathetic ganglia and adrenal medulla elicited by reserpine.' *Proc. Natl. Acad. Sci. USA*, **70**, 2767–2771.

Lipp, H.-P. and Schwegler, H. (1980). 'Improved transport of horseradish peroxidase after injection with a non-ionic detergent (Nonidet P-40) into mouse cortex and observations on the relationship between spread at the injection site and amount of transported label.' *Neurosci. Lett.*, **20**, 49–54.

Mesulam, M.-M. (1978). 'Tetramethyl benzidine for horseradish peroxidase neurohistochemistry: a non-carcinogenic blue reaction-product with superior sensitivity for visualizing afferents and efferents.' *J. Histochem. Cytochem.*, **26**, 106–117.

Mesulam, M.-M. (ed.) (1982). *Tracing Neural Connections with Horseradish Peroxidase.* IBRO Handbook Series: *Methods in the Neurosciences*. Wiley, Sussex.

Palay, S. L., McGee-Russell, S. M., Gordon, S., and Grillo, M. A. (1962). 'Fixation of neural tissues for electron microscopy by perfusion with solutions of osmium tetroxide.' *J. Cell Biol.*, **12**, 385–410.

Romeis, B. (1968). *Mikroskopische Technik*, 16. Aufl. Oldenbourg, München–Wien.

Russell, J. T., Brownstein, M. J., and Gainer, H. (1980). 'Biosynthesis of vasopressin, oxytocin, and neurophysins: isolation and characterization of two common precursors (propressophysin and prooxyphysin).' *Endocrinology*, **107**, 1880–1891.

Schwab, M. E., Javoy-Agid, F., and Agid, Y. (1978). 'Labeled wheat germ agglutinin (WGA) as a new, highly sensitive retrograde tracer in the rat brain hippocampal system.' *Brain Res.*, **152**, 145–150.

Sofroniew, M. V. (1983). 'Direct reciprocal connections between the bed nucleus of the stria terminalis and dorsomedial medulla oblongata: Evidence from immunohistochemical detection of tracer proteins.' *J. Comp. Neurol.*, in press.

Sofroniew, M. V., Eckenstein, F., Thoenen, H., and Cuello, A. C. (1982). 'Topography of choline acetyltransferase-containing neurons in the forebrain of the rat.' *Neurosci. Lett.*, **33**, 7–12.

Sofroniew, M. V. and Glasmann, W. (1981). 'Golgi-like immunoperoxidase staining of hypothalamic magnocellular neurons that contain vasopressin, oxytocin or neurophysin in the rat.' *Neuroscience*, **6**, 619–643.

Sofroniew, M. V., Madler, M., Müller, O. A., and Scriba, P. C. (1978). 'A method for the consistent production of high quality antisera to small peptide hormones.' *Fresenius Z. Anal. Chem.*, **290**, 163.

Sofroniew, M. V. and Schrell, U. (1980). 'Hypothalamic neurons projecting to the rat caudal medulla examined by immunoperoxidase staining of retrogradely transported horseradish peroxidase.' *Neurosci. Lett.*, **19**, 257–263.

Somogyi, P., Hodgson, A. J., and Smith, A. D. (1979). 'An approach to tracing neuron networks in the cerebral cortex and basal ganglia. Combination of Golgi staining, retrograde transport of horseradish peroxidase and anterograde degeneration of synaptic boutons in the same material.' *Neuroscience*, **4**, 1805–1852.

Steinbusch, H. W. M., Nieuwenhuys, R., Verhofstad, A. A. J., and van der Kooy, D. (1981). 'The nucleus raphe dorsalis of the rat and its projection upon the caudoputamen. A combined cytoarchitectonic, immunohistochemical and retrograde transport study.' *J. Physiol. Paris*, **77**, 157–174.

Sternberger, L. A. (1974). *Immunocytochemistry*. Prentice-Hall, Englewood Cliffs, NJ, USA.

Vaitukaitis, J., Robbins, J. B., Nieschlag, E., and Ross, G. T. (1971). 'A method for producing antisera with small doses of immunogen.' *J. Clin. Endocrinol. Metab.*, **33**, 988–991.

Vandesande, F., Dierickx, K., and De Mey, J. (1975). 'Identification of the vasopressin-neurophysin II and the oxytocin-neurophysin I producing neurons in the bovine hypothalamus.' *Cell Tiss. Res.*, **156**, 189–200.

Immunohistochemistry
Edited by A. C. Cuello
© 1983 IBRO

CHAPTER 17

Combined Immunohistochemistry and Autoradiography

VICTORIA CHAN-PALAY

Department of Neurobiology, Harvard Medical School, Boston, Mass. 02115

I   INTRODUCTION

These investigations provide a direct and reliable means for the demonstration of multiple transmitters or putative peptide neuromediators that coexist in the same neuron and their terminals (Chan-Palay, 1979b). Previous studies by Chan-Palay *et al.* (1978) had demonstrated that some serotonin (5-HT) neurons in the ventral medulla oblongata of rat, particularly those in the reticular formation nuclei (raphe pallidus, raphe obscurus, gigantocellularis, pars alpha, paragigantocellularis lateralis, and the interfascicularis hypoglossi) also contain the peptide substance P (SP). These studies used autoradiography after administration of ^{3}H-serotonin (^{3}H-5-HT) as well as Falck–Hillarp fluorescence for 5-HT combined with microspectrofluorimetry and immunofluorescence for SP on the same sections. Subsequent investigations by other investigators confirmed these findings using a different approach on consecutive sections (Hökfelt *et al.*, 1978). This report presents a novel approach for the demonstration of the coexistence of 5-HT and SP in single cells and terminal plexuses using simultaneous autoradiography and immunocytochemistry on the same preparation. The significance of this work is that the methods described here are: (1) readily adaptable for use for the detection of numerous other peptides, amines, and other transmitter compounds in locations elsewhere in the nervous system; and (2) utilizable for light and electron microscopy so that connections as well as the synaptology of these neurons can be studied.

For experiments described here, 5-HT was detected by application of ^{3}H-5-HT for uptake by 5-HT neurons followed by autoradiography (Chan-Palay, 1975, 1976, 1977a,b, 1979b). SP was detected by immunocytochemistry using *in vivo* injections of a characterized monoclonal SP antibody (Chan-Palay, 1979b) and the peroxidase–antiperoxidase method (PAP, Sternberger, 1979; see also Chapter 4)). *In vivo* injections of antibody provide a rapid and reliable means of marking specific immunoreactive cell groups based upon the antigen–antibody recognition and binding capacities of these cells, and studies of SP cells and their connections with light and electron microscopy have been recently reported (Chan-Palay, 1979a). Moreover, for the peptidergic neruons, where localization of cell bodies has been difficult and has necessitated the use of toxic substances such as colchicine to interfere with fast axonal flow (Hökfelt *et al.*, 1978), the *in vivo* injection method is invaluable as it reveals peptide-containing neuronal somata reliably without colchicine (Chan-Palay, 1979a). The present adaptation of *in vivo* injections of antibody in combination with autoradiography expands the range of this new technique for the exploration of many chemically specific systems in the brain and peripherally.

II METHODOLOGICAL ASPECTS

The raphe pallidus in the midline surface of the ventral medulla was used throughout for these model studies on account of its accessibility to stereotaxic and visual approaches for microinjections (Chan-Palay, 1977b; Brown *et al.*, 1977; Chan-Palay, 1979a) and its demonstrated content of 5-HT, 5-HT-SP, and SP neurons (Chan-Palay, 1977a; Chan-Palay *et al.*, 1978; Hökfelt *et al.*, 1978; Ljungdahl *et al.*, 1979). Adult rats (300–400 g body weight, Charles River Breeding Labs) were used in these experiments. The raphe pallidus was approached from the ventral aspect as previously described (Chan-Palay, 1977b; Brown *et al.*, 1977; Chan-Palay, 1979a) in rats anaesthetized with chloral hydrate (35%, 0.1 ml/100 g body weight (b.w.). The bone of the basiocciput overlying the raphe pallidus was removed and the basilar artery and ventral medulla visualized after slitting the dura. The mortality rate was less than 1% in acute experiments. Microinjections were made by pressure (Chan-Palay, 1977b) through glass micropipettes with tip diameters of approximately 10 µm. Two to five separate injections each consisting of a volume of 0.025–0.05 µl were made into the raphe pallidus per animal.

II.1 Materials

All compounds used in these experiments, with the exception of the monoclonal antibody, which was used undiluted, were dissolved in 0.9% sterile saline:

(a) tritiated serotonin (^{3}H-5-HT, 10^-7 m, specific activity, 10.8 µCi/mmol. Amersham Searle);

(b) clorgyline, a monoamine oxidase inhibitor (May and Baker, 10 mg/100 g b.w., 12 h before surgery);

(c) serotonin uptake inhibitors: GE654 (Astra, 1 mg/100 g b.w.), Zimelidine (Astra, 1 mg/100 g b.w.), Norzimelidine (Astra, 1 mg/100 g b.w.) administered 2 h before surgery;

(d) 5,6-dihydroxytryptamine creatinine sulphate (5,6-DHT. Sigma. 3.0 µg/µl, 10 µl per 100 g b.w.);

(e) reserpine (1 mg/100 g b.w. administered 12 h before surgery);

(f) monoclonal antibody against SP, used undiluted in the partially purified form after precipitation with ammonium sulphate and dialysis (Cuello *et al.*, 1979).

(g) control sera, undiluted monoclonal antibody adsorbed overnight with SP (2.5 µgs10 µl).

Three experimental paradigms were tested (Figure 1).

II.2 Double Pipette Injections

Double-barrelled micropipettes with one barrel filled with ^{3}H-5-HT and the other filled with monoclonal SP antibody were used. The tip-to-tip separation distances were not greater than 50–80 µm, and the contents of both electrodes were ejected simultaneously by the application of pressure. Each injection site received equal volumes of 0.025 µl of solution per pipette, a total of 0.05 µl per site.

II.3 Simultaneous Injection

Simultaneous injection of ^{3}H-5-HT and monoclonal SP antibody from a single pipette. An aliquot of ^{3}H-5-HT was evaporated to dryness and undiluted monoclonal SP added. A total of 2–4 µCu of ^{3}H-5-HT with a total of 0.2 to 0.3 µl of SP antibody was injected in each animal in five se ions, each containing approximately 0.5 µCi of ^{3}H-5-HT and 0.05 µl of antibody.

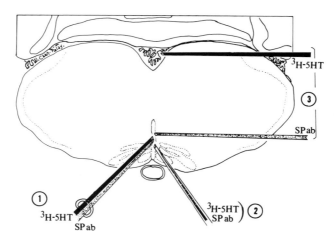

Figure 1 Diagram to illustrate three experimental paradigms and modes of delivery of the two tracers for combined immunocytochemistry and autoradiography. (1) Double pipette injection with simultaneous delivery from one pipette filled with ^{3}H–5–HT and the other with monoclonal antibody to substance P directly into raphe pallidus. (2) Single pipette injection with simultaneous delivery of ^{3}H–5–HT and monoclonal antibody to SP directly into raphe pallidus. (3) Injection of monoclonal antibody to SP into raphe pallidus with intracisternal injection of ^{3}H–5–HT

II.4   Intracisternal Infusion

Intracisternal infusion of ^{3}H-5-HT (25 µl over 5 min) administered manually by Hamilton syringe into animals, all of which were pretreated with clorgyline 12 h before. This was followed an hour later by *in vivo* injections of undiluted monoclonal SP antibody.

II.5   Control Experiments

(i) Two animals in each group of the experiments described above received injections containing monoclonal SP antibody preadsorbed overnight with SP instead of the actual antibody.

(ii) Monoamine oxidase inhibition. At least three animals in each group received previously determined effective doses of clorgyline 12 h before surgery; the remaining three did not. All animals in the ^{3}H-5-HT intracisternal infusion/SP injection experiments were pretreated with clorgyline. Monoamine oxidase inhibitors such as clorgyline used in conjunction with ^{3}H-5-HT autoradiography serve effectively to retard the metabolism of ^{3}H-5-HT into its metabolites, thus ensuring that the label in autoradiograms indicates sites of 5-HT transport and storage rather than that of 5-hydroxyindoacetic acid, 5-HIAA (Chan-Palay and Jonsson, unpublished data from thin-layer chromatography experiments).

(iii) Serotonin uptake inhibitors, GE654, Zimelidine and Norzimelidine, were used. Each substance was tried separately in groups consisting of three animals and administered 2 h before surgery. The single micropipette injections of combined ^{3}H-5-HT and SP antibody were used.

(iv) Three rats were treated with 5,6-DHT (30 µg/100 g b.w. in 10 µl) administered intracisternally 7 days prior to surgery. This neurotoxin is preferentially taken up into serotonin neurons causing their ultimate degeneration as well as a limited amount of tissue damage at the injection site (Baumgarten *et al.*, 1971). The single micropipette injections of combined ^{3}H-5-HT and SP antibody were used.

(v) Three rats were treated with reserpine in a single dose (2 g/100 g b.w., i.p.) administered 12 h before surgery. The single micropipette injections of combined ^{3}H-5-HT and SP antibody were used. Reserpine has a documented ability to deplete stored monoamines from neurons in the central and peripheral nervous system (Carlsson, 1966).

Following injections the animals were fixed, tissues were prepared for immunocytochemistry, then autoradiography. All rats were maintained for 1–2 h after injection and were then perfused with cold Tyrode's buffer (Ca^{2+} free, 50 ml) followed by 500 ml ice-cold 4% formaldehyde with 0.25% glutaraldehyde in 0.2 µ phosphate buffer, pH 7.4. Following perfusion the brain was removed and soaked in this fixative for 1–2 h, then rinsed and soaked in Tris buffer (0.05 M, pH 7.6) overnight. Horizontal sections 15–20 µm thick through the entire raphe pallidus were cut on a Vibratome into Tris buffer maintained at 10 °C. The consecutive serial sections were then treated with rabbit anti-rat immunoglobulin (IgG) diluted 1:10 in Tris–Triton X-100 0.05% reacted with rabbit PAP (1:100) and with 0.022% diaminobenzidine in Tris buffer and 0.3% hydrogen peroxide for 7 min (for details see Chan-Palay, 1979a; see also Chapter 4). Individual serial sections were examined for injection sites and cells with SP immunoreactivity. The sections were mounted in serial order onto chrom-alum (0.05%) and gelatin (0.5%) treated slides and allowed to air-dry in a clean environment. All sections were examined by phase and Nomarski interference microscopy. Attention was paid to the intensity of the immunoreactive product.

Thereafter, the slides were processed for autoradiography (see Chan-Palay, 1977b; pp. 502–504). Slides were dipped individually into nuclear track emulsion (Kodak NTB-2 diluted 1:1 with distilled water at 45 °C) in a light-tight photographic darkroom equipped with a sodium lamp having both red and yellow band filters (Thomas Duplex super safelight). The slides were dried for 6 h, placed in a light-tight box with a desiccant and exposed for 3–6 weeks prior to development in Kodak D-19 developer (undiluted, 18 °C, $4\frac{1}{2}$ min), fixed, washed, and dried. The slides were rapidly dehydrated and cleared in xylene prior to coverslipping in Permount, were cover-slipped directly. No further counterstains were employed. Success of the autoradiograms was judged by examination under dark-field and bright-field microscopy based on the specific accumulation of silver grains on identified neurons and processes at a level over that of the background. The combined study of positive SP immunoreactivity and of autoradiographic label with ^{3}H-5-HT was most convenient in bright-field microscopy.

II.6   General Comments on Technique

The sequence of demonstration of cytochemical labels for SP and 5-HT is limited in practice by several factors: the SP antigen–antibody complexes need to be localized rapidly to prevent loss by lengthy tissue preparation, and immunocytochemistry should be done before autoradiography. Once the immunoreactive material is permanently captured the lengthy exposures and harsh chemical procedures of developing and fixation in autoradiography can be carried out. Attempts to reverse the process by doing the autoradiography before immunocytochemistry have not been successful.

The major steps for ensuring or controlling the cytochemical specificity and sensitivity in terms of preservation of antigen, antigen–antibody complexes, radioactive label through tissue preservation, and subsequent preparation have been taken in these studies. A most important consideration, that of penetration of the label (^{3}H-5-HT) and of the antibody is ensured by their direct application into the region of interest under conditions that would allow for active and specific physiological uptake, recognition, and binding.

III   ANALYSIS OF RESULTS

Equivalent results in terms of 5-HT/SP labelled cells were obtained regardless of the mode of administration of the two labels: 3H-5-HT and monoclonal antibody to SP from double-barrelled pipettes, together from a single pipette, or antibody applied by pipette and intracisternal infusion of ^{3}H-5-HT. Practically, the single-barrel injections are the simplest to execute. The injection sites are sometimes recognizable by a small region of haemor-rhage with red blood cells stained a dark brown by their peroxidatic reaction, unrelated to SP immunoreactivity. The fundamental observations are sum-marized in Figure 2a–i. Neurons, dendrites, and axons with positive SP immunoreactivity have an unmistakable orange/brown reaction product. Those with heavy ^{3}H-5-HT accumulation are specifically labelled with autoradiographic silver grains, well above background. Cells and fibres with both ^{3}H-5-HT accumulation and SP immunoreactivity are stained orange/brown and have in addition a superimposed deposit of autoradiographic silver grains.

III.1 Neuronal Somata

Examples of SP immunoreactive cells are best shown in Figure 2a–c. These somata are generally small, 8–18 µm in diameter, with prominent round unstained nuclei (Figure 2b,c) and cytoplasm containing aggregates of intensely SP immunoreactive complexes (probably in lysosomal particles as described previously—Chan-Palay, 1979a). The five cells of this description illustrated in Figure 2a–c are intensely SP-positive but have a minimum of label with ³H-5-HT. Silver grains are present (arrow) over the cytoplasm and around the nuclear boundaries, but in numbers only moderately above background. It can be concluded then that these cells are mainly SP-positive with very little 5-HT. The neuropil surrounding these cells shows numerous processes and terminals of the SP immunoreactive variety with small accumulations of 5-HT grains (Figure 2a,c); the neuropil surrounding the labelled cell in Figure 2b shows no 5-HT accumulations above background. These five examples are taken from the rostral raphe pallidus, approaching the boundaries of the pons where small SP immunoreactive neurons are plentiful.

The three neuronal somata in Figure 2d–f show different cytochemical labelling characteristics. These cells are usually fusiform or multipolar and are larger, from 12 to 35 µm in diameter. All three neurons are intensely labelled with accumulations of silver grains from ³H-5-HT. In addition, they are also well labelled by SP immunoreactivity, the two cells in Figure 2d,e more intensely than that in Figure 2f. Examination of the neuropil surrounding these cells shows boutons with intensely orange SP immunoreactive product (arrows, Figure 2d–f) and individual boutons apposed directly upon the somatic surface (Figure 2f, crossed arrow). Dendrites and axons with ³H-5-HT label are also obvious. Examples of neurons such as these with considerable amounts of SP and 5-HT together are found readily throughout the middle and caudal extents of the raphe pallidus, particularly near the penetrating branches of the basilar artery.

The two neuronal somata shown in Figure 2g and 2h come from the raphe pallidus immediately next to the pars alpha portion of the reticular nucleus gigantocellularis lateralis. The majority of the neurons of the raphe and of the gigantocellularis nuclei in this region are serotonin-containing as previously demonstrated in mapping studies with ³H-5-HT (Chan-Palay, 1977b). Examination of these two cells reveals their distinctive features. They are large, from 25 to 60 µm in diameter. There is heavy labelling by accumulations of silver grains due to ³H-5–HT but no apparent SP immunoreactivity within the cell somata. These are serotonin neurons without SP. However, they are innervated or have close relations with SP immunoreactive nerve fibres (Figure 2g between pairs of arrows) that encapsulate the entire cell soma and emerging primary dendrites (Figure 2h, arrows).

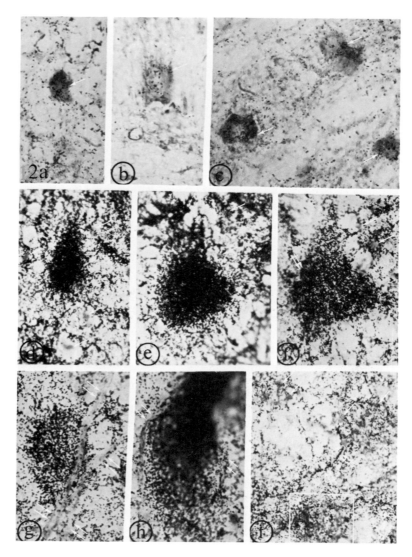

Figure 2 Photomicrographs of serotonin and SP neurons and their processes in the raphe pallidus localized by immunocytochemistry and autoradiography after simultaneous injection of ^{3}H–5–HT and monoclonal antibody to SP. a–c: Small neurons with intense SP immunoreactive staining and minimal autoradiographic label with ^{3}H–5–HT (arrows). d,e: Larger 5–HT–SP neurons with intense SP immunoreactivity as well as heavy autoradiographic label with ^{3}H–5–HT. Arrows indicate boutons or processes in the neuropil with SP immunoreactivity. F: A large neuron cell body with predominant labelling with ^{3}H–5–HT and minimal SP immunoreactivity. Crossed arrows indicate intensely reactive SP boutons upon the somatic surface and single

III.2 Nerve Fibres

Examples of dendrites of neurons with SP immunoreactivity or with
^{3}H-5-HT label, or both, are readily apparent in these preparations. Boutons
with intense SP immunoreactivity (Figure 2i, arrows) that are separate from
boutons with ^{3}H-5-HT label (Figure 2i, crossed arrows) occur in immediate
apposition. These areas can be distinguished from adjacent ones where the
two labels are intermingled, indicating a likely coexistence of SP and 5-HT
within the tangle of fibres (Figure 2i, boxed area).

III.3 Control Experiments

The control experiments designed for these studies were devised to study
the 5-HT and SP labelling properties of raphe neurons under conditions of
manipulation of the SP antibody system and then of the 5-HT system.

Injections of ^{3}H-5-HT with monoclonal antibody preadsorbed overnight
with an excess of synthetic SP resulted in no labelling in neurons of the raphe
pallidus although autoradiographic labelling with ^{3}H-5-HT was unaffected.
This observation would be expected since no effective primary antibody was
available to activate the specific SP antigen–antibody recognition and binding
system *in vivo*. Since the primary antibody was not introduced at any other
stage in the immunocytochemical procedure thereafter no specific staining
resulted. These control experiments indicate the specificity as well as the
sensitivity of the technique. There is no problem with tissue penetration since
the antibody is applied *in vivo* in the living animals.

MAO inhibitor.   Comparisons of data from these experiments conducted in
animals with and without pretreatment with monoamine oxidase inhibitors do
not show detectable differences in the quantity of autoradiographic silver
grains over neuronal somata or nerve plexuses. Since monoamine oxidase inh
ave been shown to decrease the metabolism of ^{3}H-5-HT to ^{3}H-5-HIAA
(Jonsson and Chan-Palay, unpublished data from thin-layer chromatography
experiments) it is useful for the autoradiographic portion of these experiments in order to ensure that the ^{3}H label is on the transmitter of interest

---

arrows indicate similar boutons elsewhere in the neuropil. g.h: Large neurons of the
raphe pallidus near its boundary with the gigantocellularis reticular nucleus (pars
alpha) labelled in their somata only with ^{3}H–5–HT. They are in apposition with
processes of other neurons localized by intense SP immunoreactivity (double arrows).
i: Acellular neuropil of the raphe pallidus in which boutons that are intensely SP
immunoreactive (arrows) lie next to fibres labelled by ^{3}H–5–HT (crossed arrows). In
the boxed area, the autoradiographic ^{3}H–5–HT label and the SP immunoreactive sites
are superimposed, indicating possible coexistence of both 5–HT and SP in terminals in
this region. (×260)

rather than its metabolites. One explanation for the lack of detectable differences may be the short duration of the experiment and the brief post-injection survival periods utilized.

Uptake inhibitors.   Experiments with pretreatment of animals with serotonin uptake inhibitors indicate that there is a significant reduction of autoradiographic label in all resulting preparations of raphe pallidus. The degree of depletion ranges from approximately 85 to 95%, determined by silver grain quantitations over known serotonin-rich regions. The degree of effectiveness of depletion in label depends on the uptake inhibitor utilized. It is greatest with GE654 and lower with Zimelidine and its analogue Norzimelidine. These experiments indicate that the autoradiographic label present in the experimental data described above is dependent on the selective serotonin uptake system. The SP immunoreactivity is unchanged, indicating that the antigen–antibody recognition and binding capacities are intact.

Serotonin neurotoxins.   Pretreatment of animals intracisternally 7 days prior to surgery with 5,6-DHT causes considerable degeneration in serotonin cells and fibres in the brain. The raphe pallidus of such animals injected with ^{3}H-5-HT and monoclonal SP antibody shows a significant loss of autoradiographic label as well as of SP immunoreactivity in cells and fibres, particularly in the middle and caudal aspects of this raphe nucleus. The small neurons in the rostral raphe which are mostly SP immunoreactive are less affected. These results indicate that degeneration due to 5,6-DHT can destroy serotonin neurons as well as those serotonin neurons with coexistent SP.

Reserpine.   Material from animals treated with reserpine prior to injection of the raphe pallidus with ^{3}H-5-HT and monoclonal SP antibody did not show a reduction in autoradiographic ^{3}H-5-HT label in cells or fibres. SP immunoreactivity was also not impaired. These results indicate that depletion of amine stores in 5-HT cells with or without coexistent SP does not appreciably alter their reuptake mechanisms for ^{3}H-5-HT nor their SP antigen antibody recognition and binding capacity.

IV   GENERAL ASPECTS OF THE TECHNIQUE

These studies have presented a scheme for injecting two labels, one radioactive and the other a characterized antibody into the brain for subsequent localization of the two separate transmitter systems. The technique described here utilizes ^{3}H-5-HT and monoclonal antibody to SP; however, the same technique can be used for simultaneous localization of a host of other neural mediators. For example, antibodies against transmitter enzymes may be used (e.g. tyrosine hydroxylase, dopamine-β-hydroxylase, tryptophan hydroxylase) in conjunction with radioactively labelled substances (e.g. ^{3}H-5-HT, ^{3}H-dopamine). Antibodies against a transmitter enzyme for example may be used in conjunction with a receptor ligand that is radioactively labelled. Or sequential application of antibodies against two different substances, one radioactively labelled and the other not, may be utilized as well. The present studies open vast avenues of applications for future investigation.

The present studies provide convincing evidence that the soma and processes of a single raphe neuron can contain a monoamine, 5-HT and another putative peptide transmitter SP in a single permanent preparation suitable for study with light and electron microscopy. Such neurons have been examined for their 5-HT content exhaustively. They have endogenous amine stores detectable by the Falck–Hillarp technique, verified to be 5-HT by identification of excitation and emission spectra by microspectrofluorimetry on individual cells and have 5-HT immunoreactivity. The cells have uptake systems for low-molarity ^{3}H-5-HT, are sensitive to 5-HT uptake inhibitors and monoamine oxidase inhibitors, are unaffected by reserpine, and are destroyed by 5,6-DHT. Their SP content has been identified in fixed material with animal antisera against SP by immunofluorescence and by PAP immunocytochemistry. In addition *in vivo* application of a monoclonal antibody against SP has been used to identify SP content in these cells based on their antigen–antibody recognition and binding systems in the living unfixed state. These cells are destroyed by 5,6-DHT.

Dynamic considerations in neuronal function involving multiple transmitters

Colchicine, a drug known to inhibit fast axoplasmic transport (Dahlström, 1968), causes an unphysiological accumulation of many substances including transmitters, enzymes, and precursors in the cell bodies of neurons. It has been used extensively to enhance the detectability of monoamine and peptides for cytochemical localization (see Hökfelt *et al.*, 1978). The present studies avoid the use of colchicine and succeed in demonstrating subtle differences in the somatic content of 5-HT and SP in neuronal somata.

The combined immunohistochemistry and autoradiography technique furnishes evidence to suggest that in addition to having two identified putative transmitter substances in coexistence, the amounts of each of these two substances present at any one time may vary. Individual neurons may have more of one, less of another, vice-versa, or have both in large amounts. This heterogeneity in multiple putative transmitter content was discussed briefly earlier (Chan-Palay *et al.*, 1978). Our present ideas of the concept of coexistence of putative transmitter substances may have to be expanded to encompass the two critical dimensions of time and the physiological function of the cell. It may be that neurons containing both 5-HT and SP have

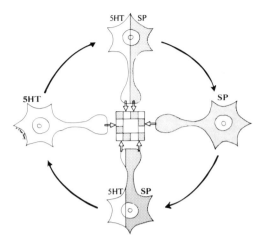

Figure 3 Schematic diagram to illustrate the concept of dynamic interrelationships between 5–HT and SP in a single neuron. A neuron with both substances in coexistence may have fluctuating levels of one or both substances depending upon parameters of rhythm, time cycle, and physiological demands for one or another mediator during specific types of phases of activity

fluctuating levels of one or both of these substances depending upon parameters of rhythm, demands for one or the other mediator during specific types or phases of activity. Such a cycle in the levels of coexistent putative transmitters is illustrated in Figure 3. It would be important for future studies to determine the factors that (a) regulate such cyclicity in neural mediators and (2) regulate the release of these substances, and (3) to determine whether the substances are released independently or concomitantly.

Our present concepts of chemical specificity in neurons must be enlarged to encompass the presence of more than one neurotransmitter or putative neuromediator within individual cells and their processes. Recognition of such a concept necessitates the search for the internal cellular machinery that can facilitate the separate manufacture, transport, storage, and release of multiple substances. In addition, the membrane-related mechanisms for the specific recognition and the differentiation of multiple neuromediators at receptors on the recipient cell's surface are critical in the identification of the intercellular message. It is not clear at present whether separate receptors are available for 5-HT and SP or whether the receptors for these two coexistent substances may be linked functionally (Figure 4). The elucidation of evidence to address these questions remains a key area for future investigation. It is necessary to point out that the existence of a potent specific uptake system of the serotonin component in the 5-HT/SP cell and the apparent lack of an equivalent uptake system in peptide-containing neurons (see Chan-Palay,

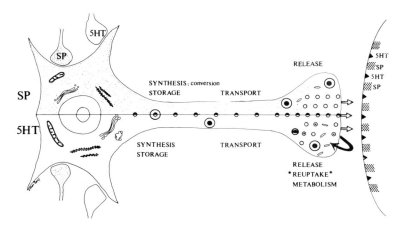

Figure 4   Schematic diagram of a neuron with 5–HT and SP in coexistence in its soma and processes. The internal cellular machinery to facilitate the synthesis, transport, storage, and release of peptide (SP, stippled upper half of cell) and amine transmitter (5–HT, clear lower half of cell) as well as the separate mechanisms required for reuptake and metabolism of the amine alone are depicted. Separate 5–HT and SP receptors are shown on the receptive cell surface to illustrate the need for further recognition/specificity. However, it is possible that some form of coupling or linkage in 5–HT and SP receptors exist for allowing for the mediation of the separate transmitters or transmitters co-released

1977a; Hökfelt *et al.*, 1976) for the putative peptide transmitter remain as the major significant differences between these two systems in the 5-HT/SP cell.

Detailed studies by electron microscope autoradiography of 5-HT neurons and their axonal projections in the mammalian brain, in locations as different as the cerebellum (Chan-Palay, 1975, 1977a,b), the supraependymal plexus (Chan-Palay, 1976), the caudate nucleus (Calas, 1976), the locus coeruleus (Mouren-Mathieu *et al.*, 1976; Pickel *et al.*, 1977a), the reticular paragigan-tocellularis lateralis nucleus (Chan-Palay, 1978c; Andrezik and Chan-Palay, 1977; Andrezik *et al.*, 1981a,b), the insulae of the external cuneate nucleus (Chan-Palay. 1978a,b) exist. These studies have shown that there is no consensus on one single constellation of ultrastructural features of the axoplasm that differentiate 5-HT axons from those of other neurons. In fact, identified 5-HT axons are different from one another in o gion of the brain and they may contain a number of different populations of synaptic vesicles when classified carefully as to size, shape, and content (see detailed discus-sion in Chan-Palay, 1977b, pp. 410–431). *Is this heterogeneity in synaptic vesicle morphology an expression of the multiplicity in their neuro-transmitter content?* A single situation has emerged from the results of studies of terminals identified with SP immunoreactivity (Pickel *et al.*, 1977b; Chan-Palay and Palay, 1977; Hökfelt *et al.*, 1977; Cuello *et al.*, 1977; Barber *et al.*, 1979) showing some differences in the synaptic vesicle populations labelled in SP axons. In the light of the present evidence for coexistence of multiple putative transmitters in 5-HT/SP neurons and their terminals, it would be wise to be cautious in discussions as to the vesicular populations primarily identifiable with SP content alone. The question of which chemical mediator for which synaptic vesicle, or if vesicles are involved at all, cannot be definitely decided on the basis of the present insufficient evidence. It must await considerably more careful investigation into the ultrastructure of nerve terminals with several of the transmitters simultaneously identified. One is reminded of the statement that 'synaptic vesicles, like chocolates, come in a variety of shapes and sizes and are stuffed with different kinds of fillings' (Palay, 1967). In addition, the content cannot be identified by the external appearance of the vesicle and more than one kind of content may be found in the one vesicle unit. Investigations with simultaneous labelling for multiple transmitter compounds are presently in progress at the electron microscope level in attempts to address these questions.

ACKNOWLEDGEMENTS

The author is grateful to Dr A. C. Cuello, Oxford University, England, for the generous donation of the monoclonal substance P antibody; Astra Company, Sweden, for the serotonin uptake inhibitors GE654, Zimelidine, and Norzimelidine; and May and Baker for clorgyline. I thank Mr H. Cook and Ms J. Hilsz for their excellent photographic and technical assistance. Supported in part by grants PHS NS 14740, NS 18539 and AFOSR 82·0328.

REFERENCES

Andrezik, A. A. and Chan-Palay, V. (1977). 'The nucleus paragigantocellularis lateralis (PGCL): definition and afferents.' *Anat. Res.*, **184**, 524–525.
Andrezik, J. A., Chan-Palay, V., and Palay, S. L. (1981a). 'The nucleus paragigantocellularis lateralis in rat: conformation and cytology.' *J. Anat. Embryol.* (In press).
Andrezik, J. A., Chan-Palay, V., and Palay, S. L. 7(1981b). 'The nucleus paragigantocellularis later7alis in rat: demonstration of afferents by the retrograde transport of horseradish peroxidase.' *J. Anat. Embryol.* (In press.)
Barber, R. P., Vaughn, J. E., Siemmon, J. R., Salvaterra, R. M., Roberts, E., and Leeman, S. E. (1979). 'The origin, distribution and synaptic relationships of substance P axons in rat spinal cord.' *J. Comp. Neurol.*, **184**, 331–352.
Baumgarten, H. G., Bjorklund, A., Lachenmeyer, L., Nobin, A., and Stenevi, U. (1971). 'Long lasting selective depletion of brain serotonin by 5,6-dihydroxytryptamine.' *Acta Physiol. Scand.* (Suppl.) **373**, 1–14.
Brown, J. T., Chan-Palay, V., and Palay, S. L. (1977). 'A study of afferent input to the interior olivary complex by retrograde axonal transport of horseradish peroxidase.' *J. Comp. Neurol.*, **176**, 1–22.

Calas, A., Besson, M. J., Gaughy, G., Alonso, G., Glowinski, J., and Cheramy, A. (1976). 'Radioautographic study of *in vivo* incorporation of ³H-monoamines in the cat caudate nucleus: identification of serotoninergic fibres.' *Brain Res.*, **118**, 1–13.

Carlsson, A. (1966). 'Drugs which block the storage of 5-hydroxytryptamine and related amines.' In Erspamer, V. (ed.), *Handbuch der experimentellen Pharmakologie, Ergänzungswerk* vol. XIX, pp. 529–592. Spring, Berlin–Heidelberg–New York.

Chan-Palay, V. (1975). 'Fine structure of labeled axons in the cerebellar cortex and nuclei of rodents and primates after intraventricular infusions with tritiated serotonin.' *Anat. Embryol.*, **148**, 235–265.

Chan-Palay, V. (1976). 'Serotonin axons in the supra- and subependymal plexuses and in the leptomeninges; their roles in local alterations of cerebrospinal fluid and vasomotor activity.' *Brain Res.*, **102**, 103–130.

Chan-Palay, V. (1977a). 'Indoleamine neurons and their processes in the normal rat brain and in chronic diet-induced thiamine deficiency demonstrated by uptake of ³H-serotonin.' *J. Comp. Neurol.*, **174**, 467–493.

Chan-Palay, V. (1977b). *Cerebellar Dentate Nucleus. Organization, Cytology, and Transmitters.* Springer, Berlin–Heidelberg–New York.

Chan-Palay, V. (1978a). 'The paratrigeminal nucleus. I. Neurons and synaptic organization including axo-axonic and dendrodendritic interrelations in the neuropil.' *J. Neurocytol.*, **7**, 405–418.

Chan-Palay, V. (1978b). 'The paratrigeminal nucleus. II. Identification and interrelations of catecholamine, indoleamine, and substance P containing axons in the neuropil.' *J. Neurocytol.*, **7**, 419–422.

Chan-Palay, V. (1978c). 'Morphological correlates for transmitter syntheses, transport, release, uptake and catabolism: a study of serotonin neurons in the nucleus paragigantocellularis lateralis.' In *Amino Acids as Chemical Transmitters*, NATO Advanced Study Symposium, pp. 1–29. Plenum Press, New York.

Chan-Palay, V. (1979a). 'Immunocytochemical detection of substance P neurons, their processes and connections by in vivo microinjections of monoclonal antibodies: Light and electron microscopy.' *Anat. Embryol.*, **156**, 225–240.

Chan-Palay, V. (1979b). 'Combined immunocytochemistry and autoradiography after *in vivo* injections of monoclonal antibody to substance P and ⁵H-serotonin: coexistence of two putative transmitters in single raphe cells and fiber plexuses.' *J. Anat. Embryol.*, **156**, 241–254.

Chan-Palay, V. and Palay, S. L. (1977). 'Ultrastructural identification of substance P cells and their processes in rat sensory ganglia and their terminals in the spinal cord by immunocytochemistry.' *Proc. Natl. Acad. Sci. USA,* **74**, 4050–4054.

Chan-Palay, V., Jonsson, G., and Palay, S. L. (19778). 'Serotonin and substance P coexist in neurons of the rat's central nervous system.' *Proc. Natl. Acad. Sci. USA,* **75**, 1582–1586.

Cuello, A. C., Galfré, G., and Milstein, C. (1979). 'Detection of substance P in the central nervous system by a monoclonal antibody.' *Proc. Natl. Acad. Sci. USA,* **76**, 3532–3536.

Cuello, A. C., Jessell, T. M., Kanazawa, T., and Iversen, L. C. (1977). 'Substance P: localization in synaptic vesicles in rat central nervous system.' *J. Neurochem.*, **29**, 747–751.

Dahlström, A. (1968). 'Effect of colchicine on transport of amine storage granules in sympathetic nerves of rat.' *Eur. J. Pharmacol.*, **5**, 111–112.

Hökfelt, T., Elde, R., Johansson, O., Luft, R., Nilsson, G., and Arimura, A. (1976). 'Immunohistochemical evidence for separate populations of somatostatin-containing and substance P-containing primary afferent neurons in the rat.' *Neuroscience*, **1**, 131–136.

Hökfelt, T., Johansson, O., Kellerth, J.-O., Ljungdahl, A., Nilsson, G., Nygards, A., and Pernow, B. (1977). 'Immunohistochemical distribution of substance P.' In von Euler, U.S. and Pernow, B. (eds), *Substance P*, pp. 117–143. Raven Press, New York.

Hökfelt, T., Ljungdahl, A., Steinbusch, H., Verhafstad, A., Nilsson, G., Brodin, E., Pernow, B., and Goldstein, M. (1978). 'Immunohistochemical evidence of substance P-like immunoreactivity in some 5-hydroxytryptamine-containing neurons in the rat central nervous system.' *Neuroscience*, **3**, 517–538.

Ljungdahl, A., Hökfelt, T., and Nilsson, G. (1979). 'Distribution of substance P-like immunoreactivity in the central nervous system of the rat. I, Cell bodies and nerve terminals.' *Neuroscience*, **3**, 861–875.

Mouren-Mathieu, A. M., Leger, L., and Descarries, L. (1976). 'Radioautographic visualization of central monoamine neurons after local instillation of tritiated serotonin and norepinephrine in adult cat.' *Soc. Neurosci. Abstr.*, **II** (Part 1), 497.

Palay, S. E. (1967). 'Principles of cellular organization in the nervous system.' In Quarton, G. C. (ed.), *The Neurosciences*, pp. 24–31. Rockefeller University Press, New York.

Pickel, V. M., Joh, T. H., and Reis, D. J. (1977a). 'A serotonergic innervation of noradrenergic neurons in nucleus locus coeruleus: demonstration by immunocytochemical localization of the transmitter specific enzymes tyrosine and tryptophan hydroxylase.' *Brain Res.*, **131**, 197–214.

Pickel, V., Reis, D. J., and Leeman, S. E. (1977b). 'Ultrastructural localization of substance P in neurons of rat spinal cord.' *Brain Res.*, **122**, 534–540.

Sternberger, L. A. (1979). *Immunocytochemistry*, 2nd edn. Wiley, New York.

Immunohistochemistry
Edited by A. C. Cuello
© 1983 IBRO

CHAPTER 18

Transmitter Specific Mapping of Neuronal Pathways by Immunohistochemistry combined with Fluorescent Dyes

L. SKIRBOLL and T. HÖKFELT

Department of Histology, Karolinska Institute, S-10401 Stockholm, Sweden; and NIMH, Biological Psychiatry Branch, Bldg 10, Rockville Pike, Bethesda, MD 20205, USA

I INTRODUCTION

In the last decade there has been a rapid development of more advanced techniques for the delineation of projections in the nervous system. In particular, horseradish peroxidase and autoradiography have proved to be powerful tools in the retrograde and anterograde tracing of neuronal pathways (Kristensson and Olsson, 1971; LaVail and LaVail, 1972; see Cowan and Cuenod, 1975). Both of these methods depend upon the ability of neurons to take up these markers and transport them along the axon. However, since principally all neurons seem to possess this ability, these techniques are relatively 'non-specific'. That is, they permit the mapping of the pathway, but provide no information regarding, for example, the specific neurotransmitters involved.

The last 10 years have also seen a remarkable increase in the number of putative transmitters described in the central nervous system. Thus, cholinergic and monoaminergic transmission have been joined by a growing number of neuropeptide transmitter candidates (see Snyder, 1980). In this regard, immunocytochemistry has evolved as an extremely useful technique for the visualization of putative transmitters and/or their synthesizing enzymes and has provided a means by which neuronal populations can be defined both anatomically and on the basis of their chemical content (see Geffen *et al.*, 1969; Cuello, 1978; Hökfelt *et al.*, 1980). Attempts to demonstrate connectivity immunocytochemically, however, have been limited. Although indirect immunofluorescence permits visualization of a substance in question both at nerve terminals and cell bodies, low transmitter content along axon processes makes it difficult to describe exact projections with confidence, i.e. the specific projection of a single cell or group of cells. For the most part, transmitter identification of pathways has relied on the ability or inability of chemical, electrolytic, or knife lesions to reduce immunohistochemical staining at nerve terminals and/or cell bodies or to alter biochemical measures in areas proximal or distal to the lesion (see Chapter 19). These approaches are often insufficient in that they rely on negative evidence and/or require massive damage to fibre tracts to produce detectable changes in transmitter levels.

There is, therefore, a demand for a method by which precisely traced neuronal pathways can simultaneously be characterized on the basis of their transmitter content. To this end, immunocytochemistry has been combined with horseradish peroxidase techniques with some limited success (Ljungdahl *et al.*, 1975). This method has, however, several serious problems which make its use difficult on a regular basis; for example, ultraviolet illumination of immunoreactivity inactivates the peroxidase which can lead to considerable difficulty in visualizing the tracing enzyme. Several other groups have made similar attempts to combine peroxidase with formaldehyde-induced fluorescence or monoamine oxidase histochemistry (Satoh *et al.*, 1977; Berger *et al.*, 1978; Blessing *et al.*, 1978; Smolen *et al.*, 1977, 1979).

Recently, Kuypers and co-workers have introduced a number of dyes which are retrogradely transported and which also fluoresce at a variety of emission spectra (Kuypers *et al.*, 1974, 1977, 1980; Bentivoglio *et al.*, 1979, 1980a,b; Van der Kooy *et al.*, 1978). Subsequently, several groups have described the simultaneous use of these immunofluorescent retrograde dyes and/or formaldehyde-induced fluorescence histochemistry for tracing precisely identified monoamine and peptide pathways in the CNS (Björklund and Skagerberg, 1979; Hökfelt *et al.*, 1979; Van der Kooy and Wise, 1980; Steinbusch *et al.*, 1980; Sawchenko and Swanson, 1981). Immunocytochemistry has several advantages over other techniques in that it permits the visualization of principally any substance against which an antiserum can be raised. Since the fluorescence characteristics of these retrograde dyes can, in several cases, be separated from fluorophores attached to the second antibody in the indirect immunofluorescent procedure, these dyes permit visualization of a single labelled cell, and in some cases its dendritic arborization, and allow conjunctive and/or simultaneous identification of immunofluorescent staining in the *same* cell. Thus, by combining the retrograde tracing of these dyes with transmitter specific immunocytochemistry, a method has been developed by which neuronal pathways can be mapped and at the same time, their chemical content characterized. The present article is a summary of work carried out in our laboratory. Further details of the technique will be given elsewhere (Skirboll *et al.*, 1983; Hökfelt *et al.*, 1983).

II METHODOLOGY

II.1 Fluorescent Tracers

The dyes tested for combined retrograde tracing and immunocytochemistry were selected on the basis of screening experiments carried out by Kuypers and collaborators. Several of the dyes were obtained from Dann and collaborators (Dann *et al.*, 1970, 1971, 1973, 1975; Schnedl *et al.*, 1977). The following dyes were tested:

(A) *True blue* (code 150/129) trans-1,2-bis(5-amidino-2-benzofuranyl) ethylene-2HCl (5%).
(B) *Fast blue* (code 253/50) a diamidino compound related to *True blue* (5%).
(C) *Nuclear yellow* (Hoechst S 769121) 2-(-4-sulphamylphenyl)-6-(6-4-methypiperazinol)-2-benzimidazolyl)benzimidazole trishydrochloride (1%)
(D) *Propidium iodide* (Sigma Chemical Co., St Louis, MO, USA) (3%)
(E) *Bisbenzimide* (Hoechst 33258) (Latt and Stetten, 1976; Loewe and Urbanietz, 1974) (1%)
(F) *Primuline* (Eastman 1039) (Kuypers *et al.*, 1977) (5%)

All compounds were dissolved or suspended in distilled water. Some of the dyes were stored at −20 °C over several months prior to injection, but in no case did this affect the fluorescence intensity or the retrograde transport of the dye. *True blue* and *Nuclear yellow* were relatively insoluble and were, therefore, sonicated for 30 min after initial mixture and sonication was repeated for at least 5 min before each use.

Each of these dyes demonstrated different histological characteristics and thus any attempt to combine them with immunohistochemistry required that many parameters be tested.

II.2 Injection

Male albino rats (150–200 g b.w.) were injected unilaterally with dye either into the caudate nucleus (A 8380 µm; L 3500 µm and ventral 5000 µm according to the atlas of König and Klippel, 1963) or into the spinal cord approximately at the level of C2. Dyes were either injected by hand via a 5 µl

Hamilton syringe in a volume of about 0.2–0.3 μl, or via a glass micropipette. Pipettes were pulled and broken to a tip diameter of 25–50 μm and attached to a Medical Systems Pump (Great Neck, NY) which permitted the delivery of small volumes of drug via pressure injection. Although this method permitted a more precise ejection of dye and limited the volume of dye delivered, it could not be used for the ejection of either *True blue* or *Nuclear yellow*. The insolubility of these two dyes invariably clogged the pipette and prohibited efficient dye ejection.

Examination of sections cut from the site of injection revealed no differences between the dyes, except as determined by the volume of dye injected. In most cases the primary site of injection contained a central core of necrosis. Perhaps the greatest problem associated with this technique, however, results from the movement of the dye back up the tract of the injecting instrument. This can result in the deposit of dye in structures adjacent to the target, and can subsequently lead to 'false' labelling of cell bodies not associated with the target structure. This problem can be limited somewhat by lowering the instrument very slowly into place and leaving it for a minimum of 5 min following the completion of injection. The use of glass pipettes produces a smaller tract and can thus also limit non-specific dye spread.

II.3 Survival Times

The times required between dye injection and animal sacrifice to produce optimal retrograde transport and minimal non-specific labelling have been described in detail by Kuypers and collaborators (for references see above). These times may vary from several hours to several days depending upon the dye in question and the length of the pathway being traced. Survival time does, however, prove to be a limiting factor in the combination of retrograde tracing with immunohistochemistry. Immunocytochemical visualization of neuropeptides most often requires that the animal receives colchicine 24 h before sacrifice; this agent serves to arrest axonal transport and permit accumulation of the peptide in the cell body. It would be expected that colchicine would also arrest retrograde transport of the dye. This is, in fact, the case; virtually no cells are dye-labelled if the dye and colchicine are injected simultaneously. Thus, these studies required a two-step procedure. Initially, the animals were injected with the appropriate dye and allowed to recover for the time period sufficient to permit maximal retrograde transport (24–72 h). At the end of this period colchicine was injected into the lateral ventricle (60–120 μg in 20 μl) and the animal was sacrificed 24 h later. This technique proved effective when applied to *Propidium iodide*, *True blue*, *Fast blue*, and *Primuline*. However, both *Bisbenzimide* and *Nuclear yellow* move rapidly out of the cell bodies and into neighbouring glial tissue if the animals are not sacrificed at least 6 h after dye injection. Since, in most cases, it is necessary to follow dye injection with a 24 h colchicine treatment, a total survival time of 30 h (6 h dye + 24 h colchicine) invariably leads to massive labelling of surrounding glial tissue (and perhaps adjacent cells). Under such circumstances it is usually not possible to be certain whether or not any given *Bisbenzimide* or *Nuclear yellow* stained cell has been labelled only by retrograde transport.

II.4 Preparation of Tissue and Immunohistochemistry

Rats were perfused with ice-cold formalin (10%) following which the brains were dissected out and immersed in buffered 5% sucrose for 24 h prior to being cut on a cryostat (for details, see Hökfelt *et al.*, 1973). Brains in which dye was injected into the caudate nucleus were sectioned both at the level of the substantia nigra (A 2580–1760 μm according to the atlas of König and Klippel, 1963) and the dorsal raphe nucleus (P 290 μm). Following spinal cord injections, sections were cut through the lower brain stem. Sections processed for immunohistochemistry were stained with one of two antisera; antiserum raised against the classical transmitter 5-hydroxytryptamine (5-HT) (Steinbusch *et al.*, 1978) and antiserum to tyrosine hydroxylase, the rate-limiting enzyme in catecholamine synthesis used as a marker for dopamine (Markey *et al.*, 1980) (for details see Section III).

Since immunocytochemical procedures require that tissues not only be washed several times but also exposed to several temperature changes, it was necessary to determine to what degree each of the dyes was retained after immunocytochemistry. To this end, the number of dye-labelled cells in a particular section were compared before and after immunocytochemistry. There are, however, several problems which confound this approach. For example, once the sections are cut, mounting them in glycerol and buffer or xylene prior to microscopic examination can enhance movement of the dye out of the cell and into neighbouring glia or simply reduce dye intensity. Although mounting in Entallan or oil prevents such diffusion problems, the use of these media do preclude or make any subsequent immunocytochemistry difficult. Thus, in order to obtain an accurate cell count, sections were taken directly from the cryostat and viewed *unmounted* under the microscope.

Another more serious detriment to accurate cell counting comes from fading. *True blue*, *Fast blue*, *Bisbenzimide*, and *Nuclear yellow* fade rapidly under exposure to ultraviolet light. Evaluative studies with these dyes thus required that adjacent sections be examined; the number of dye-labelled cells could be counted in one section and compared to an adjacent *unexposed* section which was stained for immunocytochemistry. This procedure was not necessary when examining either *Propidium iodide* or *Primuline*. Since neither of these dyes was markedly subjected to fading or diffusion even after somewhat prolonged (several minutes) ultraviolet exposure, the same section could be examined before and after immunocytochemistry. Quantitation revealed that about 80% of *True blue* and *Fast blue* labelled cells survived the immunocytochemical procedure, while a full 98–100% of *Propidium iodide* and *Primuline* labelled cells survived similar conditions. In contrast, only 1–2% of *Nuclear yellow* and *Bisbenzimide* labelled cells retained dye after being submitted to the immunocytochemistry.

Because of the fading which accompanies exposure to ultraviolet light and the tendency for immunocytochemistry to 'wash out' dye (particularly in weakly labelled cells), any careful matching of retrogradely labelled cells with immunostained cells requires a two-step procedure for some of the dyes: (1) a photograph should be made of the dye-labelled cells in the 'fresh', un-mounted section and (2) a matching photograph should then be taken after immunocytochemistry of the immunostained cells. By comparing the two photographs, cells which contain both dye and transmitter can be delineated and separated from cells which contain only dye or only immunofluorescent stain. This two-step procedure is recommended when employing *True blue*, *Fast blue, Nuclear Yellow*, or *Bisbenzimide*. In contrast, the stability of *Propidium iodide* and *Primuline* suggests that it is possible to photograph both the dye and immunofluorescence in the same session. The latter dyes are therefore particularly valuable, since they allow the omission of the tedious photography of cells only containing the retrograde tracer.

II.5   Visualization

The emission and activation maxima of each of the fluorescent dyes have been examined in detail by Björklund and Skagerberg (1979). In several cases their emission and excitation characteristics allow effective separation from the fluorophores conjugated to the second antibody of the immunocyto-chemical process, i.e. fluorescein isothiocyanate (FITC) or rhodamine (for detailed account of use of filters see Chapter 2). Thus, in some cases excitation of the same section at different wavelengths allows separation of dye-labelling from immunofluorescent staining. Furthermore, the differential emission characteristics of the dyes results in clear differences in fluorescence colour of these substances: *Propidium iodide* and rhodamine both fluoresce orange-red; *True blue* and *Fast blue* show an ice-blue colour, *Bisbenzimide* is whitish-yellow, while FITC fluoresces green. Thus, the selection of appropri-ate microscopic filter combinations makes it possible to examine a *single* section and visualize the dye using one filter combination and the immuno-fluorescent staining using another (for details see Section III).

The ability to differentiate between dye and immunofluorophore is depen-dent upon choosing the right combination of dye, conjugated second anti-body, and filter. For example, although one cannot see FITC fluorescence through a filter used to visualize *True blue* or *Fast blue*, the blue fluorescence does 'shine through' the FITC filters. Thus, viewing a section in which a cell is strongly *Fast blue*-labelled under FITC filters might give rise to a 'false-positive' for immunoreactivity. This problem can be remedied by using a rhodamine-conjugated second antibody in experiments in which either *Fast blue* or *True blue* are used as the retrograde dye. The difference between the emission characteristics of, on the one hand, rhodamine, and on the other hand, *True* and *Fast blue* are sufficiently large such that these two substances can be seen in the same section with the appropriate filters as different colours. This same technique can be effectively employed with *Propidium iodide* by using FITC as opposed to rhodamine as the second antibody conjugate (for differential use of FITC and rhodamine-conjugated antibodies, see Chapter 2).

III RECOMMENDED PROCEDURE

Of the compounds tested *Fast blue*, *True blue*, *Propidium iodide*, and *Primuline* are the ones best suited for combination with immunocytochemistry. Thus, the procedure described below will be directed towards the application of these three dyes.

(a) Dyes are injected either using a 5 µl Hamilton syringe or a glass micropipette attached to pressure ejection unit (Medical Systems, Great Neck, NY, USA). Efforts should be made to limit the volume of dye injected to reduce the spread to adjacent structures not associated with the target neuronal population. The injection instrument should be left in place for 5–10 min after the completion of dye injection to reduce reflux of dye up the injection tract.

(b) For all three recommended dyes, a 48–72 h survival time is sufficient to permit optimal dye transport for short (caudate to substantia nigra and/or raphe) or long (spinal cord to brain stem) projections. This may vary, however, between species and depending upon the length of the pathway being traced.

(c) In the case of immunocytochemical identification of substances present in low concentrations in cell bodies (such as is the case with many of the neuropeptides), the animal receives an intraventricular colchicine injection (60–120 µg in 20 µl for rats) 24 h prior to sacrifice. It is important to remember that colchicine treatment must follow transport of the dye and should not be administered on the same day of dye delivery.

(d) Animals are perfused through the ascending aorta with 10% ice-cold formalin (40 g paraformaldehyde dissolved in 1000 ml of 0.1 M phosphate buffer according to Pease, 1962) for 30 min. The brains are then dissected out, immersed in the same fixative for 90 min, and rinsed in 0.1 M

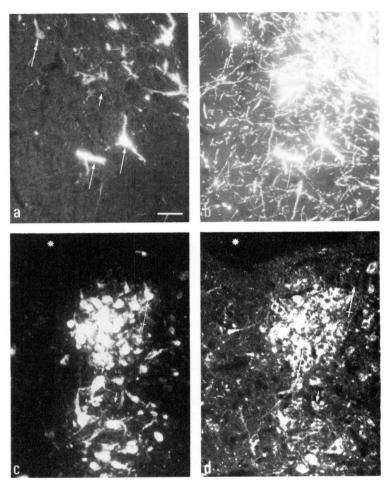

Figure 1 (a–d) Fluorescence micrographs of the substantia nigra, zona compacta
(a,b), and dorsal raphe nucleus of the pontine mesencephalic periaqueductal central
grey (c,d) after injection of *Fast blue* (a) and *Propidium iodide* (c) into the caudate
nucleus of the rat and subsequent processing for indirect fluorescence with antiserum
to tyrosine hydroxylase (b) and 5-hydroxytryptamine (d). (a,b) After photography of
zona compacta cells retrogradely labelled with *Fast blue* (a), the section was processed
for indirect immunofluorescence using a rhodamine-conjugated second antibody (b).
Note that many cells are both *Fast blue* and tyrosine hydroxylase-positive (long
arrows). Short arrows point to a tyrosine hydroxylase-positive and *Fast blue*-negative
cell. (c,d) This section was directly processed for indirect immunofluorescence using
an FITC-conjugated second antibody. The cells labelled by retrogradely transported
Propidium iodide (c) and immunostained with antiserum to 5-hydroxytryptamine (d)
could be visualized separately by changing excitation and stop filters. Long arrows
point to 'double-labelled' cell; crossed arrows to *Propidium iodide*-positive and
5-hydroxytryptamine-negative cell, and short arrows to 5-hydroxytryptamine-positive
and *Propidium iodide*-negative cell. Asterisks indicate aqueduct. (Bar = 50 μm; all
micrographs have the same magnification.) These black-and-white micrographs have
been reproduced from colour photos supplied by the authors.

phosphate buffer with 5% sucrose added. After at least 24 h rinsing, the brains can be cut on a cryostat (section thickness set at 10 or 15 µm). For *Fast blue*, sections should be immediately viewed unmounted under the microscope and photographed. In some cases, in order to get a sharper photograph, it may be necessary to *briefly* mount the section with xylene. After photography the sections can be processed for immunocytochemistry. For *Primuline* and *Propidium iodide*, the sections can be taken directly from the cryostat and processed since neither of these dyes are subject to 'wash out' through the immunocytochemical procedure. If it is necessary to store the sections between cutting and immunocytochemistry, the dye is well retained if sections are stored *unmounted* at room temperature.

(e) Sections are processed for the indirect immunofluorescence procedure of Coons (1958), essentially as described previously (Hökfelt *et al.*, 1973). Briefly, the sections are incubated with the appropriate antiserum, for example tyrosine hydroxylase or 5-HT, at 4 °C for 24–48 h, rinsed in phosphate buffered saline (PBS), incubated with FITC (for use with *Propidium iodide* or rhodamine for use with *Primuline, True Blue* or *Fast Blue*) conjugated antibodies for 30 min at 37°C, rinsed in PBS, mounted in a mixture of glycerol and PBS (3:1), and examined in a fluorescence microscope equipped with an oil dark-field condenser.

(f) For visualization of dyes and immunofluorophores in a Zeiss fluorescence microscope the following filters can be used: *Fast blue* fluorescence can be analysed using a Schott UG-1 filter for activation and a Zeiss 41 as a secondary filter, as recommended by Björklund and Skagerberg (1979). *Propidium iodide* and rhodamine fluorescence can be examined using a Schott B546 as a primary filter and a LP 590 as a secondary filter. FITC fluorescence is best seen with a KP 500 excitation filter and LP 520 stop filter. Scopix RP 1 black and white film (Gevaert, Belgium) is used for *Fast blue*, *Primuline* and FITC photography, while Agfapan 400 black and white film (Agfa-Gevaert, West Germany) serves best for *Propidium iodide* and rhodamine. For colour photography, Kodak High Speed Ektachrome (160 Tungsten, Eastman Kodak Corp., Rochester, NY, USA) can be used (see also Chapter 2; for filter selection also contact microscope manufacturers' representatives).

ACKNOWLEDGEMENTS

The present study was supported by the Swedish Medical Research Council (SMRC) 04X-2887, Magnus Bergvalls Stiftelse, Knut och Alice Wallenbergs Stiftelse, and Ollie and Elof Ericssons Stiftelse. L.S. was a Fogarty–SMRC post-doctoral fellow. We also thank the SMRC for travel funding for L.S. We thank Ms J. Backman, Ms A. Edin, Ms V. Hiort, Ms U. Lindefelt, and Ms G. Norell for excellent technical assistance. The expert secretarial help of Mrs Birgit Frideen is gratefully acknowledged.

The results presented in this article are taken from an original publication in preparation (Skirboll *et al.*, 1983); the authors gratefully acknowledge the assistance of the co-authors in supplying antibodies (tyrosine hydroxylase, Professor Menek Goldstein, Department of Psychiatry, New York University, Medical Center, New York, NY, USA; 5-hydroxytryptamine, Drs Harry Steinbusch and Albert Verhofstad, Department of Anatomy and Embryology, Katholic University, Nijmegen, The Netherlands) and fluorescent dyes (Professors Otto Dann, Institut fur Pharmazie und Lebensmittelchemie des Friedrich-Alexander-Universität, Erlangen, West Germany and H. Kuypers, Department of Anatomy, Erasmus University, Rotterdam, The Netherlands).

REFERENCES

Bentivoglio, M., Kuypers, H. J. G. M., Catsman-Berrevoets, C., and Dann, O. (1979). 'Fluorescent retrograde neuronal labeling in rat by means of substances binding specifically to adenine-thymine rich DNA.' *Neurosci. Lett.*, **12**, 235–240.

Bentivoglio, M., Kuypers, H. G. J. M., and Catsman-Berrevoets, C. (1980a). 'Retrograde neuronal labeling by means of bisbenzimide and nuclear yellow (Hoechst S 769121). Measures to prevent diffusion of the tracers out of retrogradely labelled cells.' *Neurosci. Lett.*, **18**, 19–24.

Bentivoglio, M., Kuypers, H. G. J. M., Catsman-Berrevoets, C., and Dann, O. (1980b). 'Two new fluorescent retrograde neuronal tracers which are transported over long distances.' *Neurosci. Lett.*, **18**, 25–30.

Berger, B., Nguyen-Legros, J., and Thierry, A. (1978). 'Demonstration of horseradish peroxidase and fluorescent catecholamines in the same neuron.' *Neurosci. Lett.*, **9**, 297–302.

Björklund, A. and Skagerberg, G. (1979). 'Simultaneous use of retrograde fluorescence tracers and fluorescence histochemistry for convenient and precise mapping of monoaminergic projections and collateral arrangements in the CNS.' *J. Neurosci. Methods*, **1**, 261–277.

Blessing, W. W., Furness, J. B., Costa, M., and Chalmers, J. P. (1978). 'Localization of catecholamine fluorescence and retrogradely transported horseradish peroxidase within the same nerve cell.' *Neurosci. Lett.*, **9**, 311–315.

Coons, A. H. (1958). 'Fluorescent antibody methods.' In Danielli, J. F. (ed.), *General Cytochemical Methods*, pp. 239–259. Academic Press, New York.

Cowan, W. M. and Cuenod, M. (eds) (1975). *The Use of Axonal Transport for Studies of Neuronal Connectivity*. Elsevier, Amsterdam.

Cuello, A. C. (1978). 'Immunocytochemical studies of the distribution of neurotransmitters and related substances in CNS.' In Iversen, L. L. *et al.* (eds), *Handbook of Psychopharmacology*, vol. 9, pp. 69–137. Plenum Press, London.

Dann, O., Bergen, G., Demant, E., and Volz, G. (1971). 'Trypanocide diamidine des 2-Phenyl-benzofurans, 2-Phenyl-idens und 2-Phenyl-idols.' *Liebigs Ann. Chem.*, **749**, 68–91.

Dann, O., Fick, H., Pietzner, B., Walkenhorst, E., Fernbach, R., and Seh, D. (1975). 'Trypanocide Diamidine mit drei isoleirten Ringsystemen.' *Liebigs Ann. Chem.*, 160–194.

Dann, O., Hieke, E., Hahn, H., Miserre, H-H., Lürding, G., and Rössler, R. (1970). 'Trypanocide Diamidine des 2-Phenyl-thionaphthens.' *Liebigs Ann. Chem.*, **734**, 23–45.

Dann, O., Volz, G., Demant, E., Pfeifer, W., Bergen, G., Fick, H., and Walkenhorst, E. (1973). 'Trypanocide Diamidine mit vier Ringer in einem order zwei Ringsystemen.' *Liebigs Ann. Chem.*, 1112–1140.

Geffen, L. B., Livett, D. G., and Rush, R. A. (1969). 'Immunohistochemical localization of protein components of catecholamine storage vesicles.' *J. Physiol. (Lond.)*, **204**, 593–605.

Hökfelt, T., Fuxe, K., Goldstein, M., and Joh, T. (1973). 'Immunohistochemical localization of three catecholamine synthesizing enzymes: aspects on methodology.' *Histochemie*, **33**, 231–254.

Hökfelt, T., Johansson, O., Ljungdahl, Å., Lundberg, J. M., and Schultzberg, M. (1980). 'Peptidergic neurons.' *Nature*, **284**, 515–521.

Hökfelt, T., Phillipson, O., Kuypers, H. G. M., Bentivoglio, M., Catsman-Berre-voets, C., and Dann, O. (1979). 'Tracing of transmitter histochemically identified neuron projections: immunohistochemistry combined with fluorescent retrograde labeling.' *Neurosci. Lett.*, Suppl. 3, 342.

Hökfelt, T., Skagerberg, G., Skirboll, L. and Björklund, A. (1983). Combination of retrograde tracing and neurotransmitter histochemistry. In Björklund, A. and Hökfelt, T. (eds.) *Handbook of Chemical Neuroanatomy*, Vol. 1. Elsevier, Amsterdam, in press.

König, J. F. and Klippel, R. A. (1963). *The Rat Brain: A Stereotaxic Atlas of the Forebrain and Lower Parts of the Brain Stem*. Williams & Wilkins, Baltimore.

Kristensson, K. and Olsson, Y. (1971). 'Retrograde axonal transport of protein.' *Brain Res.*, **29**, 363–365.

Kuypers, H. G. J. M., Bentivoglio, M., Catsman-Berrevoets, C., and Baros, A. T. (1980). 'Double retrograde neuronal labeling through divergent collaterals, using two fluorescent tracers with the same excitation wavelength which label different features of the cell.' *Exp. Brain Res.*, **40**, 383–392.

Kuypers, H. G. J. M., Bentivoglio, M., Van der Kooy, D., Catsman-Berrevoets, C. (1974). 'Retrograde transport of bisbenzimide and propidium iodide through axons to their parent cell bodies.' *Neurosci. Lett.*, **12**, 1–7.

Kuypers, H. G. J. M., Catsman-Berrevoets, C., and Padt, R. E. (1977). 'Retrograde axonal transport of fluorescent substances in rats forebrain.' *Neurosci. Lett.*, **6**, 127–135.

Latt, S. A. and Stetten, G. (1976). 'Spectral studies on 33258 Hoechst and related bisbenzamidazole dyes useful for fluorescence detection of deoxyribonucleic acid synthesis.' *J. Histochem. Cytochem.*, **24**, 24–33.

LaVail, J. H. and LaVail, M. (1972). 'Retrograde axonal transport in the central nervous system.' *Science*, **176**, 1416–1417.

Ljungdahl, Å., Hökfelt, T., Goldstein, M., and Park, D. (1975). 'Retrograde peroxidase tracing of neurons combined with transmitter histochemistry.' *Brain Res.*, **84**, 313–319.

Loewe, H. and Urbanietz, J. (1974). 'Basisch substituierte 2,6-Bisbenzamidazolderivate, neine neue chemotherapeutisch aktive Körperklasse.' *Arzneim. Forsch.*, **24**, 1927–1933.

Markey, K. A., Kondo, S., Shenkman, L., and Goldstein, M. (1980). 'Purification and characterization of tyrosine hydroxylase from a clonal pheochromocytoma cell line.' *Mol. Pharmacol.*, **17**, 79–85.

Pease, D. C. (1962). 'Buffered formaldehyde as a killing agent and primary fixative for electron microscopy.' *Anat. Rec.*, **142**, 342.

Satoh, K., Tokyama, M., Yamamoto, K., Sakumoto, T., and Shimizu, N. (1977). 'Noradrenaline innervation of the spinal cord studied by horseradish peroxidase method combined with monoamine oxidase staining.' *Exp. Brain. Res.*, **30**, 175–186.

Sawchenko, P. and Swanson, L. (1981). 'A method for tracing biochemically defined pathways in the central nervous system using combined fluorescence retrograde transport and immunohistochemical techniques.' *Brain Res.*, **210**, 31–52.

Schnedl, W., Midelsaar, A.-V., Breitenbach, M., and Dann, O. (1977). 'DIPI and DAPI: fluorescence banding with only negligible fading.' *Hum. Genet.*, **36**, 167–172.

Skirboll, L. R., Hökfelt, T., Kuypers, H. G. J. M., Bentivoglio, M., Catsman-Berrevoets, C., Goldstein, M., Steinbusch, H., Verhofstad, A., Terenius, L., and Phillipson, O. (1983). 'A method for combining immunohistochemistry with retrogradely transported dyes: transmitter specific mapping of neuronal pathways.' (To be submitted)

Smolen, A., Glazer, E. G., and Ross, L. L. (1977). 'Localization of avian bulbospinal monoaminergic neurons by fluorescence histochemistry and retrograde transport of HRP.' *Neurosci. Abstr.*, **3**, 261.

Smolen, A. J., Glazer, E. J., and Ross, L. L. (1979). 'Horseradish-peroxidase histochemistry combined with glyoxylic acid induced fluorescence used to identify brain stem, catecholaminergic neurons which project to thoracic spinal cord.' *Brain Res.*, **160**, 353–357.

Snyder, S. H. (1980). 'Brain peptides as neurotransmitters.' *Science*, **209**, 976–983.

Steinbusch, H. W., Van Der Kooy, D., Verhofstad, A. A., and Pellegrino, A. (1980). 'Serotonergic and non-serotonergic projections from the nucleus raphe dorsalis to the caudate-putamen complex in the rat, studied by a combined immunofluorescence and fluorescence retrograde axonal labeling technique.' *Neurosci. Lett.*, **19**, 137–142.

Steinbusch, H. W. M., Verhofstad, A. A. J., and Joosten, H. W. J. (1978). 'Localization of serotonin in the central nervous system by immunohistochemistry: description of a specific and sensitive technique and some applications.' *Neuroscience*, **3**, 811–819.

Van Der Kooy, D., Kuypers, H. G. J. M., and Catzman-Berrevoets, C. (1978). 'Single mamillary body cells with divergent axon collaterals. Demonstration by a simple fluorescent retrograde double labeling technique in the rat.' *Brain Res.*, **158**, 189–196.

Van Der Kooy, D. and Wise, R. (1980). 'Retrograde fluorescent tracing of substantia nigra neurons combined with catecholamine histofluorescence.' *Brain Res.*, **183**, 447–452.

CHAPTER 19

Combined Immunohistochemistry with Stereotaxic Lesions

A. CLAUDIO CUELLO, MARINA DEL FIACCO-LAMPIS and
GEORGE PAXINOS

Neuroanatomy-Neuropharmacology Group, Departments of Pharmacology and Human Anatomy, Oxford University, Oxford, UK; Department of Anatomy, University of Cagliari, Cagliari, Sardinia, Italy; and Department of Psychology, The University of New South Wales, Kensington, New South Wales, Australia

I INTRODUCTION

Neuroanatomy has been revolutionized on one hand because of the explosion of new techniques to investigate neuronal connections (see Heimer and Robarts, 1981) and on the other hand by the plethora of newly discovered neuroactive substances and the emergence of highly sensitive biochemical procedures to detect them. This will, no doubt, result in an increased knowledge of the neurotransmitters and neuroactive substances involved in classical and newly found neuronal pathways. Examples of this are given by the increasing number of combined neuroanatomical biochemical studies in many areas of the brain. Immunocytochemistry is playing a crucial role in this task, as this technique can very effectively reconcile neuroanatomy with biochemistry by detecting, at cellular and subcellular levels, immunoreactive sites of neurally relevant substances. Nevertheless, immunocytochemistry *per se* generally does not solve the problem of whether immunoreactive substances are present in local circuit or projecting neurons. This is largely due to the fact that in most cases immunoreactivites for neurotransmitters and their markers are restricted to terminal and preterminal networks (see Cuello, 1978; Hökfelt *et al.*, 1980). To circumvent this problem colchicine has been widely applied to demonstrate immunoreactivities in cell bodies. This, nevertheless, still falls short of relating immunoreactive cell bodies with immunoreactive fibre networks. It is therefore necessary to apply other procedures. In Chapter 18 the use of retrogradely transported fluorescent dyes combined with immunocytochemistry is discussed. Other procedures, such as the combination of retrogradely transported HRP and PAP immunohistochemistry, have been tried recently (Bowker *et al.*, 1981: Priestley *et al.*, 1981). In this chapter we will discuss the use of kainic acid, colchicine, and microknife deafferentations, according to the experience gathered in our laboratory, to investigate neurotransmitter specific pathways. There are no standard protocols for the use of these techniques in conjunction with immunohistochemistry. They have to be tailored for the specific system to be explored. In order to facilitate this task we will comment on some of the principles involved, and also on the parameters and conditions used to investigate defined neuronal circuits.

II   USE OF TOXINS COMBINED WITH IMMUNOCYTOCHEMISTRY

II.1   Colchicine

Blockers of the axonal transport have been used in neuroanatomical research to cause a proximal accumulation of substances which are synthesized in the perikaryon and subsequently conveyed to the nerve terminals. The antimitotic drug colchicine binds to protein subunits of microtubules (Wilson, 1970), causing their disruption. This mechanism, first observed for the filaments of the mitotic spindle, has also been reported in relation to neuroplasmic proteins (Borisy and Taylor, 1967). It has been suggested that neurotubules take part in the fast axonal transport (Schmitt, 1968) and their disruption by the local application of colchicine has been consequently regarded as the reason for its arrest (Dahlström, 1968). Increase of noradrenaline-induced fluorescence following colchicine treatment has been shown in sympathetic ganglia and peripheral adrenergic axons (Dahlström, 1968) as well as in the central nervous system (Sorimachi *et al.*, 1977). The intraventricular adminstration of the drug has been successfully used to improve the visualization of immunoreactive cell bodies in the central nervous system (see Hökelt *et al.*, 1980). However, the effects of intraventricularly injected colchicine appear to be restricted to areas of the brain most closely related to the ventricular or subarachnoid spaces, and therefore the areas more accessible to the drug.

Local application of cotton pellets soaked with colchicine (Ljungdahl *et al.*, 1978) or stereotaxic microinjections of the drug (Del Fiacco and Cuello, 1980; Del Fiacco *et al.*, 1982) result in a powerful tool to reveal otherwise unreactive peptide-containing cell bodies and nerve fibre tracts in the central and peripheral nervous system.

II.2 Kainic Acid

Kainic acid is a rigid analogue of glutamic acid with potent excitatory effects on neurons of the mammalian central nervous system (Shinozaki, 1978). Intracerebral injections of small amounts of kainic acid result in a widespread degeneration of neuronal cell bodies in the area without damaging axons passing through, or nerve terminals present in the region (Olney, 1978). The extent of the loss of neurons and the neuronal populations affected seem to vary from region to region, and due controls using conventional histology should be carried out before embarking on combined neurotoxin–immunocytochemical experiments (see Olney and de Gubareff, 1978; Nadler *et al.*, 1978).

Examples of the use of kainic acid in neurochemical research, where the drug has caused lesions restricted to neuronal somata, can be found in the work of Coyle and Schwarcz (1976) and Di Chiara and collaborators (1977). McGeer and collaborators (1978) have discussed the advantages of this type of lesion as compared with classical electrolytic lesions. In immunocytochemistry we have found that very small amounts of the toxin delivered in small volumes (0.5 μl), in defined stereotaxic locations produce restricted spread and equally restricted lesions. This allows the investigation of topographic relations of projecting neurons by the comparison of the injection sites with the loss of immunoreactive material present in terminal networks of projecting neurons (Del Fiacco *et al.*, 1982).

III STEREOTAXIC INJECTIONS OF NEUROTOXINS: PROCEDURES AND EXPERIMENTAL RESULTS

For the delivery of small volumes of neurotoxins in defined nuclear areas or fibre tracts in the mammalian CNS it is necessary to be familiar with stereotaxic procedures. For most of our work in rodents we have alternatively used the atlas of Konig and Klippel (1963), and Pellegrino *et al.* (1979). It is

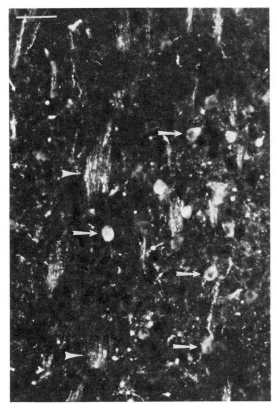

Figure 1 Enkephalin-immunoreactive cell bodies (arrows) in the cudate-putamen after intrapallidal microinjections of colchicine. Arrowheads indicate bundles of enkephalin-immunoreactive nerve fibres. No immunoreactive cell bodies were seen in the globus pallidus. (Scale bar = 50 μm.) (Reproduced by permission Springer-Verlag from Cuello *et al.*, 1981)

distribution of immunoreactive material in the lesioned side. As the neuro-toxic actions of kainic acid develop very rapidly (Olney, 1978) short survival times are indicated for combined lesion–immunocytochemical studies. For most purposes a survival time of 48 h is recommended.

IV   THE USE OF STEREOTAXIC KNIFE CUTS COMBINED WITH IMMUNOCYTOCHEMISTRY

Since originally introduced by Halasz and Pupp (1965) knife deafferenta-tions with rigid and, later, retractable microknives have been used primarily in neuroendocrinological research. This technique has more recently been applied in neurochemical and behavioural research. Here we will discuss the

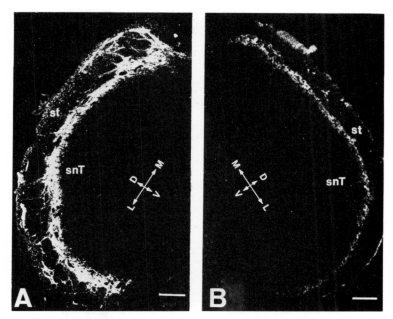

Figure 2 Substance P immunoreactivity in the lower medulla oblongata of the rat following the intraganglionar application of colchicine. Note in A the intense immunofluorescence in the fibre tract (st, spinal tract) and in the terminal network of the untreated side as compared with B, treated side. DMVL denotes spatial orientation (dorsal, medial, ventral, lateral). snT, spinal trigeminal nucleus. (Scale bar = 200 μm.) (From Del Fiacco and Cuello, 1981)

potential applications of this tool in combination with neurotransmitter (or neurotransmitter markers) immunocytochemistry for tracing transmitter-specific neuronal pathways. The knife we have applied is a modified version of that described by Voloschin *et al.* (1968), Sclafani and Grossman (1969), and Gold *et al.* (1973). Retractable knives, in which the cutting wire lies inside the guiding cannula while the knife is stereotaxically positioned, have the advantage of not producing widespread damage along their insertion track. In combined lesion–immunocytochemical studies the microknife usually leads to a depletion of the immunoreactivity in the nerve terminal fields of severed axons and a proximal build-up of the immunoreactivity indicating the direction of the projection, while seldom affecting immunoreactivity of cell somata.

IV.1 The Construction of Microknives

Microknives can be constructed with 30 gauge tubing (Small Parts, Florida, USA) bent at one end so that a 0.13 mm diameter tungsten wire forced

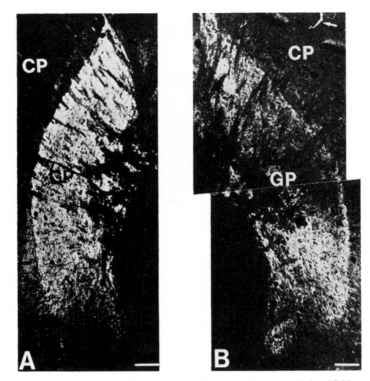

Figure 3   Enkephalin immunofluorescence of the rat globus pallidus (GP) as revealed in a horizontal section. A, control, untreated side. B, Ipsilateral side to localized microinjection of kainic acid in medial portions of the caudate-putamen (CP). Arrow points to non-specific fluorescence. (Scale bar = 200 μm.) (Reproduced by permission from Del Fiacco *et al.*, 1982)

through the tubing extends in the direction of the curved end. To construct the knife a 60 mm long piece of 30 gauge tubing is cut. The ends of the tubing should be filed to produce a circular lumen. Filing and cutting of the tubing can be accomplished by using a sanding disc mounted on a rotating dental drill. The debris of metal at the ends of the lumen can be removed by rotating the tapered portion of a thin needle in the lumen. Then with the aid of pliers, one end of the cannula is bent to the desired angle. The greater the angle to which the tubing is bent the smaller the distance the wire will travel before curving upwards. To avoid the collapse of the cannula walls at the point of the bend, a wire should be inserted in the cannula. This wire has to be filed to a needle-point tip before it can be forced through the cannula lumen and can be the same as that used for the extendable part of the knife (0.13 mm diameter tungsten or stainless steel wire: G.E. Co. Cleveland Wire Operation, PO Box

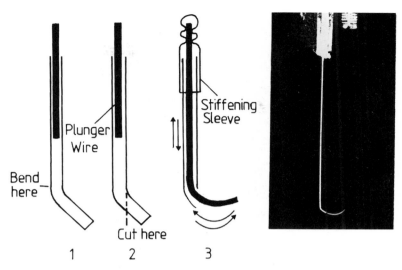

Figure 4 Drawings 1–3 represent stages of assembly of retractable microknife as described in text. Photograph shows a knife mounted in an electrode holder

3030, Cleveland, Ohio 44117). As noted by Gold *et al.* (1973), the bent portion of the cannula guide can be shortened. However, if the bent part is trimmed off completely, then the extended wire will swerve considerably. Finally, a piece of tungsten or stainless steel wire is forced through the cannula to the desired extent.

The described knife can be used as it is. However the following modification greatly facilitates the extension and withdrawal of the wire. A piece of 24 (or 23) gauge cannula is fitted over the 30 gauge cannula. The upper portion of the 24 gauge cannula is compressed with pliers so that the cannula walls collapse and grasp the tungsten wire. Once the cannula guide has been attached to the stereotaxic instrument holder, the wire knife can be withdrawn or extended by pulling or pushing the 24 gauge cannula (see Figure 4).

In order to facilitate the extension and withdrawal of the knife, and to accurately control the length to which the knife wire extends, we have attached a rack-and-pinion mechanism with a vernier scale on the stereotaxic electrode holder. This system is illustrated in Figure 5. In this modified version of the retractable knife the guiding tube is firmly secured to a standard electrode holder device, with a layer of masking tape or similar material to cushion the pressure on the tubing walls. A chuck with a taper adjustment holds the outermost tubing (see Figure 4) which in turn grasps the inner cutting wire. Displacement of this unit, with the help of the rack-and-pinion mechanism, in relation to the electrode holder results in 0.1 mm precision extension and retraction of the cutting wire.

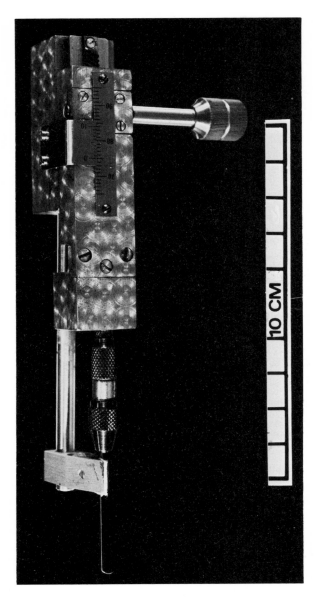

Figure 5 Retractable knife, constructed as in Figure 4, mounted in a David Kopf electrode holder. A rack-and-pinion mechanism with a vernier is also mounted in the electrode holder connected with a chuck having a taper adjustment. This chuck secures the outermost cannula which is connected with the inner cutting wire. Displacements of the rack-and-pinion mechanism result in extension or withdrawal of the inner cutting wire. (Scale = 10 cm in 1 cm divisions)

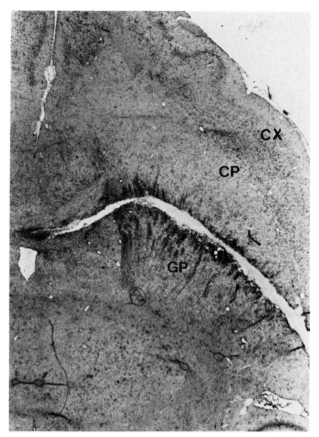

Figure 6 Horizontal section of the rat brain. Deafferentation of the globus pallidus (GP) using a Halasz type of stereotaxic knife. The section was stained with the Gomori technique (Pearse, 1968) for acid phosphatase. Black tracts represent lysosomal acid phosphatase in degenerating axon bundles in the caudate-putamen (CP) and which are more abundant in the globus pallidus. CX, cortex. (Cuello and Paxinos, 1978)

IV.2   The Production and Localization of Microknife Lesions

The general comments on the use of stereotaxic techniques discussed in Section III apply also for microknife deafferentation.

To make a knife lesion it is essential to study the appearance of the area to deafferentate in conventional stereotaxic atlases, attempting to reconstruct the possible position of the shaft of the knife and the arc described by the wire according to the length it will be extended. In making a knife cut, the guide cannula (or tubing) is inserted in the brain with the wire withdrawn. When the tip of the cannula reaches the desired depth, the wire is extended and the electrode holder lowered to produce the cut. If the intended cut should reach the bottom of the brain, the knife can be advanced until the cannula is seen to bow as the wire hits the base of the skull. This operation is facilitated by the use of a stereomicroscope.

Horizontal cuts can be made by inserting the knife horizontally through the occipital bone at the back of the cerebellum. Oblique insertions are on occasions required to cut some tracts perpendicularly.

For the histological reconstruction of the cut, as well as for the examination of accumulation of immunoreactive material in interrupted axons, the brain should be sectioned in planes perpendicular to that of the knife cut. In combined lesion–immunocytochemical studies we have found that horizontal sections of the brain facilitate the comparative analysis of immunoreactivity in control and lesioned sides by having both sides in the same section. For a precise identification of the cut it is advisable to process, alternatively, sections for immunocytochemistry and conventional histology (Nissl staining or equivalent). When the extent of the non-specific damage is to be assessed, sections should be processed to reveal acid phosphatase activity (Pearse, 1968) as an indication of lysosomal activity (see Figure 6).

Ideal survival times for immunocytochemical studies are 72 h for build-up of axonally transported immunoreactive material and 7 days for depletion. For most purposes a compromise of 4 days survive is adequate.

IV.3 Examples of Stereotaxic Knife Cuts combined with Immunocytochemistry

Example 1   Neurotensin immunoreactivity was detected in interrupted fibres descending in the hypothalamic fornix of the rat. In order to obtain this microknife cut the guide cannula was inserted into the brain 7 mm anterior to the interaural plane and 2.5 mm lateral to the midline with the skull positioned following Konig and Klippel (1963). The knife was lowered until the bottom of the wire could, if extended, reach 3.0 mm above the interaural plane. The cutting wire was then forced out of the guide tubing (cannula) tip for 2.5 mm in a coronal plane towards the midline. The cannula with the extended wire was then lowered until the tip of the cannula was seen to bow as the wire hit the skull. After a 4-day survival period the perfused fixed brain was sectioned horizontally and processed to demonstrate neurotensin immunoreactivity, as illustrated in Figure 7, neurotensin-positive fibres were detected 'descending' in the fornix. They could be traced back to the most superficial layers of the hippocampal formation. This illustrates how this technique can be applied to reveal immunoreactive material within a fibre tract as well as showing the direction of the projection.

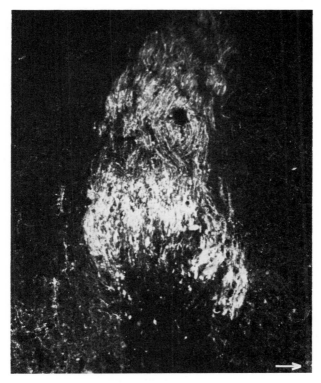

Figure 7 Neurotensin immunoreactivity build-up at the point of knife transection of the hypothalamic fornix. Horizontal section of the rat brain, arrow points medially. Immunofluorescence is detectable in the hippocampal side of the lesion. (From Paxinos, Butcher, and Cuello, in preparation)

Example 2 The fasciculus retroflexus of the rat was interrupted unilaterally by a knife cut perpendicular to its trajectory from the diencephalon to the midbrain. Depletion of substance P immunoreactivity was observed in the ipsilateral side of the interpeduncular nucleus and ventrotegmental area (Cuello *et al.*, 1978b) (see Figure 8). In order to insert the cannula in an oblique trajectory and to sever the axons of the fasciculus retroflexus, the incisor bar was lowered 7.0 mm below the horizontal interaural plane. The guide cannula was inserted in the brain at an angle of 30° to the vertical and 3.0 mm lateral to midline, and then lowered until the bottom of the arc of the cutting wire, if extended, would reach 0.5 mm posterior to the anterior–posterior stereotaxic zero. The wire was then forced through the cannula to a length of 3.00 mm from the cannula tip. The cut was made by lowering the cannula with the extended wire at a distance of 5.7 mm.

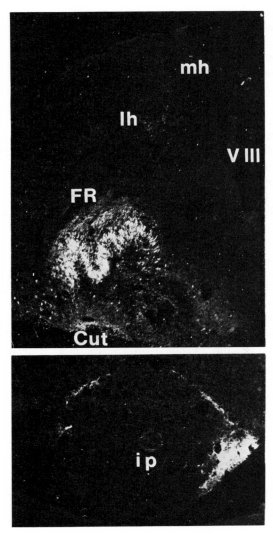

Figure 8 Upper: section of the rat brain in the plane of the trajectory of the fasciculus retroflexus (FR). Knife cut was performed in a perpendicular plane (lower, left). Observe the build-up of substance P immunofluorescent material in the severed axons of the fasciculus retroflexus. lh: lateral habenula; mh: medial habenula; V III: third ventricle. Bottom: Depletion of substance P in the external borders of the nucleus interpeduncularis (ip) ipsilateral to knife cut as above. Coronal section of the brain

Example 3 Complete and partial deafferentations of the globus pallidus from its connections with the caudate-putamen in the rat were performed with the original Halasz and Pupp (1965) knife and with the retractable version described above. The complete deafferentation was performed with the rigid Halasz–Pupp knife constructed in such a way that the first 3.5 mm of the cutting wire was perpendicular to the guiding cannula while the remaining distal part (3.8 mm) was parallel to it. The animals were placed in the stereotaxic apparatus in a flat-skull position; i.e. with bregma and lambda at the same vertical level. The zero reference point used was bregma, midline, and skull surface reference points for AP (anterior–posterior), L (lateral), and V (vertical) planes. The tip of the knife was inserted into the brain at AP: 0.0 and L: 1.9 mm. The cannula was lowered until the tip of the knife reached 8.0 mm below the surface of the skull and the tungsten wire rotated 180°, following the anterior and lateral borders of the globus pallidus. This rotation inscribed the top and sides of an hemicylinder (see Figures 6 and 9). Such a cut produced a total depletion of the immunoreactivity to Leu-enkephalin in the globus pallidus (Cuello and Paxinos, 1978) which was accompanied by a continuous build-up of enkephalin immunoreactivity in axons present in the caudate-putamen side of the cut (Del Fiacco *et al.*, 1982; Cuello and Paxinos, 1978) (see Figure 9). Partial deafferentation was performed with the retractable type of microknife with the rat brain positioned as described above.

Figure 10 illustrates one cut performed in the anterior third of the caudate-putamen with the cutting wire extended 4.0 mm from the tip of the guiding cannula, effectively separating that position of the corpus striatum from the corresponding globus pallidus. This resulted in a loss of the immunoreactivity in the globus pallidus which was limited to the area normally receiving afferents from the caudate putamen (see Figure 10) while the areas still connected with the neostriatum remained unaffected. The build-up of enkephalin immunoreactivity, on the other hand, was limited to the sectioned axons and the caudate-putamen side of the cut.

V CONCLUSIONS

Generalized axonal blockade produced by colchicine, administered either parenterally or stereotaxically into ventricular or cisternal spaces, leads to the accumulation of immunoreactive material in cell somata in central and peripheral neurons. The procedure is applicable for the mapping of cell groups containing a particular antigenic site, but does not allow pathway tracing. Localized injections produced regional effects and demonstrated immunoreactive fibre tracts in addition to cell bodies. This procedure also led to some more evident loss of immunoreactivity in the terminal areas. Kainic acid, on the other hand, tends to destroy cell bodies while sparing nerve terminals and passing by fibres; nevertheless the sensitivity to the drug may vary from region to region. Focal injections of this compound result in the loss of immunoreactivity in terminal fields of affected projecting neurons.

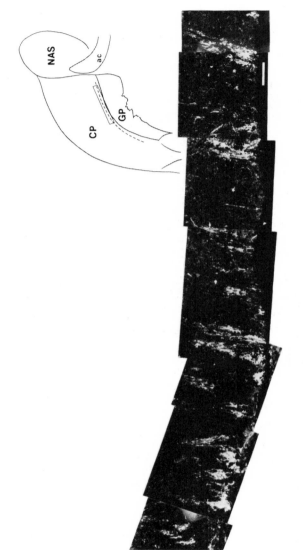

Figure 9 Build-up of enkephalin immunoreactivity in the neostriatal side of a knife cut, which isolates the globus pallidus (GP) from the caudate-putamen (CP). Horizontal sections of the rat brain, perpendicular to plane of cut. Cut similar to that represented in Figure 5. (Scale bar = 50 μm). In the insert, the dashed line indicates the knife cut and rectangle shows approximate field of photomontage. (Reproduced by permission from Del Fiacco *et al.*, 1982)

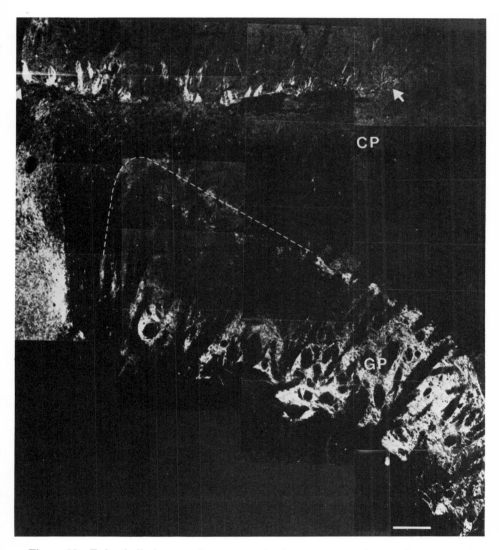

Figure 10 Enkephalin immunofluorescence in the rat corpus striatum after a coronal cut placed in the caudate-putamen (CP), anterior to the globus pallidus. Build-up of enkephalin-immunoreactive material is observed in the anterior side of the cut while a marked loss of specific fluorescence is seen in the antero-medial part of the globus pallidus (GP). Horizontal section of the brain, perpendicular to plane of knife cut. Arrow points to lateral extremity of cut. Dashed line indicates approximate limits of the globus pallidus. (Scale bar = 200 μm.) (Reproduced by permission from Del Fiacco *et al.*, 1982)

Rigid and retractable knife cuts can be applied successfully in combination with immunocytochemistry. Although this procedure requires some stereotaxic skills it allows the rapid exploration of major projecting tracts in the CNS by the analysis of the direction of the build-up in fibre tracts and the loss of immunoreactive material in nerve terminal fields.

These procedures are complementary among themselves and with other procedures such as the retrograde transport of fluorescent dyes (see Chapter 18) or horseradish peroxidase (Bowker *et al.*, 1981; Priestley *et al.*, 1981) combined with immunocytochemistry. While the neurotoxins and microknife injections are mostly indicated for the exploration of possible overall connections of neurotransmitter (or neurotransmitter marker)-containing neurons, the methods based on a combination of immunocytochemistry with retrograde transport are more appropriate for detailed analysis of such connections.

ACKNOWLEDGEMENTS

The technical assistance of Mr Bramwell, and the art and photographic work of Mr B. Archer, Mr T. Richards, Mr T. Barclay, and Miss J. Lloyd is gratefully acknowledged, as well as the preparation of instruments by Mr J. Glozier. We would like to thank Mrs E. Iles and Miss J. Ballinger for efficient secretarial assistance. This work has been supported by grants from the Wellcome Trust and the E. P. Abraham Cephalosporin Trust (Oxford) to A.C.C. and by grant ARGC D1 80 15 147 I to G.P.

REFERENCES

Avrith, D. and Mogenson, G. J. (1978). 'Reversible hyperphagia and obesity following intracerebral microinjections of colchicine into the ventromedial hypothalamus of the rat.' *Brain Res.*, **153**, 99–107.

Avrith, D., Hass, H. L., and Mogenson, G. (1977). 'Behavioural and electrophysiological changes following microinjections of colchicine in the substantia nigra.' *Proc. XXVII Int. Congr. Physiol. Sci., Paris*, **XIII** (39), abstract 97.

Barry, J., Dubois, M. P., Poulain, P., and Leonardelli, J. (1973). 'Caractérisation et topographie des neurones hypothalamiques immunoréactifs avec des anticorps anti-LRF de synthèse.' *C.R. Acad. Sci. (Paris)*, Serie D, **276**, 3191–3193.

Borisy, G. G. and Taylor, E. W. (1967). 'The mechanism of action of colchicine.' *J. Cell Biol.*, **34**, 525–533.

Bowker, R. M., Steinbusch, H. W. M., and Coulter, J. D. (1981). 'Serotonergic and peptidergic projections to the spinal cord demonstration by a combined retrograde HRP histochemical and immunocytochemical staining method.' *Brain Res.*, **211**, 412–417.

Coyle, J. T. and Schwarcz, R. (1976). 'Lesion of striatal neurones with kainic acid provides a model for Huntington's chorea.' *Nature*, **263**, 244–246.

Cuello, A. C. (1978). 'Immunocytochemical studies of the distribution of neurotransmitters and related substances in the CNS. In Iversen, L. L. *et al.* (eds), *Handbook of Psychopharmacology*, vol. 9, pp. 69–137. Plenum Press, New York.

Cuello, A. C. and Paxinos, G. (1978). 'Evidence for a long Leu-enkephalin striopallidal pathway in the rat brain.' *Nature*, **271**, 178–180.

Cuello, A. C., del Fiacco, M., and Paxinos, G. (1978a). 'The central and peripheral ends of the substance-P containing neurones in the rat trigeminal system.' *Brain Res.*, **152**, 499–509.

Cuello, A. C., Emson, P. C., Paxinos, G., and Jessell, T. (1978b). 'Substance P containing and cholinergic projections from the habenula.' *Brain Res.*, **149**, 413–429.

Cuello, A. C., Del Fiacco, M., Paxinos, G., Somogyi, P., and Priestley, J. V. (1981). 'Neuropeptides in striato-nigral pathways.' *J. Neural Transmission*, **51**, 83–96.

Dahlström, A. (1968). 'Effect of colchicine on transport of amine storage granules in sympathetic nerves of rat.' *Eur. J. Pharmacol.*, **5**, 111.

Del Fiacco, M. and Cuello, A. C. (1980). 'Substance P and enkephalin-containing neurones in the rat trigeminal system.' *Neuroscience*, **5**, 803–815.

Del Fiacco, M., Paxinos, G., and Cuello, A. C. (1982). 'Neostriatal enkephalin, immunoreactive neurones project to the globus pallidus.' *Brain Res.*, **231**, 1–17.

Di Chiara, G., Olianas, M., Del Fiacco, M., Spano, P. F., and Tagliamonte, A. (1977). 'Intranigral kainic acid is evidence that nigral non-dopaminergic neurons control posture.' *Nature*, **268**, 743–745.

Gold, R. M., Kapatos, G., and Carey, P. J. (1973). 'A retracting wire knife for stereotaxic brain surgery made from a microliter syringe.' *Physiol. Behav.*, **10**, 813–815.

Halasz, B. and Pupp, L. (1965). 'Hormone secretion of the anterior pituitary gland after physical interruption of all nervous pathways to the hypophysiotrophic area.' *Endocrinology*, **88**, 553–562.

Heimer, L. and Robarts, M. J. (eds) (1981). *Neuroanatomical Tract-tracing Methods.* Plenum Press, New York.

Hökfelt, T., Johansson, O., Ljungdahl, A., Lundberg, J. M., and Schultzberg, M. (1980). 'Peptidergic neurones.' *Nature*, **289**, 515–521.

Konig, J. F. R. and Klippel, R. A. (1963). *The Rat Brain.* Williams & Wilkins, Baltimore.

Ljungdahl, A., Hökfelt, T., and Nilsson, G. (1978). 'Distribution of substance P-like immunoreactivity in the central nervous system of the rat.' *Neuroscience*, **3**, 861–943.

Moore, R. Y. (1978). 'Surgical and chemical lesion techniques.' Iversen, L. L. *et al.* (eds), *Handbook of Psychopharmacology*, vol. 9, pp. 1–39. Plenum Press, New York.

Moore, R. Y. (1981). 'Methods for selective, restricted lesion placement in the central nervous system.' In Heimer, L. and Robarts, M. J. (eds), *Neuroanatomical Tract-Tracing Methods*, pp. 55–89. Plenum Press, New York.

McGeer, P. L., McGeer, E. G., and Hattori, J. (1978). 'Kainic acid as a tool in neurobiology.' McGeer, E. G. *et al.* (eds), *Kainic Acid as a Tool in Neurobiology*, pp. 123–138. Raven Press, New York.

Nadler, J. V., Perry, B. W., and Cotman, C. W. (1978). 'Preferential vulnerability of hippocampus to intraventricular kainic acid.' In McGeer, E. G. (*ed.*), *Kainic Acid as a Tool in Neurobiology*, pp. 219–237. Raven Press, New York.

Olney, J. W. (1978). 'Neurotoxicity of excitatory amino acids.' In McGeer, E. G. *et al.* (ed.), *Kainic Acid as a Tool in Neurobiology*, pp. 95–121. Raven Press, New York.

Olney, J. W. and de Gubareff, T. (1978). 'Extreme sensitivity of olfactory corticol neurons to kainic acid toxicity.' In McGeer, E. G. (ed.), *Kainic Acid as a Tool in Neurobiology*, pp. 201–217. Raven Press, New York.

Paxinos, G., Watson, C. R. R., and Emson, P. C. (1980). 'AChE-stained horizontal sections of the rat brain in stereotaxic coordinator.' *J. Neurosci. Methods*, **3**, 129–149.

Pearse, A. G. E. (1968). *Histochemistry Theoretical and Applied*. Churchill Livingstone, London.

Pellegrino, L., Pellegrino, A. S., and Cushman, A. L. (1979). *A Stereotaxic Atlas of the Rat Brain*. Plenum Press, New York.

Priestley, J. V., Somogyi, P., and Cuello, A. C. (1981). 'Neurotransmitter-specific projection neurons revealed by combining PAP immunohistochemistry with retrograde transport of HRP.' *Brain Res.*, **220**, 231–240.

Sar, M., Stumpf, W. E., Miller, R. J., Chang, K.-J., and Cuatrecasas, P. (1978). 'Immunohistochemical localization of enkephalin in rat brain and spinal cord.' *J. Comp. Neurol.*, **182**, 17–38.

Schmitt, F. O. (1968). 'Fibrous protein—neuronal organelles.' *Proc. Natl. Acad. Sci, USA*, **60**, 1092–1104.

Sclafani, A. and Grossman, S. P. (1969). 'Hyperphagia produced by knife cuts between the medial and lateral hypothalamus in the rat.' *Physiol. Behav.*, **4**, 533–537.

Shinozaki, H. (1978) 'Discovery of novel actions of kainic acid and related compounds.' In McGeer *et al.* (eds), *Kainic Acid as a Tool in Neurobiology*, pp. 17–35. Raven Press, New York.

Sorimachi, M., Hino, O., and Tsunekawa, K. (1977). 'Colchicine may interfere with the axonal transport of noradrenaline in the central noradrenergic neurons.' *Experientia*, **33**, 649–650.

Voloschin, L., Joseph, S. A., and Knigge, K. M. (1968). 'Endocrine function in male rats following complete and partial isolation of the hypothalamo-pituitary unit.' *Neuroendocrinology*, **3**, 387–397.

Wilson, L. (1970). 'Properties of colchicine binding protein from chick embryo brain. Interactions with vinca alkaloids and podophyllotoxin.' *Biochemistry*, **9**, 4999–5007.

Index